ADVANCES IN

Pediatrics

Editor-in-Chief
Carol D. Berkowitz, MD, FAAP, FACEP

Chief, Division of General Pediatrics,
Department of PediatricsAurora,
Harbor-UCLA Medical Center,
Distinguished Professor of Pediatrics,
David Geffen School of Medicine at UCLA,
Torrance, California

ELSEVIER

PHILADELPHIA LONDON TORONTO MONTREAL SYDNEY TOKYO

ADVANCES IN
Pediatrics

VOLUMES 1 THROUGH 66 (OUT OF PRINT)

VOLUME 67

Publishing Director, Medical Reference: Dolores Meloni
Editor: Kerry Holland
Developmental Editor: Diana Ang

Editorial Office:
Elsevier
1600 John F. Kennedy Blvd,
Suite 1800
Philadelphia, PA 19103-2899

International Standard Serial Number: 0065-3101
International Standard Book Number: 13: 978-0-323-81379-2

ADVANCES IN
Pediatrics

CONTRIBUTORS

CRAIG A. ALTER, MD, Professor of Clinical Pediatrics, Perelman School of Medicine, University of Pennsylvania, Division of Endocrinology, The Children's Hospital of Philadelphia, Philadelphia, Pennsylvania, USA

RAYMEN R. ASSAF, MA, MD, MPH, Clinical Instructor, David Geffen School of Medicine at UCLA, Los Angeles, California, USA; Pediatric Emergency Medicine, Fellow, Department of Emergency Medicine, Harbor-UCLA Medical Center, Torrance, California, USA

KATHERINE M. BARTOLETTA, MD, MS, Resident, Department of Pediatric and Adolescent Medicine, Mayo Clinic, Rochester, Minnesota, USA

BROOKE C. BAVINGER, MD, Department of Pediatrics, Division of General Pediatrics, University of South Florida Morsani College of Medicine, Tampa, Florida, USA

CAROL D. BERKOWITZ, MD, FAAP, Chief, Division of General Pediatrics, Department of Pediatrics, Harbor-UCLA Medical Center, Distinguished Professor of Pediatrics, David Geffen School of Medicine at UCLA, Torrance, California, USA

MICHELLE A. BLANCO, MD, Department of Pediatrics, Division of General Pediatrics, University of South Florida Morsani College of Medicine, Tampa, Florida, USA

ALEXIS N. BOWDER, MD, MPH, Division of Pediatric Surgery, Department of Surgery, Medical College of Wisconsin, Milwaukee, Wisconsin, USA

MARISSA A. BRUNETTI, MD, Assistant Professor of Clinical Anesthesiology, Critical Care Medicine, and Pediatrics, Perelman School of Medicine, University of Pennsylvania, Attending Intensivist, The Children's Hospital of Philadelphia, Philadelphia, Pennsylvania, USA

TIFFANY CHENNEVILLE, PhD, Professor and St. Petersburg Campus Chair, Marie E. and E. Leslie Cole Endowed Chair in Ethics, Department of Psychology, University of South Florida, St Petersburg, Florida, USA

LAURIE E. COHEN, MD, Associate Professor of Pediatrics, Division of Endocrinology, Boston Children's Hospital, Harvard Medical School, Boston, Massachusetts, USA

JANAN DIETRICH, PhD, Director of Biobehavioural Research, Perinatal HIV Research Unit, Faculty of Health Sciences, University of Witwatersrand, Johannesburg, Gauteng, South Africa, Health Systems Research Unit, South African Medical Research Council, Cape Town, South Africa

M. DENISE DOWD, MD, MPH, Professor of Pediatrics, University of Missouri–Kansas City School of Medicine, Clinical Professor of Pediatrics, University of Kansas School of Medicine, Associate Director for Research, Division of Emergency Medicine, Children's Mercy Kansas City, Kansas City, Missouri, USA

JOHN S. FUQUA, MD, Professor of Clinical Pediatrics, Indiana University School of Medicine, Riley Hospital for Children, Indianapolis, Indiana, USA

KEMESHA GABBIDON, PhD, Assistant Professor, Department of Psychology, University of South Florida, St Petersburg, Florida, USA

SAMIR K. GADEPALLI, MD, MS, Section of Pediatric Surgery, Department of Surgery, University of Michigan, Mott Children's Hospital, Susan B. Meister Child Health Evaluation and Research Center, Michigan Medicine, Ann Arbor, Michigan, USA

SARA GARCIA, MD, Department of Pediatrics, Division of General Pediatrics, University of South Florida Morsani College of Medicine, Tampa, Florida, USA

MATTHEW GATES, MD, Department of Pediatrics, Clinical Instructor of Pediatrics, University of South Florida Morsani College of Medicine, Tampa, Florida, USA

JULIA E. GRABOWKSI, MD, Division of Pediatric Surgery, Assistant Professor, Department of Surgery, Ann & Robert H. Lurie Children's Hospital of Chicago, Northwestern University Feinberg School of Medicine, Chicago, Illinois, USA

RUPAL C. GUPTA, MD, Interim Director, Division of General Academic Pediatrics, Children's Mercy Kansas City, Assistant Professor of Pediatrics, University of Missouri–Kansas City School of Medicine, Clinical Assistant Professor of Pediatrics, University of Kansas School of Medicine, Kansas City, Kansas, USA

MICHELLE P. HOJNICKI, DO, Department of Pediatrics, Division of General Pediatrics, University of South Florida Morsani College of Medicine, Tampa, Florida, USA

STEFANIE HORNSCHUH, MSc, Senior Researcher, Perinatal HIV Research Unit, Faculty of Health Sciences, University of Witwatersrand, Johannesburg, Gauteng, South Africa

AUDREY D. KAMZAN, MD, FAAP, Chief, Division of Pediatric Hospital Medicine, Mattel Children's Hospital, Associate Professor, David Geffen School of Medicine at UCLA, Los Angeles, California, USA

MARIA E. KNAUS, MD, Pediatric Surgery Research Fellow, Center for Surgical Outcomes Research, Abigail Wexner Research Institute, Nationwide Children's Hospital, Columbus, Ohio, USA

DAVE R. LAL, MD, MPH, Professor, Division of Pediatric Surgery, Department of Surgery, Medical College of Wisconsin, Milwaukee, Wisconsin, USA

CAROL M. LILLY, MD, MPH, Department of Pediatrics, Division of General Pediatrics, University of South Florida Morsani College of Medicine, Tampa, Florida, USA

NINA S. MA, MD, Kerr Family Endowed Chair in Endocrinology, Director, Bone and Mineral Metabolism Program, Section of Endocrinology, Children's Hospital Colorado, Associate Professor of Pediatrics, University of Colorado School of Medicine, Aurora, Colorado, USA

DEBORAH McCURDY, MD, Clinical Professor of Pediatrics, Division of Allergy/Immunology/Rheumatology, Fellowship Director of Pediatric Rheumatology, David Geffen School of Medicine at UCLA, Mattel Children's Hospital, Los Angeles, California, USA

MELINDA MURPHY, MD, FAAP, Assistant Professor, Department of Pediatrics, University of South Florida Morsani College of Medicine, Tampa, Florida, USA

ELAYNA NG, MD, FAAP, David Geffen School of Medicine at UCLA, Pediatric Hospital Medicine Fellow, Mattel Children's Hospital, Los Angeles, California, USA

PATRICIA O'BRIEN, MD, PhD, FAAP, Assistant Professor, Department of Pediatrics, University of South Florida Morsani College of Medicine, Tampa, Florida, USA

MIRIAM F. PARSA, MD, MPH, Pediatric Rheumatology, Cottage Children's Medical Center, Santa Barbara, California, USA; Volunteer Clinical Faculty, Division of Allergy/Immunology/Rheumatology, David Geffen School of Medicine at UCLA, Mattel Children's Hospital, Los Angeles, California, USA

KURLEN S.E. PAYTON, MD, Assistant Professor of Pediatrics, Department of Pediatrics, Division of Neonatology, Cedars-Sinai Medical Center, Associate Professor of Pediatrics, David Geffen School of Medicine at University of California Los Angeles, Los Angeles, California, USA

KIMBERLY A. RANDELL, MD, MSc, Associate Professor of Pediatrics, University of Missouri–Kansas City School of Medicine, Clinical Associate Professor of Pediatrics, University of Kansas School of Medicine, Division of Emergency Medicine, Children's Mercy Kansas City, Kansas City, Missouri, USA

NATHAN S. RUBALCAVA, MD, Section of Pediatric Surgery, Department of Surgery, University of Michigan, Mott Children's Hospital, Ann Arbor, Michigan, USA

RACHEL L. SEWELL, MD, Children's Hospital Colorado, Department of Pediatrics, University of Colorado School of Medicine, Aurora, Colorado, USA

KARUNA V. SHEKDAR, MD, Assistant Professor of Clinical Radiology, Perelman School of Medicine, University of Pennsylvania, Division of Radiology, The Children's Hospital of Philadelphia, Philadelphia, Pennsylvania, USA

STEPHANIE R. STARR, MD, Associate Professor, Department of Pediatric and Adolescent Medicine, Mayo Clinic, Rochester, Minnesota, USA

LINDSEY A. WARNER, MD, MS, Children's Hospital Colorado, Department of Pediatrics, University of Colorado School of Medicine, Aurora, Colorado, USA

KELLY D. YOUNG, MD, MS, Health Sciences Clinical Professor of Emergency Medicine, David Geffen School of Medicine at UCLA, Los Angeles, California, USA; Program Director, Pediatric Emergency Medicine, Department of Emergency Medicine, Harbor-UCLA Medical Center, Torrance, California, USA

CONTENTS VOLUME 68 • 2021

When Less is More: The Role of Overdiagnosis and Overtreatment in Patient Safety

Audrey D. Kamzan and Elayna Ng

Antibiotic Stewardship in Pediatrics

Kurlen S.E. Payton and Marissa A. Brunetti

Pituitary Tumors in Children

Craig A. Alter, Karuna V. Shekdar, and Laurie E. Cohen

Adrenal Tumors in Childhood

John S. Fuqua

Advances in Pediatrics 68 (2021) xix–xxi

ADVANCES IN PEDIATRICS

INTRODUCTION

Life Goes On: Health Care Systems, Complex Medical Conditions, and Newer Trends in Health Care: Post Pandemic

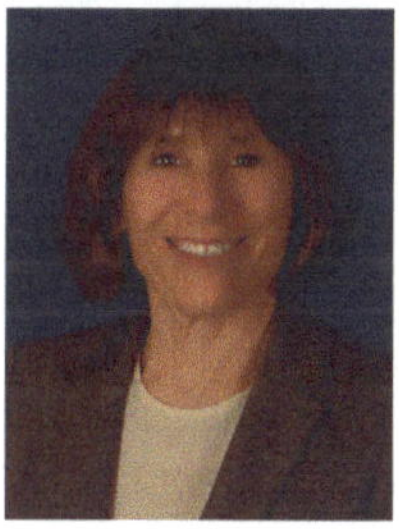

Carol D. Berkowitz, MD, FAAP

In my introduction to the 67th issue of *Advances in Pediatrics*, I commented how the issue had been crafted before the COVID pandemic struck, but that as we were going to press in the spring of 2020, things were improving. How naïve a comment that was! But by then, all the authors and topics for the 68th issue had been selected, and once again, the needs of children and pediatricians went beyond the emerging issues of school closures, virtual learning, COVID vaccination, and the appearance of new COVID-related pediatric diseases, such as multisystem inflammatory disease.

Overarching health care and health care systems are addressed in several articles in this latest issue of *Advances in Pediatrics*. Leading off is a discussion of Health Systems Science, the third branch of medicine along with Basic Science and Clinical Medicine. Health Systems Science evaluates the evolution of medicine from solo practice and small medical groups to large complex health systems, and the economics of health care and the medical home. Also included is the impact of COVID-19 on health care and resources and the effect the large-scale social unrest that our society witnessed during the pandemic had. In a similar vein, "When Less Is More: The Role of Overdiagnosis in Pediatric Patient Safety" details how overuse, including overdiagnosis and overtreatment, contributes to the high cost of health care, waste, and patient harm in the form of adverse effects. Avoidance of the inappropriate use of antibiotics is provided

https://doi.org/10.1016/j.yapd.2021.05.016
0065-3101/21/© 2021 Published by Elsevier Inc.

through antibiotic stewardship, allowing infectious disease experts to monitor the prescribing of antibiotics and advise medical staff on the appropriate choice and duration of therapy. The involvement of pediatric patients in medical decisions related to their care often requires acknowledging the balance between children as vulnerable individuals requiring protection and their need to be autonomous. Use of the Chenneville protection-autonomy model provides a framework for how best to involve minors in treatment and research. In caring for children, clinicians must remain cognizant of the many antecedent factors that affect a child's life and their health, and how parental adverse childhood experiences as well as the child's traumatic experiences have lasting effects.

On a positive note, improved medical care has allowed children with chronic medical conditions to survive well into adulthood. These children are often followed in complex care clinics by multidisciplinary teams that provide options for addressing challenges that children and families face. When children are admitted to the hospital, care is facilitated not just by the skilled surgical teams but also by the hospitalists who assess the risk for conditions like respiratory problems, venous thromboembolism, and pain management. Although the list of these complex medical conditions is long, we provide an update on inflammatory bowel disease and juvenile idiopathic arthritis.

Controversies exist around vitamin D, and these resurfaced during COVID. Vitamin D in pediatrics also has unresolved questions, including the lack of a standard definition of optimal vitamin D status. Less controversial is the importance of a breast exam in pediatric patients, particularly teens. While most breast masses are benign, patients as well as their parents are often concerned. When to observe, when to do an ultrasound, and when to do a fine needle biopsy are some of the issues to consider when a patient complains of a breast lump. While breast masses may be detected by physical examination, tumors in other areas, such as the pituitary or the adrenal gland, may present with an array of symptoms, including alterations in growth and development, or as an incidental finding when imaging studies are done for unrelated reasons. The assessment and management of endocrine tumors depend on the associated studies and findings that are detailed in their respective articles.

As is always the case, *Advances in Pediatrics* reports on children across the entire age spectrum from infancy through late adolescence. We are able to see the latest approach to esophageal atresia, including diagnosing any associated syndromes. We also learn about the "Trends in Recreational Drug Use and Ingestion" and the wide sometimes perplexing picture with which these patients present. This year, as in the past, there remain new developments in how health care is delivered and, in the diagnosis and management of the many conditions that affect the pediatric population.

Carol D. Berkowitz, MD, FAAP
Division of General Pediatrics
Department of Pediatrics
Harbor–University of California
Los Angeles Medical Center
David Geffen School of Medicine at UCLA
1000 West Carson Street
Torrance, CA 90509, USA

E-mail address: cberkowitz52@gmail.com

Advances in Pediatrics 68 (2021) 1–19
ADVANCES IN PEDIATRICS

Health Systems Science

Katherine M. Bartoletta, MD, MS,
Stephanie R. Starr, MD*

Department of Pediatric and Adolescent Medicine, Mayo Clinic, 200 First Street Southwest, Rochester, MN 55905, USA

Keywords

• Health systems science • Systems thinking • Medical home • Telehealth
• Population health • Social determinants of health • Health policy
• Health economics

Key points

- Health systems science (HSS) is the study of how health care is delivered, including how health professionals collaborate and how the health care system can improve patient care and health care delivery.
- A foundational understanding of the HSS framework can aid pediatric professionals of all backgrounds to identify and close existing and emerging pediatric health and health care gaps.
- The pediatric medical home is a prime setting to close health care delivery gaps through longitudinal care, with strategies including care coordination, advocacy, and incorporation of telehealth.
- Pediatric health professionals must have an understanding of pediatric-relevant health economics and health policy, as well as the structural and social determinants of health, to meaningfully improve the health of children, especially in the setting of the COVID-19 (coronavirus disease 2019) pandemic.

HEALTH PROFESSIONS EDUCATION REQUIRES A NEW APPROACH

Gaps in United States health and the health care system

The term US health care system is a misnomer, because it did not evolve in a deliberate, evidence-based, coordinated manner focused on maximizing societal health. Our current system has evolved over time, without a singular vision, to become a complex web of hospitals, clinics, health care professionals, payment

*Corresponding author. *E-mail address:* starr.stephanie@mayo.edu

https://doi.org/10.1016/j.yapd.2021.05.001

models, and policies. Although historically there has not been a single unifying vision for US health care, this changed in 2008 when the Institute for Healthcare Improvement (IHI) published its Triple Aim, which seeks to improve patients' experience of care and population health outcomes while minimizing or decreasing per capita costs [1]. The Quadruple Aim expanded on this by including improved clinician work-life integration [2].

The complex US health care system performs poorly compared with similar nations, and this gap is even more stark when contrasting performance with health care spending [3]. Socioeconomic factors and health behaviors have a greater impact than the health care systems on the health of patients and society [4]. For example, individuals living in the same city but in a different zip code area can have tragically wide variation in life expectancy [5].

Existing and emerging pediatric health problems

Infants, children, and adolescents face growing health threats that affect their ability to meet their human potential. Approximately 1 out of every 5 children in the United States has a special health care need [6]. In 2017 to 2018, nearly 25% of US households had 1 or more children with special health care needs [6]. In 2015, an estimated 3 million children witnessed a shooting annually, and in 2018 firearms were the leading cause of death for children and teens [7,8]. Adverse childhood experiences (ACEs) are common, preventable, lead to chronic health conditions, and disproportionally affect the most vulnerable children [9]. Children face increasing health threats from accelerating climate change and from ongoing environmental threats such as lead toxicity [10,11].

The year 2020 brought new challenges to all children, their families, and communities because no one has been untouched by the COVID-19 (coronavirus disease 2019) pandemic. Immigrant and other vulnerable communities have been disproportionately affected [12,13]. Vulnerable students unable to attend schools because of stay-at-home orders and hybrid learning models experienced decreased access to food, requiring emergency strategies to fill the need [14]. Millions of US children lost their health insurance as unemployment increased in 2020, because roughly half of children have employee-sponsored health insurance [13].

The pandemic also highlighted the importance of understanding the connectedness among multiple entities across the broadest definition of the health care system, including personal protective equipment supply chain issues, cascading systems failures, and a laying bare of the US health economics and payment system [15,16]. Numerous systems failures have negatively affected children, families, pediatric health professionals, and their care teams. The pandemic has exacerbated health professional burnout, but, despite this, pediatricians and other health professionals have flexed their adaptive expertise muscles and rapidly innovated to meet the needs of pediatric patients in the areas of telehealth, prioritizing staff as well as patient safety, and partnering with public health in new ways [17]. Some pediatricians met the needs of their local communities by joining inpatient medicine teams to care for hospitalized adults with COVID-19 [18].

The death of George Floyd in May 2020 and many other black citizens by law enforcement brought significant social unrest and amplified the health impact of structural racism on children, families, and communities. This social unrest and emphasis has generated calls to dismantle structural racism in clinical, educational, and research systems in medicine as well as in communities. It has also highlighted the additional negative impact on minority health professionals [19]. Individual actions alone are insufficient, and a systems approach must be taken to address structural racism in addition to existing and other more recent health issues such as COVID-19.

Physicians have historically been trained in the basic (eg, microbiology, pharmacology, pathophysiology) and clinical (eg, history taking, physical examination) sciences to improve child health. Over several decades and before 2020, there has been an increasing call for physicians and physician trainees to learn new concepts and skills to help close the widening gap between the pace of change in clinical practice and that in medical education and professional development [20,21,22]. These new competencies include a focus on patient needs and experiences, thinking with a systems view, population health, measuring performance, managing change, optimizing teamwork, leveraging new technology, and eliminating waste [23,24]. They extend beyond existing competencies and accreditation requirements in undergraduate and graduate medical education, and have been incrementally added over time with significant variation in speed and breadth. The COVID-19 pandemic, evolving societal recognition of structural racism and its impact on health, and worsening climate issues further emphasize the importance of these new competencies.

Third science is needed to close current and future gaps in child health

This burning platform (US health care system performance, impact of other factors on health beyond traditional health care, and the malalignment between pace of change in practice vs medical education), superimposed on existing and emerging threats to child health, require the health professions to embrace a third science in medical education and practice to complement basic and clinical science [25]. Many third-science concepts and skills have been introduced over time in piecemeal fashion, making it difficult to conceptualize and see relationships across the full complement of concepts and skills needed to adapt to existing and emerging health threats. The lifelong learning of all clinicians, including those who care for children, ideally includes a 3-science approach. This third science has been termed health systems science (HSS).

HEALTH SYSTEMS SCIENCE AS THE THIRD SCIENCE

Definition and framework

HSS is the study of how health care is delivered, including how health professionals collaborate and how the health care system can improve patient care and health care delivery [26]. This framework was developed from the work of medical schools who sought to help close gaps between clinical practice (health and health care gaps experienced by patients) and medical education (Fig. 1) [26].

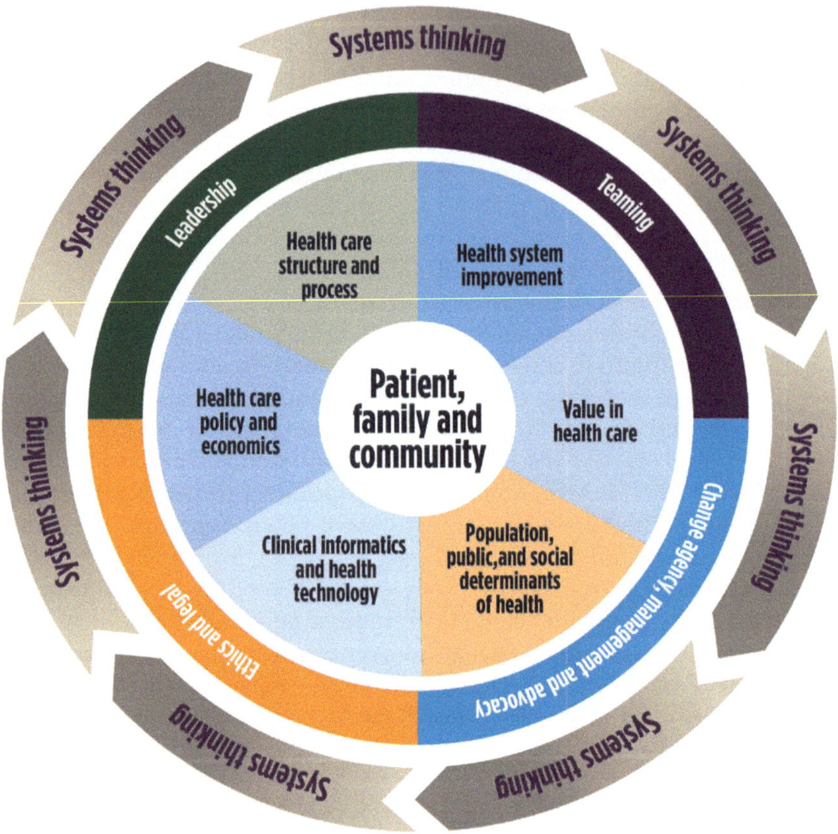

Fig. 1. Core functional, foundational, and linking domains for HSS. (*From* What is health systems science? Building an integrated vision. In: Skochelak SE, Hammoud MM, Lomis KD, et al., editors. Health Systems Science, 2nd edition. Philadelphia: Elsevier; 2020. p.9. Used with permission of the American Medical Association. ©Copyright American Medical Association 2020. All rights reserved.)

At the core of HSS are the patient, family, and community. For the additional aspects of the framework to be effective, pediatric providers must consider the impact actions will have on the patient, family, and community. The inner circle includes the core functional domains of HSS: health care structures and processes; health system improvement; value in health care; population health, public health, and social determinants of health; clinical informatics and health technology; and health care policy and economics. The middle circle represents the foundational domains that relate to more than 1 core domain: leadership; teaming; change agency, management, and advocacy; and ethics and legal. The linking domain for all other domains is systems thinking.

The breadth of topics in this third science and their categorization can be represented in other ways and domains, but the HSS framework is the most common framework used by multiple medical schools, GME programs, and (increasingly) health systems seeking to become learning health care systems (systems that align science, informatics, incentives, and culture for continuous improvement and innovation, best practices seamlessly embedded in the care process, patients and families as active participants in all elements, and new knowledge captured as an integral by-product of care) [27,28].

Systems citizenship

Health professionals must do more than learn HSS concepts and skills. They must enable themselves and their colleagues to recognize their responsibility to see and close gaps in the system as part of their professional identify. This process has been described as systems citizenship [29,30,31]. Health professionals can use the HSS framework (and, within it, the concepts and skills) to categorize gaps and identify leverage points and strategies to intervene.

There may be no better pediatric example of systems citizenship and advocacy in recent years than the story of lead toxicity in the Flint, Michigan, drinking water. Dr. Mona Hanna-Attisha was first alerted to the threat of lead toxicity for children in her community during a conversation with a high school friend and environmental engineer who shared that the water treatment was missing an important chemical to control corrosion, potentially increasing the concentration of lead in the drinking water. She believed she had a professional obligation to improve the system in order to improve the health of children in her community [32].

It is easy for trainees and clinicians to feel overwhelmed by the gaps and systems challenges they, their teams, and their patients face. Moving beyond seeing gaps to categorizing them and choosing those within their scope of influence or control to help address (eg, via advocacy, quality improvement, community engagement) may enable pediatric health professionals to see, categorize, and act on gaps based on their roles, their passions, their skill sets, and the needs of local children in the community. Clinicians who work on systems to reduce administrative burden for teams can help mitigate burnout for their colleagues [33,34]. Systems thinking, the linking domain in HSS, is required for all clinicians to meet their professional responsibility as systems citizens.

SYSTEMS THINKING

Systems thinking is the HSS linking domain that brings together the core functional and foundational domains of HSS. Systems thinking is essential to developing a holistic and comprehensive view of patient care, the broader health care system, and challenges in health care. Systems thinking depicts the importance of not solely considering each domain in a silo but instead recognizing cause-and-effect relationships and the dynamic integration of each domain to positively affect health care. With this framework, providers can use tools and skills as well as a unique perspective to change and improve the system.

The Waters Center for Systems Thinking has developed resources to aid in learning and developing problem-solving skills, including systems thinking habits and tools [35]. The habits and tools have been introduced into medical school curricula and can be used by pediatric providers in training and in practice. Fig. 2 provides a summary of each of the 14 habits of a systems thinker. An application of systems thinking to a pediatric clinical case is presented in Table 1, and detailed descriptions of each systems thinking habit with clinical examples and case studies have also been published [26].

All individuals who seek to improve child health can put systems thinking into active practice. This expansive community includes pediatric primary care providers, subspecialists, nurses, respiratory therapy, psychologists, social work, physical therapy, occupational therapy, community and county services, and schools. By collaborating across disciplines, clinicians can create active change and improvement in pediatric health.

The rest of this article highlights selected HSS domains and their relevance to current pediatric health and health care challenges.

HEALTH CARE STRUCTURES AND PROCESSES

Dr Avedis Donabedian [36] was the first to study US health care quality. In 1988, he published a model for measuring quality in health care, describing the importance of measuring not only health outcomes but also the health

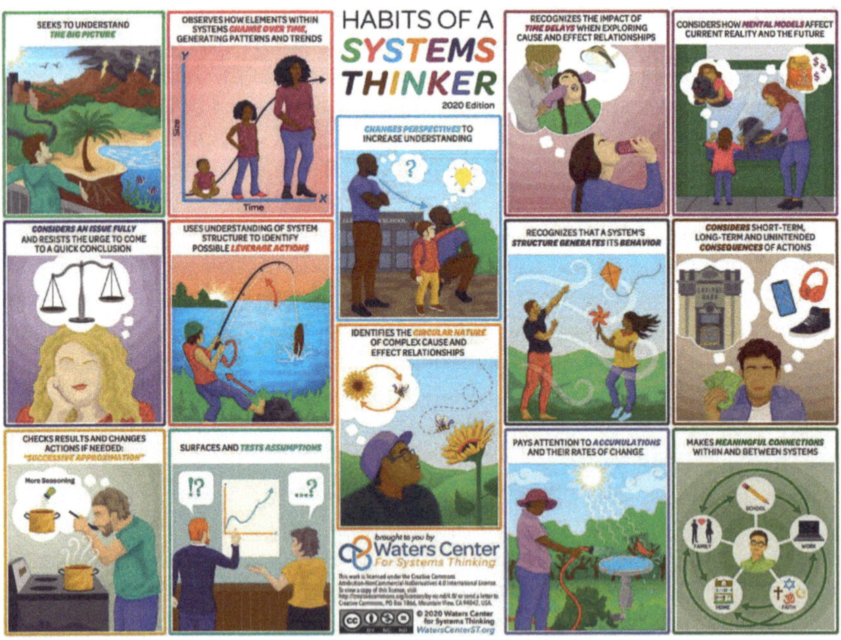
HABITS OF A
SYSTEMS
THINKER
2020 Edition
SEEKS TO UNDERSTAND THE BIG PICTURE
OBSERVES HOW ELEMENTS WITHIN SYSTEMS CHANGE OVER TIME, GENERATING PATTERNS AND TRENDS
Y
Size
Time
X
CHANGES PERSPECTIVES TO INCREASE UNDERSTANDING
?
RECOGNIZES THE IMPACT OF TIME DELAYS WHEN EXPLORING CAUSE AND EFFECT RELATIONSHIPS
CONSIDERS HOW MENTAL MODELS AFFECT CURRENT REALITY AND THE FUTURE
$ $ $
CONSIDERS AN ISSUE FULLY AND RESISTS THE URGE TO COME TO A QUICK CONCLUSION
USES UNDERSTANDING OF SYSTEM STRUCTURE TO IDENTIFY POSSIBLE LEVERAGE ACTIONS
IDENTIFIES THE CIRCULAR NATURE OF COMPLEX CAUSE AND EFFECT RELATIONSHIPS
RECOGNIZES THAT A SYSTEM'S STRUCTURE GENERATES ITS BEHAVIOR
CONSIDERS SHORT-TERM, LONG-TERM AND UNINTENDED CONSEQUENCES OF ACTIONS
CHECKS RESULTS AND CHANGES ACTIONS IF NEEDED: "SUCCESSIVE APPROXIMATION"
More Seasoning
SURFACES AND TESTS ASSUMPTIONS
!?
...?
PAYS ATTENTION TO ACCUMULATIONS AND THEIR RATES OF CHANGE
MAKES MEANINGFUL CONNECTIONS WITHIN AND BETWEEN SYSTEMS
SCHOOL
FAMILY
WORK
HOME
FAITH
brought to you by
Waters Center
For Systems Thinking
© 2020 Waters Center for Systems Thinking
WatersCenterST.org

Fig. 2. Habits of a systems thinker. (*From* The Waters Center for Systems Thinking, 2020, with permission.)

Table 1
Applying habits of a systems thinker to a clinical case

You are a pediatric hospitalist. You are discharging a 3-y-old patient with history of liver transplant home today following hospitalization for dehydration secondary to viral gastroenteritis. The patient has occasionally used ondansetron for management of nausea in the hospital. You have electronically prescribed a short course of ondansetron to the hospital pharmacy and have discussed the home use, risks, and benefits of this medication with the family. The child and family return home. The following night, you receive a call that the child had an episode of emesis following the immunosuppressive medication. They mention they were never able to pick up the ondansetron because it was not ready at the pharmacy when they left the hospital. As a systems thinker, you adapt to the situation at hand and critically think about the underlying system that created this gap in patient care to help prevent similar gaps in the future.

Which systems thinking habits might you apply in this situation? What actions might you take that would show systems thinking?

Habit	Potential Actions
Changes perspectives to increase understanding	• Recognize the emotional, financial, and social challenges families face when a child is hospitalized • Identify family challenges in accessing care, including obtaining prescriptions before discharge
Considers short-term, long-term, and unintended consequences of actions	Identify potential consequences for this patient • Short-term: patient may be readmitted to the hospital, poor symptom management at home • Long-term: family may think they were not adequately prepared for discharge home, may affect perception of health care system • Unintended: family may have to find ways to get to a pharmacy in the night, find childcare, and/or transportation
Considers an issue fully and resists the urge to come to a quick conclusion	• Collect data on pediatric hospital discharges with discharge medications not filled in the previous 6–12 mo • Collaborate with pharmacy colleagues on strategies to help ensure medication prescriptions are filled • Consider implementing a quality improvement project
Uses understanding of system structure to identify possible leverage actions	After developing an understanding of the hospital prescribing process, brainstorm ideas to adjust your practice • Collaborate with nursing colleagues to have families and patients physically go to the hospital pharmacy to ensure they are able to obtain prescriptions before discharge • Add step on discharge checklist that notes discharge medications have been filled • Connect with pharmacy if patients are unable to obtain the prescription before discharge to devise an alternative plan • Adapt to anticipating discharge needs as the hospital course evolves and send prescriptions as early as feasible to ensure they are ready for patients before discharge

Data From What Is Systems Thinking? Waters Center for Systems Thinking. Published 2020. Accessed November 21, 2020. Available at https://waterscenterst.org/systems-thinking-tools-and-strategies/what-is-systems-thinking/.

care processes (steps in health care work) and structures (the personnel, materials, physical spaces, and so forth needed for health care work) required to achieve ideal health outcomes [36]. This Donabedian (structure-process-outcome) model, with the addition of other measures such as patient experience, remains the benchmark for measuring health care quality. Highlighted next are 2 pediatric structures that serve important functions toward achieving ideal health for children: the pediatric medical home and schools.

Pediatric medical home

The American Academy of Pediatrics (AAP) defines the pediatric medical home as "delivery of advanced primary care with the goal of addressing and integrating high-quality health promotion, acute care, and chronic condition management in a planned, coordinated, and family-centered manner" [37]. Successful pediatric medical homes must include patients and their families at the center, similar to the HSS framework. The pediatric medical home, a model for comprehensive primary care, centers on the partnership between the family, a pediatric clinician, and the multidisciplinary team to establish ongoing care and facilitate access to services such as behavioral health and subspecialty care, care coordination, education, and surgical and inpatient services.

Pediatric medical homes ideally recognize the impact of social determinants of health as greater than the impact of the health care system, and therefore prioritize effective connections for families with community pediatric-relevant health structures such as local organizations, public health departments, facilities for children with complex care needs, hospitals, and schools. Medical home teams can advance population health via community partnerships such as community mass vaccinations and school clinics. The COVID-19 pandemic highlighted the importance of effective interactions across pediatric health structures, including medical homes, hospitals, public health, and schools.

Schools

Schools became an increasingly important partner in caring for children during the COVID-19 pandemic, incorporating new methods to optimize child, family, and community health. Some schools are now providing virtual counseling appointments. Early childhood intervention programs are completing initial assessments via virtual visits. Pediatric clinicians can advocate for child health by collaborating with schools on several levels. As community members, they can assist with appropriate school reopening plans. Providers can become part of research projects that are focused on safe schools and work alongside county public health and school nurses to ensure children have access to medical care and medications. Most importantly, pediatric clinicians must share essential resources with families and schools that address emerging family needs (eg, nutrition and food access, mental health resources, and child safety).

Application in clinical practice

You see a 14-year-old boy with attention-deficit/hyperactivity disorder (ADHD) and major depression in your clinic. You have been his primary care pediatrician for several years and know the family well. His father is worried about his mood. He attends school virtually at home because of the COVID-19 pandemic. Most days he is home alone because his father and mother are both working. He helps his younger brother during the school day as well and is struggling with focusing on a computer for several hours daily, feels isolated from peers, has decreased appetite, and is not sleeping well. He has not been able to follow with a community outpatient therapist because of the pandemic and associated costs.

Application of systems thinking with knowledge of existing pediatric health care structures and processes can help you develop a broad list of possible interventions for this boy and his family within the limits of the COVID-19 pandemic. You are aware of many community resources that have adapted during this time, and want to improve his health in a way that aligns with his family's preferences and values.

- You enroll him in your clinic's integrated behavioral health care management program for adolescents with depression. A team member will call him each week, and monthly follow-up virtual visits will be established with you or a colleague.
- You encourage him to contact his high school counselor as a resource to optimize his success in school, focusing on classes, and completing homework in a timely manner. You print information from the school's Web site to help him secure an appointment.
- You share with the family the contact information for an adolescent peer support group led virtually by a certified nurse at the county public health department.
- You provide details on local community organization programs that provide an encouraging learning environment for students engaged in virtual learning, and whose parents are working outside the home during business hours.

POPULATION, PUBLIC, AND SOCIAL DETERMINANTS OF HEALTH

Pediatric clinicians and health systems have been closely connected with their public health counterparts for some time. Population health is a fairly new term in pediatric practice. Although public health works to protect and improve community health via policy, education, outreach, and research, population health provides "an opportunity for healthcare systems, agencies and organizations to work together in order to improve the health outcomes of the communities they serve" [38] . In the past, many clinicians thought that improving the health of each individual improves population health, but the importance of improving population health (including those who do not regularly access care) to improve the health of individuals is now recognized.

Social determinants of health as part of structural competency

Fig. 3 shows the relationships between health structures, social determinants of health, and health disparities. Collectively these topics and their relationships have been defined as structural competency, or the structural determinants of the social determinants of health [39].

Structural competency includes 5 core competencies [40]:

1. Recognizing the structures that shape clinical interactions
2. Developing an extraclinical language of structure
3. Rearticulating cultural formulations in structural terms

4. Observing and imagining structural interventions
5. Developing structural humility

Pediatric clinicians in medical homes have the opportunity to discuss social determinants of health with patients and their families, implement education on implicit bias, advocate for child health through using the HSS framework, and be agents of change. Pediatric providers can promote equity by developing a culturally safe medical home, train staff in culturally competent care, develop language support services, and create a standard screening tool for social determinants of health [41]. Some educators are teaching learners to identify structural determinants of social determinants of health by applying cause-and-effect (fishbone) diagrams to published social medicine teaching cases [42]. Clinical teams might consider using this approach to applying systems thinking habits (such as "use understanding of system structure to identify possible leverage actions") in order to identify action steps for improving the care of individual patients.

Pediatric health professionals can also participate in population health initiatives to address disparities, and advocate for health care policy at the local, state, and national levels that affects safe housing, grocery store access, and safe schools, and reduces the health effects of structural racism [41,43].

CLINICAL INFORMATICS AND HEALTH TECHNOLOGY: TELEHEALTH

Telehealth is critical to ensuring access to high-quality care, particularly through the pediatric medical home. Its use grew rapidly during the COVID-19 pandemic [44]. Telehealth incorporates telehealth and e-health, including video visits, patient portal messages, telephone care, remote patient monitoring, and subspecialty electronic consults [45]. A prepandemic survey of AAP pediatricians in 2016 suggested that only 15% of pediatricians reported any form of telehealth use in the previous 12 months, with barriers to incorporation including insufficient payment and billing challenges [46]. Many barriers were reduced as part of the COVID-19 response, although long-term financial support is still unclear.

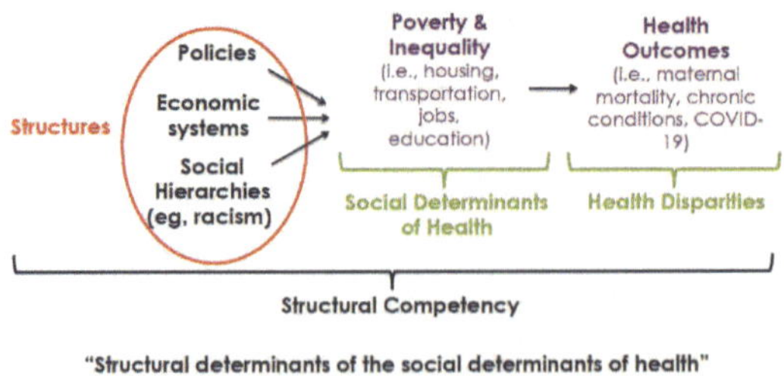

Fig. 3. Structural determinants of the social determinants of health. (*From* Health Outreach Partners and the Structural Competency Working Group, with permission.)

The selection of telehealth tools and processes depends on the type of pediatric care, health care delivery setting, and patient preferences for care [47]. Fiks and colleagues [48] provided a recent broad view of potential pediatric primary care benefits of telehealth with the Quadruple Aim in mind, which are summarized in Fig. 4. Alongside benefits, challenges remain, including ensuring equitable access to telehealth for patients and families and exploring payment models. Before the pandemic, Tomines [47] described how urgent care telehealth within the pediatric medical home may be an alternative to in-person acute care visits. With numerous options for connecting with patients of all ages, the medical home may ultimately be able to reach more patients along the care continuum, as has been learned in part by innovations during the pandemic.

HEALTH CARE POLICY AND ECONOMICS

The Health care policy and economics domain includes these major areas of content [30]:

1. Health policy
2. Health care financing
3. The impact of policy on insurance and reimbursement
4. Incentives for clinicians and health systems within different payment models

Health policy is defined as laws, regulations, procedures, administrative actions, incentives, or voluntary practices of governments or other institutions that have implications for or relate to health [49]. Health economics is the study of decisions (including incentives that lead to decisions, and consequences from those decisions) as they relate to production, distribution, and consumption of goods and services related to health when resources are limited and have alternative uses [50].

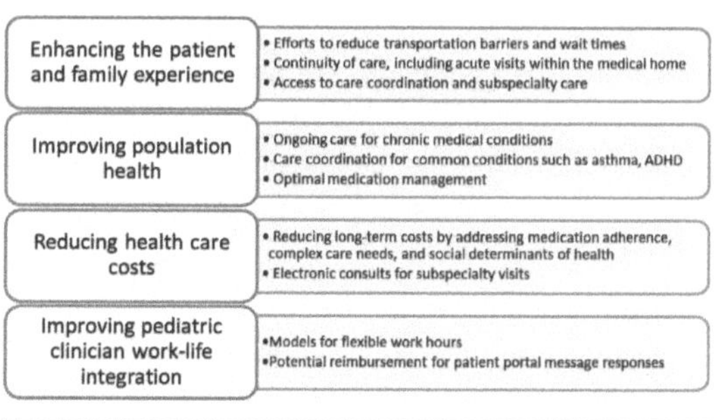

Fig. 4. Benefits of Incorporating telehealth into the pediatric medical home. The Quadruple Aim tenets are listed on the left, with examples of potential benefits to patients, families, and clinicians. (Content from Fiks AG, Jenssen BP, Ray KN. A Defining Moment for Pediatric Primary Care Telehealth. *JAMA Pediatr.* 2020 Jul 13. https://doi.org/10.1001/jamapediatrics.2020.1881. Epub ahead of print. PMID: 32658256.)

Pediatric clinicians in any system should have a basic understanding of health care payment models, including employment-based and government health insurance, and their potential impact on patients and their families. Pediatric clinicians within and beyond the medical home who understand the basics of these concepts are better positioned to improve the health care and health of the patients and families they serve, and to advocate locally and regionally to improve access to care via new payment models and other strategies.

Health policy and health insurance that enable health

The percentage of children without health insurance was increasing before 2020, in part because of the increasing cost of employer-sponsored insurance [13]. Many families experienced loss of employment during the COVID-19 pandemic, leaving more individuals without employer-sponsored insurance. Because of these changes, Medicaid and the Children's Health Insurance Program (CHIP) now need to provide coverage to a growing number of pediatric patients who are uninsured [13].

The public charge rule may keep immigrant families from enrolling their children in Medicaid or CHIP. The public charge rule is a part of federal immigration policy that is used to determine immigration or residency status [51]. Recent changes to the definition of public charge were made that resulted in negative consequences for applicants using public benefits such as Medicaid, the Supplemental Nutrition Assistance Program, or government housing, because use of government-supported resources can be used against individuals when determining permanent residency status [51]. This association left many families choosing not to enroll in government-based insurance for their children. Several physician associations, including the AAP, joined to oppose the public charge rule on the basis that it creates a significant barrier to health care and the well-being of children [52].

Innovative ideas for acting on the changes to the public charge rule and developing both short-term and long-term plans to strengthen Medicaid and CHIP will be necessary to ensure the continued success of these programs and ensure children have access to essential health care.

It is important that practices consider the broader health care system and the insurance they accept to eliminate health care disparities and increase access to care. Researchers and clinicians can collaborate to investigate health barriers and health outcomes within their population and use this information to implement change to eliminate disparities.

Payment system reform for children

The COVID-19 pandemic has reinforced the importance of health care payment system reform for children. The current system focuses on a fee-for-service payment model, with many advocating for a transition toward a value-based payment model in primary care to better address population health and social determinants of health. Current reform models have focused almost solely on adult health care because pediatric care overall is less costly and therefore reform may not lead to significant short-term savings [53]. However, this focus on adult care leaves vulnerable children with limited comprehensive care and has long-term societal costs (eg, untreated effects of ACEs) [53]. Focusing on reforming health care for children and investing in early childhood health would have a long-term impact on population health outcomes and cost savings.

There have been several potential effective models to integrate children into health care payment reform from accountable care organizations to bundled payments. The pediatric medical home model is adequately equipped to successfully incorporate evidence-based reform models, including providing behavioral health within the medical home; integrating community health workers; and screening, intervening, and ensuring a successful referral to organizations for treatment of ACE-related health conditions [53].

It is imperative that pediatric clinicians play a role in payment system reform for children. Pediatric clinicians can collaborate with community organizations and county public health to aid in enrolling children eligible for Medicaid and CHIP, and to increase opportunities for children to receive medical care in the community through advocating at the legislative level. By working within the pediatric medical home and beyond, pediatric clinicians can see the system with a broader view to advocate for both short-term and long-term change and new health care delivery and payment models at the local, state, and national levels.

CHANGE AGENCY, MANAGEMENT, AND ADVOCACY

Every pediatric clinician and leaders at all levels experienced major changes in their daily work during the COVID-19 pandemic. Pediatric and other clinical leaders were required to communicate volumes of information at a pace of change and during a time of significant, unprecedented uncertainty. Leaders also balanced the needs of patients and their communities while supporting their workforce and frontline clinical teams. This domain includes all of the content, knowledge, and skills needed by clinicians to be effective change agents to improve systems of care for patients [26].

Advocacy

There has always been a special emphasis on advocacy in pediatric medical education and practice given shared care of vulnerable individuals without a legal voice [54]. This emphasis was amplified in 2020 following the pandemic's onset and renewed, widespread efforts to address structural causes of racism and its effect on children. The pandemic heightened awareness of structural racism and accelerated opportunities and efforts to advocate for children [55]. The earlier review of other HSS domains shared multiple opportunities to advocate for children to improve their health, including advocacy for individual children and their families, populations of patients (by demographics and/or health condition), and via local, regional, and national health policy advocacy.

Table 2
Applying multiple health systems science concepts and skills to a clinical case

You care for a 10-y-old girl with moderate persistent asthma that is poorly controlled. You know her family well and call them because she has missed 2 recent follow-up appointments. Her father answers and says he recently became unemployed. He no longer has employer-sponsored insurance and was nervous to bring his daughter to the scheduled visit because of visit costs. You talk with her father about her poorly controlled asthma, looking for opportunities to help their family identify and address additional barriers to care. Her father shares barriers including transportation, cost of visits and medications, time, lack of insurance, and access to an inhaler with spacer device at school.

Using a systems thinking approach, you consider the number of ways you can apply HSS concepts and skills to improve asthma care and outcomes for this girl and other children in your practice

Potential Actions	HSS Domains
Collaborate with social worker to connect with the family to start discussing enrollment in Medicaid	• Health care policy and economics • Population, public, and social determinants of heath • Teaming
Enroll your patient in your asthma care coordination, enabling nurses reach out on a scheduled basis to assess her asthma control, challenges with adherence to her asthma treatment plan, and access to her written, individualized asthma action plan at both home and school	• Value in health care • Health care structure and process • Teaming
Share community resources for receiving timely and equitable health care and resources for transportation to appointments	• Value in health care • Population, public, and social determinants of health • Teaming
Review your office scheduling procedures to ensure appointments are being offered at times that facilitate access for families with a variety of schedules	• Value in health care • Leadership • Population, public, and social determinants of health • Change agency, management, and advocacy
Consider developing a quality improvement project designed to increase the percentage of patients with asthma in your practice with optimal asthma control and access to asthma action plans	• Health system improvement • Value in health care • Population, public, and social determinants of health • Change agency, management, and advocacy
Consider opportunities to work with local health leaders (schools, public health) to improve health outcomes for children with asthma	• Health system improvement • Value in health care • Population, public, and social determinants of health • Change agency, management, and advocacy

SUMMARY

Care is a verb, and caring is the cornerstone of all health professions. An evidence-based approach to caring for patients and their families must also include caring for the systems that affect the health of children. The current performance of the US health care system, the impact of structural and social determinants on health outcomes, the poor alignment between pace of change in practice and in medical education, and existing and emerging threats to child health require pediatric health professionals to embrace a third science in addition to basic and clinical science. The HSS framework gives pediatric clinicians and their teams a conceptual framework and common language to recognize and enact change to improve access and the care of pediatric patients, their families, and their communities. Table 2 summarizes opportunities to apply concepts and skills in the HSS domains described earlier using a clinical case as an example.

Pediatric health professionals and their multidisciplinary teams who incorporate systems thinking into practice are well positioned to improve health and health care for the infants, children, and adolescents they serve. The medical home is a key structure to improving population health, and teams within the medical home can continue to improve health and health care via telehealth, engaging in advocacy efforts, and learning strategies to help mitigate the negative impact of health economics and payment on children and families.

CLINICS CARE POINTS (EVIDENCE-BASED PEARLS AND PITFALLS FOR POINT OF CARE)

- All pediatric health teams should ensure all members understand and commit to their 2 essential roles in advancing the health of children: direct clinical care and their work to improve the system.
- All clinical teams caring for children should commit to and engage in ongoing work to ensure equitable care for all children rooted in cultural humility and culturally sensitive care.
- Pediatricians, other pediatric health professionals, and their interprofessional teams should screen for social determinants of health and ACEs during hospitalizations and outpatient visits.
- Clinicians providing acute, emergency, and specialty care for children should confirm the medical home for every child, helping to establish a connection for those without one.
- All pediatric medical homes should work to ensure high-quality, accessible telehealth for their pediatric patients and families.
- All pediatric health professionals can identify opportunities to improve the health of children in their population and/or community. Opportunities include population medicine efforts (eg, care management for children with chronic diseases), quality improvement initiatives, policy or other local/regional advocacy, and partnerships with schools and public health departments.

- Pediatric health professionals should understand how health care payment models affect the financial impact on families for the common tests and treatments they order as part of their approach to discussing effectiveness, cost, and families' preferences and values.
- Pediatric health teams should consider incorporating HSS principles such as systems thinking to closing clinical gaps and addressing practice challenges.

Disclosure

Dr K.M. Bartoletta has no disclosures. Dr S.R. Starr received an honorarium as faculty for the American Medical Association's Health Systems Academy Scholars' Program. She is coeditor of the Elsevier textbook *Health Systems Science, Second Edition* and coauthored an American Medical Association Health Systems Science online module but does not receive compensation from the book or the module.

References

[1] Berwick DM, Nolan TW, Whittington J. The triple aim: care, health, and cost. Health Aff (Millwood) 2008;27(3):759–69.

[2] Bodenheimer T, Sinsky C. From triple to quadruple aim: care of the patient requires care of the provider. Ann Fam Med 2014;12(6):573–6.

[3] Schneider EC, Sarnack DO, Squires D, et al. For the Commonwealth Fund. Mirror, Mirror 2017: International Comparison Reflects Flaws and Opportunities for Better U.S. Health Care. 2017. Available at: https://interactives.commonwealthfund.org/2017/july/mirror-mirror/. Accessed November 22, 2020.

[4] County Health Rankings & Roadmaps. University of Wisconsin Public Health Institute. Available at: https://www.countyhealthrankings.org/explore-health-rankings/measures-data-sources/county-health-rankings-model. Accessed November 21, 2020.

[5] Life expectancy: could where you live influence how long you live? Robert Wood Johnson Foundation. 2020. Available at: https://www.rwjf.org/en/library/interactives/whereyouliveaffectshowlongyoulive.html. Accessed November 21, 2020.

[6] Children with Special Health Care Needs: National Survey of Children's Health Data Brief. Health Resources and Services Administration Maternal and Child Health. 2020. Available at: https://mchb.hrsa.gov/sites/default/files/mchb/Data/NSCH/nsch-cshcn-data-brief.pdf. Accessed November 22, 2020.

[7] The Impact of Gun Violence on Children and Teens. Everytown Research & Policy. 2019. Available at: https://everytownresearch.org/report/the-impact-of-gun-violence-on-children-and-teens/. Accessed November 21, 2020.

[8] Leading Causes of Death and Injury - PDFs|Injury Center|CDC. 2020. Available at: https://www.cdc.gov/injury/wisqars/LeadingCauses.html. Accessed November 26, 2020.

[9] Adverse Childhood Experiences. Violence Prevention. Centers for Disease Control and Prevention. 2020. Available at: https://www.cdc.gov/violenceprevention/aces/index.html. Accessed November 21, 2020.

[10] Climate Change and Public Health - Climate Effects on Health | CDC. 2020. Available at: https://www.cdc.gov/climateandhealth/effects/default.html. Accessed November 26, 2020.

[11] Children's Environmental Health Module. 2020. Available at: https://ephtracking.cdc.gov/showChildEHTopics. Accessed November 26, 2020.

[12] Clark E, Fredricks K, Woc-Colburn L, et al. Disproportionate impact of the COVID-19 pandemic on immigrant communities in the United States. PLoS Negl Trop Dis 2020;14(7):e0008484.
[13] Millions Of Children Have Lost Their Health Insurance—What's Our Plan? | Health Affairs Blog. 2020. Available at: https://www.healthaffairs.org/do/10.1377/hblog20200729.620204/full/. Accessed November 21, 2020.
[14] Jablonski BBR, Casnovsky J, Clark JK, et al. Emergency Food Provision for Children and Families during the COVID-19 Pandemic: Examples from Five U.S. Cities. Applied Economic Perspectives and Policy 2021;43(1):169–84.
[15] Tomaskovic-Devey D. The COVID-19 pandemic: normal accidents and cascading system failures (inequality, poverty, and mobility). American Sociological Association; 2020. Available at: https://www.asanet.org/news-events/footnotes/may-jun-2020/research-policy/covid-19-pandemic-normal-accidents-and-cascading-system-failures-inequality-poverty-and-mobility. Accessed November 21, 2020.
[16] Schwartz SA. COVID-19 and the documented failure of the American illness profit system — We have to stop treating our doctors, nurses, healthcare workers, and ourselves this way. Explore (NY) 2020;16(4):210–3.
[17] Hartzband P, Groopman J. Physician Burnout, Interrupted. N Engl J Med 2020;382(26): 2485–7.
[18] Giordano M. Children's doctors in the world of adults. The Hospitalist. 2020. Available at: https://www.the-hospitalist.org/hospitalist/article/226687/pediatrics/childrens-doctors-world-adults. Accessed November 21, 2020.
[19] Manning KD. When grief and crises intersect: perspectives of a black physician in the time of two pandemics. J Hosp Med 2020;15(9):566–7; https://doi.org/10.12788/jhm.3481.
[20] Irby DM, Cooke M, O'Brien BC. Calls for reform of medical education by the Carnegie Foundation for the Advancement of Teaching: 1910 and 2010. Acad Med 2010;85(2): 220–7.
[21] Skochelak SE. A decade of reports calling for change in medical education: what do they say? Acad Med 2010;85(9 Suppl):S26–33.
[22] Crosson FJ, Leu J, Roemer BM, et al. Gaps in residency training should be addressed to better prepare doctors for a twenty-first-century delivery system. Health Aff (Millwood) 2011;30(11):2142–8.
[23] Lucey CR. Medical education: part of the problem and part of the solution. JAMA Intern Med 2013;173(17):1639–43.
[24] Berwick DM, Finkelstein JA. Preparing medical students for the continual improvement of health and health care: Abraham Flexner and the new "public interest". Acad Med 2010;85(9 Suppl):S56–65.
[25] Gonzalo JD, Haidet P, Papp KK, et al. Educating for the 21st-century health care system: an interdependent framework of basic, clinical, and systems sciences. Acad Med 2017;92(1): 35–9.
[26] Skochelak SE, Hammoud MM, Lomis KD, et al. Health systems science. 2nd edition. Philadelpia: Elsevier; 2020.
[27] Yong PL, Olsen L, McGinnis JM. Value in health care: accounting for cost, quality, safety, outcomes, and innovation. Institute of Medicine: roundtable on value & science-driven health care: charter and vision statement. Washington, DC: National Academies Press; 2010. Available at: https://www.ncbi.nlm.nih.gov/books/NBK50934/. Accessed November 21, 2020.
[28] Institute of Medicine. Best care at lower cost: the path to continuously learning health care in America. The National Academies of Sciences, Engineering, Medicine. Washington, DC: National Academies Press; 2013. Available at: https://www.nap.edu/catalog/13444/best-care-at-lower-cost-the-path-to-continuously-learning. Accessed November 22, 2020.

[29] Aron DC, Headrick LA. Educating physicians prepared to improve care and safety is no accident: it requires a systematic approach. Qual Saf Health Care 2002;11(2):168–73.
[30] Gonzalo JD, Wolpaw T, Wolpaw D. Curricular transformation in health systems science: the need for global change. Acad Med 2018;93(10):1431–3.
[31] Hafferty FW, Levinson D. Moving beyond nostalgia and motives: towards a complexity science view of medical professionalism. Perspect Biol Med 2008;51(4):599–615.
[32] Lead was poisoning the water in Flint, Michigan: Dr. Mona Hanna-Attisha put her reputation on the line to prove it. USA Today. 2020. Available at: https://www.usatoday.com/in-depth/life/women-of-the-century/2020/08/11/19th-amendment-flint-water-crisis-elevated-dr-mona-hanna-attisha/5535823002/. Accessed November 21, 2020.
[33] National Academies of Sciences, Engineering, and Medicine. Taking action against clinician burnout: a systems approach to professional well-being. The National Academies of Sciences, Engineering, Medicine. Washington, DC: National Academies Press; 2019. Available at: https://www.nap.edu/catalog/25521/taking-action-against-clinician-burnout-a-systems-approach-to-professional. Accessed November 22, 2020.
[34] Perlo J, Balik B, Swensen S, et al. IHI framework for improving joy in work. IHI white paper. Cambridge (MA): Institute for Healthcare Improvement; 2017. Available at: http://www.ihi.org:80/resources/Pages/IHIWhitePapers/Framework-Improving-Joy-in-Work.aspx. Accessed November 21, 2020.
[35] What Is Systems Thinking? Waters Center for Systems Thinking. 2020. Available at: https://waterscenterst.org/systems-thinking-tools-and-strategies/what-is-systems-thinking/. Accessed November 21, 2020.
[36] Donabedian A. The quality of care: how can it be assessed? JAMA 1988;260(12):1743–8.
[37] Medical Home. American Academy of Pediatrics. Available at: http://www.aap.org/en-us/professional-resources/practice-transformation/medicalhome/Pages/home.aspx. Accessed November 21, 2020.
[38] What is population health? Milken Institute School of Public Health. The George Washington University; 2015. Available at: https://onlinepublichealth.gwu.edu/resources/what-is-population-health/. Accessed November 22, 2020.
[39] Health Outreach Partners and the Structural Competency Working Group. 2020. Available at: https://www.structcomp.org. Accessed November 22, 2020.
[40] Metzl JM, Hansen H. Structural competency: theorizing a new medical engagement with stigma and inequality. Soc Sci Med 2014;103:126–33.
[41] Trent M, Dooley DG, Dougé J, et al. The impact of racism on child and adolescent health. Pediatrics 2019;144(2):e20191765.
[42] Hassan I, Bui T. Developing social medicine cases using a structural competency framework. Workshop presented at AMA ChangeMedEd Conference; September 18, 2019; Chicago, IL.
[43] Kuo AK, Summers NM, Vohra S, et al. The promise of precision population health: reducing health disparities through a community partnership framework. Adv Pediatr 2019;66:1–13.
[44] Marcin JP, Rimsza ME, Moskowitz WB. The use of telehealth to address access and physician workforce shortages. Pediatrics 2015;136(1):202–9.
[45] Telehealth and telemedicine: a research anthology of law and policy resources. Health professionals gateway. Centers for Disease Control and Prevention; 2019. Available at: https://www.cdc.gov/phlp/publications/topic/anthologies/anthologies-telehealth.html. Accessed November 22, 2020.
[46] Sisk B, Alexander J, Bodnar C, et al. Pediatrician attitudes toward and experiences with telehealth use: results from a national survey. Acad Pediatr 2020;20(5):628–35.
[47] Tomines A. Pediatric telehealth: approaches by specialty and implications for general pediatric care. Adv Pediatr 2019;66:55–85.

[48] Fiks AG, Jenssen BP, Ray KN. A defining moment for pediatric primary care telehealth. JAMA Pediatr 2020; https://doi.org/10.1001/jamapediatrics.2020.1881.
[49] Definition of Policy. Office of the associate director for policy and strategy. Centers for Disease Control and Prevention; 2015. Available at: https://www.cdc.gov/policy/analysis/process/definition.html. Accessed November 22, 2020.
[50] Public health economics. Public Charge Rule and Its Impact on Child Health: A Call to Action. Pediatrics 2020;146(6); https://doi.org/10.1542/peds.2020-001495.
[51] Patel N, Reddy S, Wilson N. Public Charge Rule and Its Impact on Child Health: A Call to Action. Pediatrics 2020;146(6).
[52] Joint Statement of America's Frontline Physicians Opposing Public Charge Final Rule. 2019. Available at: https://www.psychiatry.org/newsroom/news-releases/joint-statement-of-america-s-frontline-physicians-opposing-public-charge-final-rule. Accessed November 21, 2020.
[53] Health Care Payment and Delivery System Reform for Children as a Tool to Improve the Health of Vulnerable Communities. Families USA and Futures Without Violence. 2020. Available at: https://familiesusa.org/wp-content/uploads/2020/07/CHI_Kids-System-Transformation_FINAL.pdf. Accessed November 22, 2020.
[54] Chamberlain LJ, Kelly N. Child Advocacy in the Twenty-first Century. Adv Pediatr 2015;62(1):91–103.
[55] COVID-19 Response: Advocacy Report. American Academy of Pediatrics. 2020. Available at: https://downloads.aap.org/DOFA/COVID-19%20Advocacy%20Report%205.0.pdf. Accessed November 22, 2020.

Advances in Pediatrics 68 (2021) 21–35
ADVANCES IN PEDIATRICS

When Less is More
The Role of Overdiagnosis and Overtreatment in Patient Safety

Audrey D. Kamzan, MD[a,b,*], Elayna Ng, MD[a,b]
[a]Division of Pediatric Hospital Medicine, Mattel Children's Hospital, 10833 LeConte Avenue, A2-383 MDCC, Los Angeles, CA 90095, USA; [b]David Geffen School of Medicine at the University of California, Los Angeles, 10833 Le Conte Avenue, A2-383 MDCC, Los Angeles, CA 90095, USA

Keywords
• Overuse • Overdiagnosis • Overtreatment • Waste • Low-value care
• Patient safety

Key points

- Overuse (including overdiagnosis and overtreatment), also referred to as low-value care, is a major contributor to waste in health care and causes harm to patients.
- Overuse can be measured either directly—by comparing the care provided to established guidelines—or indirectly—by measuring unexplained variability in care that cannot be explained by population differences.
- Overdiagnosis is the detection of abnormalities that are unlikely to cause harm. It often leads to overtreatment, in which the harms of treatment outweigh the benefits.
- The motivations driving overuse are multifactorial and include physician attitudes, patient factors, industry influence, and others.
- Solutions to prevent overuse include increasing provider education and awareness programs (such as the Choosing Wisely campaign), changing institutional priorities to focus on preventing overuse, and improving patient-provider communication.

*Corresponding author. David Geffen School of Medicine at the University of California, Los Angeles, 10833 Le Conte Avenue, A2-383 MDCC, Los Angeles, CA 90095, USA.
E-mail address: akamzan@mednet.ucla.edu

https://doi.org/10.1016/j.yapd.2021.05.013

INTRODUCTION

A bedrock tenet of the practice of medicine, immortalized in the Hippocratic oath, is the principle, "first, do no harm." Yet, in the endeavor to diagnose, prevent, and treat illness, providers often provide care that has no hope of benefitting the patient and may even cause harm. In the United States, the rate of usage of health care services varies significantly by region [1,2]. Although it might be assumed that greater usage would lead to better population health, more not always is better. Studies show that in regions where more health services are provided, certain outcomes are worse [3]. Why is it that providers so often find themselves providing care that is of no benefit to, and even harms, patients? This article describes the scope of the problem of health care overuse, explores the complex motivations that lead to overdiagnosis and overtreatment, and proposes solutions that may help mitigate the tendency toward overuse. As providers seek to lower health care expenditures and protect patients from harm, they must understand that each test ordered and each treatment prescribed represents a potential for harm. Sometimes the best way to avoid harm from medical interventions is to avoid the intervention in the first place and to instead ask, "How can providers safely do less?"

BACKGROUND

In 1999, the Institute of Medicine released "To Err is Human," a report that revealed that 44,000 to 98,000 people died each year in United States hospitals due to medical errors and adverse events (some estimates are 2–3 times higher) [4]. This staggering revelation has triggered countless quality improvement and patient safety initiatives as well as the birth of the Agency for Healthcare Research and Quality. Although some individual measures have demonstrated modest success, there is little evidence that the past 20 years of efforts have, in the aggregate, reduced harm to patients [5].

The pediatric population is particularly vulnerable to harm and medical errors in many ways that differ from adults [6]:

- Childhood development: errors may lead to harm that has an impact on a child's development, often in ways that are not initially apparent. For example, pediatric asthma patients who are not prescribed inhaled corticosteroids may be overprescribed systemic steroids, which can have an impact on growth over time [7].
- Demographics: children of different ages require different care, adding a layer of complexity to their care.
- Reliance on caregivers: pediatric patients are often unable to report their own needs and are dependent on caregivers to decide what treatment is appropriate.
- Not just small adults: children often are treated in environments designed primarily for adults (eg, adult emergency departments), where providers may lack knowledge about the different disease processes and manifestations in children [8,9].

- Prescribing of medications: pediatric dosing is weight-based, which demands added complexity of systems, such as computerized physician order entry. Even though medication error rates are similar between adults and pediatrics, potentially harmful errors occur 3 times as often in pediatric patients [10].

Health care in the United States is among the most expensive in the world; in 2014, the United States spent 16.4% of the gross domestic product (approximately $9034 per capita) on health care, compared with the global Organisation for Economic Co-operation and Development (OECD) average of 8.7%. The US life expectancy in that same year, however, was 81.3 years, compared with the OECD average of 83.1 years, and the number of avoidable deaths in the United States was 5.8 per 100,000 people versus the OECD average of 4.3 per 100,000 [11,12]. When examining the relationship between health care expenditures and life expectancy (Fig. 1) or unavoidable deaths (Fig. 2), the correlation is only weakly positive. Thus, more health care dollars spent do not always translate to better health.

Where are these health care dollars going, if not to improving patient health? Waste, at its lowest estimates, constitutes up to 20% of all US health care expenditures [13]. Waste comes in many forms, including failures of care delivery, failures of care coordination, administrative complexity, fraud, and overuse/overtreatment. This article explores this last category of waste: the problem of overuse and overtreatment. In 2019, overtreatment accounted for $75.7 billion to $101.2 billion in waste–approximately 28% to 40% of all waste [14]. The recognition of the burden of overuse has led to a movement of "safely doing less."

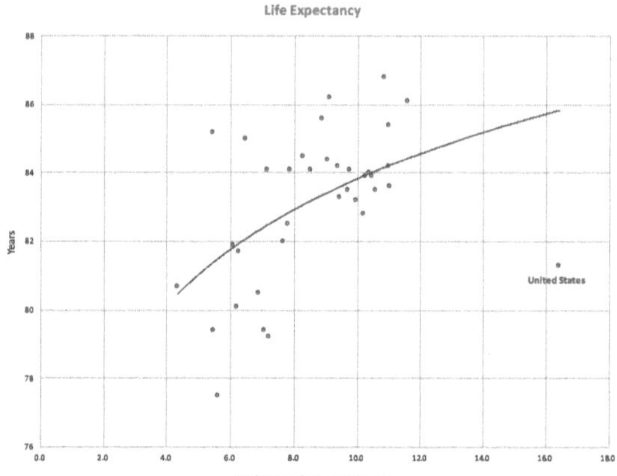

Fig. 1. Linear regression demonstrating correlation between OECD nations' life expectancy in years per 100,000 people and percent of gross domestic product (GDP) spent on health care. *Data from* OECD 2014, *Health Expenditure* and *Health Status*, https://stats.oecd.org/. Accessed November 20, 2020.

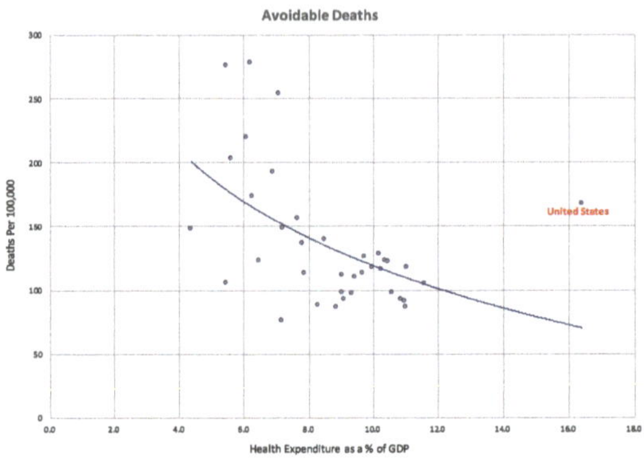

Fig. 2. Linear regression demonstrating correlation between OECD nations' avoidable deaths and percent of gross domestic product (GDP) spent on health care. *Data from* OECD 2014, *Health Expenditure* and *Health Status*, https://stats.oecd.org/. Accessed November 20, 2020.

DEFINITIONS OF OVERUSE, OVERDIAGNOSIS, AND OVERTREATMENT

Patient safety is defined as the "freedom from accidental injury" during medical care, such as adverse drug events or health care–associated infections [4]. One threat to patient safety is *overuse* (also known as *low-value care*), defined as the provision of medical services that are more likely to cause harm than good or that a fully informed patient would not want [15]. Overuse is often difficult to identify, however, because it requires a clear definition of what use is appropriate. What may be right for 1 patient may not be right for another patient, and often there is insufficient scientific evidence to know what is appropriate. Some treatments may be considered universally helpful, whereas others are universally ineffective or harmful; everything else lies in the gray zone in-between, where the benefit may be scant, the degree of benefit depends on patient characteristics, or there is little evidence to decide (Fig. 3) [16]. Furthermore, a patient may find an intervention valuable whereas the physician does not or vice versa. Even physicians who think they are providing treatment in accordance with their patients' values

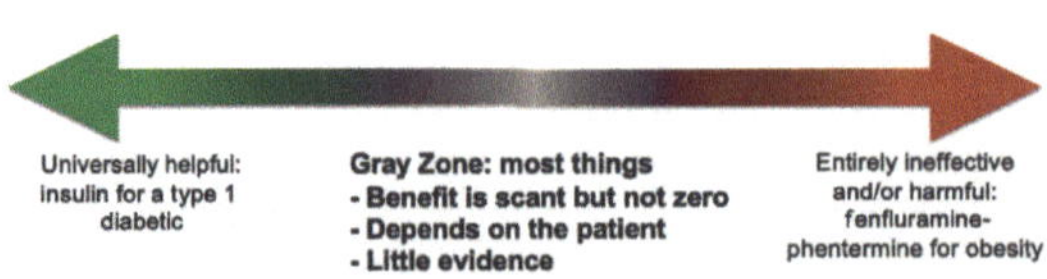

Fig. 3. Gray zone services: when determining what is considered overuse, some treatments are universally beneficial and others universally ineffective or harmful; however, most fall in the gray zone in-between, making the definition of overuse complicated in many situations. *From* Brownlee S, Chalkidou K, Doust J, et al. Evidence for overuse of medical services around the world. Lancet. 2017 Jul 8;390(10090):156-168; with permission of Elsevier.

often are not–a phenomenon termed *preference misdiagnosis*. For example, doctors treating breast cancer patients believe 71% of patients rate keeping their breast a top priority, when in fact only 7% do [17]. There are times when the values of a physician and patient may appear to align, but, if better informed about risks and benefits, the patient's values would be different [18]. All these factors make overuse difficult to define.

The complexities of determining what constitutes overuse also make it difficult to measure. Overuse can be measured either directly or indirectly:

- Direct measurement: scientific evidence or consensus dictates what is appropriate, and deviation from this is tracked and measured (eg, despite published guidelines recommending amoxicillin for the management of community-acquired pneumonia, the most commonly prescribed outpatient pediatric antibiotics are macrolides and broad-spectrum antibiotics) [19].
- Indirect measurement: unexpected variation in health care utilization is measured, and increased utilization not attributable to population differences is presumed to be due to overuse (eg, rates of elective percutaneous coronary interventions vary 10-fold within the state of California) [20].

Overuse is closely related to *overdiagnosis*, defined as the overdetection or overdefinition of disease [21]. Overdiagnosis is distinct from misdiagnosis–whereas misdiagnosis is the incorrect identification of disease, overdiagnosis identifies a true abnormality, but one that if left untreated causes no harm to the patient. Overdiagnosis may occur when diagnostic technology, such as laboratory testing and imaging, becomes more sensitive, identifying abnormalities that ultimately will not harm the patient. It also may occur when the definition threshold of a diagnosis is lowered, without clear added benefit to the patient. For example, the diagnostic criteria for attention-deficit/hyperactivity disorder (ADHD) have broadened over time to include children 4 years to 18 years of age (instead of 6–12 years), making ADHD one of the most common pediatric diagnoses [22]. It is yet unclear that this broadened definition has led to an overall benefit for patients, but a diagnosis of ADHD does present a potential for harm in the form of medication side effects, costs, and even altered perceptions of the patient by their teachers, peers, parents, and self [23]. In Canada, where the birthday cutoff for school entry is December 31, a study found that children born in December were significantly more likely to receive a diagnosis of ADHD than children born in January [24]. The implication is that children who are younger and perhaps less developmentally mature than their peers are more likely to receive a diagnosis of ADHD. Furthermore, the broadened age criteria to children as young as 4 years of age has led to the prescription of stimulants to more than 10,000 children 2 years to 3 years of age, a phenomenon known as *diagnostic creep* [25].

Overdiagnosis in turn leads to *overtreatment*, defined as treatment where there is no evidence of net benefit. This includes treatment that is futile or excessive in complexity, duration, or cost. The rates of diagnosis and treatment of neonates for hyperbilirubinemia have increased significantly, whereas mortality due to kernicterus has remained unchanged since 1979 [26]. Parents of infants who had jaundice or phototherapy were more likely to seek medical attention after resolution, to perceive subsequent illnesses as moderate or severe, and to fear leaving their infant with a caregiver [27]. Thus, even treatments perceived as very low risk, such as phototherapy, may come with hidden costs to the patient and family.

THE SCOPE OF HARM

The impact of overuse is often described in terms of rising health care costs and wasted resources; although this is accurate, it represents only 1 aspect of the detriment of overuse. The impact on the health care system at large may not be the most powerful argument against overuse. After all, physicians tend to feel their first responsibility is to the individual patient rather than the system as a whole [28], and patients often are skeptical of measures aimed at cutting costs [29,30]. A more powerful case to patients and providers against unnecessary testing and treatment may be the potential for overuse to directly harm patients.

Korenstein and colleagues [31] have developed a framework for understanding the negative impacts of overuse on patients, which include physical effects, psychological effects, treatment burden (such as the time required to travel to appointments), social effects (such as altered identity or status due to a new diagnosis), financial effects, and overall dissatisfaction with health care. Physical effects are the harms best described in the literature, but other types of harm are likely more prevalent than known, because they likely are underrecognized by providers. Importantly, low-value care has been found to affect minority groups disproportionately, in particular racial minorities; Black and Hispanic Medicare recipients were more likely to receive unnecessary cardiac screening, preoperative testing, and other low-value care [32]. Racial minorities, long known to be less likely to receive care that is necessary and beneficial, are also more likely to be subjected to care that is ineffectual or harmful. Thus, low-value care appears to be one of many contributors to ongoing health care disparities.

CASE STUDY IN OVERUSE: NEUROBLASTOMA SCREENING

From 1995 to 2000, Germany implemented a neuroblastoma screening program in which 6 of the 16 German states screened infants for neuroblastoma with urine catecholamines [33]. The other 10 states did not adopt the screening protocol and served as a control group (all states had similar baseline neuroblastoma rates). More cases were detected in the screened group than in the control group; however, despite increased detection of cases, there ultimately was no difference in the incidence of stage 4 neuroblastoma or mortality rates. This likely was because some neuroblastomas spontaneously regress. Any benefit of early diagnosis was outweighed by the harms of treatment–the 3 deaths in the screening group were due to complications of treatment (2 from complications of surgery and 1 from complications of chemotherapy). Based on rates of disease in the control area, it was estimated that approximately two-thirds of the detected cases likely would have spontaneously regressed and never been detected had they not been screened; in other words, two-thirds of cases represented overdiagnosis. Similar screening efforts were undertaken in Quebec, Canada, with similar results [34]. Japan also performed neuroblastoma screening until concerns were raised about the potential for overdiagnosis of tumors that otherwise would have regressed spontaneously [35]. Since the Japanese screening program was halted in 2004, the mortality rate and incidence of advanced-stage disease appears to have remained unchanged [36]. The case study of neuroblastoma screening is a clear example of a well-intended effort to save lives that, while increasing the rates of cancer detection, unfortunately likely only resulted in harm to patients rather than helping them.

WHY DO PROVIDERS DO MORE WHEN LESS IS BEST?

As providers seek ways to reduce overuse in health care, 1 question persists: Why do providers do more when doing more is unhelpful, or even harmful? The forces that drive decision-making are complex and multifactorial:

Culture of medicine

- In medicine, there often is a high value placed on certainty and finding answers. The expectations placed on physicians to be right often means that physicians have discomfort with admitting uncertainty to others [37]. There may be a tendency to do more treatment and testing as a way of avoiding missing something important. Studies have demonstrated higher antibiotic overuse in cultures where there is a greater tendency toward uncertainty avoidance [38].

Clinician attitudes and beliefs

- Physician personalities and biases have an impact on the tendency toward low-value testing and treatment. A study by Cutler and colleagues [39] explored physician beliefs regarding adult end-of-life care; based on surveys, physicians were characterized as *cowboys* (those who consistently favored aggressive life-saving measures beyond what guidelines would recommend) and *comforters* (those who prioritized comfort and palliation). They found that geographic areas with a higher percentage of cowboys tended to have higher Medicare expenditures.
- Past experiences likely also play a role in physician decision-making; the sentiment, "I got burned once," is a familiar feeling to all physicians. Whether consciously or subconsciously, a memorable experience of a missed diagnosis or failure in management can color future physician behavior. Some of this past experience provides value, but in other cases it may cause practitioners to perform extra testing or unnecessary treatment in the hopes of not missing a particular outcome, however improbable. Kahneman and Tversky [40], famed psychologists who studied judgment and decision-making, found through their research that an outcome of a negative nature, even when of equal intensity to an outcome of a positive nature, tends to have greater psychological impact. Thus, the 1 time a physician missed a diagnosis may guide a physician's decision-making more heavily than all the times he or she helped a patient by finding the correct diagnosis.

- Fear of litigation, also known as the practice of defensive medicine, also may play a role in overtreatment. One component of the rising costs of health care is due to care provided in physicians' attempt to avoid lawsuits [41]. Furthermore, errors of omission—in which a patient is harmed by missing a diagnosis or failing to treat—tend to be punished more frequently by litigation than errors of commission—in which a patient is harmed by an unnecessary test or treatment [42].

Practice environment

- Most reimbursement structures in the United States are based on a fee-for-service model, so there is an inherent reward in doing more; this culture may put subtle pressure on care providers to perform more testing and services than they might otherwise. In areas where reimbursements for services increase, provision of care by physicians also tends to increase [43].
- Ordering fewer tests is not always easier; when provider time is a limited resource, it may be easier to order additional testing or therapies than provide the additional vigilance and effort that would be required instead. In cases of a work-up already performed at another institution, it may require less effort to reorder the same testing than to attempt to obtain medical records.
- Quality measures in pediatric ambulatory and emergency department settings tend to focus more on problems of underuse (ie, encouraging providers to test or treat more) than problems of overuse [44]. Implementation of these metrics often has unintended consequences of overuse and overdiagnosis. A quality improvement project in Delaware designed to expedite cardiac catheterizations for ST-segment elevation myocardial infarctions (STEMIs) did succeed in reducing door-to-balloon time from 76 minutes to 61 minutes [45]. On further analysis, however, this intervention was found to increase false-positive STEMI diagnoses, from 7.7% to 16.5%. Thus, when quality metrics are implemented, it is important to look at counterbalancing measures as a potential source of overuse.

Patient factors and experiences

- Physicians often cite pressure from patients as a reason for doing more. In a study of pediatric patients with minor head injuries, providers acknowledged the influence of parental anxiety in their decision-making for whether or not to perform computerized tomography testing [46].
- Testing often is done in order to reassure patients. In many cases, however, it fails to achieve that goal. In a systematic review, low-yield testing done "to reassure patients" for benign conditions (eg, dyspepsia, palpitations, and back pain) had no effect on patient worry, nonspecific anxiety, or symptom persistence [47].
- When testing yields ambiguous results, patients may experience a phenomenon called *investigation momentum*, in which inconclusive testing begets further testing. In a study of men undergoing prostate-specific antigen screening, those who received inconclusive results were more likely to desire prostate biopsy than those who had not been screened. Both patient groups were left with similar uncertainty, but only those who had had the initial testing desired further work-up [48].

Culture of health care consumption

- In the United States, patients pay significant out-of-pocket costs for insurance premiums, copayments, and more. Patients are encouraged to be advocates for themselves, which may lead them to pursue additional treatment and testing with the sense that "you get what you pay for."

Publication bias

- The concept of publication bias in scientific literature has been well documented: studies demonstrating positive findings are much more likely to achieve publication than studies demonstrating negative findings [49]. Physicians therefore must rely on studies that tend to find in favor of testing and treatment without being balanced by studies demonstrating a lack of benefit of interventions.

Culture of medical education

- Most medical schools utilize problem-based learning curricula in which students studying a case must uncover a relatively rare disease, which encourages a shotgun approach of extensive diagnostic testing. This culture rewards students for guessing rare diagnoses and for engaging in possibilistic—rather than probabilistic—thinking.

Industry influence

- Several diseases have had their diagnostic criteria broadened in recent years, such as ADHD, Alzheimer disease, depression, hypercholesterolemia, and hypertension. Moynihan and colleagues [50] investigated the panels that established new, expanded diagnostic criteria and found that, on average, 75% of panel members had ties to the pharmaceutical and device industry. Although it is impossible to determine to what extent these panelists' industry ties biased the formation of the diagnostic criteria, these relationships must be considered a potential cause of broadened definitions of disease, and in turn an increase in testing and prescribing practices.

WHAT CAN BE DONE?

How can providers work toward decreasing overtreatment and overdiagnosis as a way of reducing health care waste? One solution has been to work to increase awareness and education of physicians, as well as the public, on the risks of overuse.

The Choosing Wisely campaign

In 2012, the American Board of Internal Medicine established the Choosing Wisely campaign; the campaign's main goals were to reduce wasteful care, encourage conversations about treatment between physicians and patients, and debunk the notion that more is better [51]. Part of this effort was to create a list of low-value tests and treatments that patients should question. The themes highlighted by Choosing Wisely have inspired many scholarly efforts and quality improvement initiatives: in the first year since its inception, there already were 160 peer-reviewed articles published that mentioned the Choosing Wisely campaign [52]. More than 80 specialty societies [53] have partnered to create their own lists, including the American Academy of Pediatrics (Fig. 4) [54] and many pediatric subspecialty societies. Choosing Wisely partnered with Consumer Reports in order to disseminate the information in a way that was more accessible to patients. The campaign created materials specifically for patients and families to increase their education and empowerment during health care visits, including “5 Questions to Ask Your Doctor Before You Get Any Test, Treatment or Procedure” (Fig. 5) [55]. These resources are offered on the Choosing Wisely web site in low health literacy language as well as for non-English speakers.

Changes in institutional priorities

Another potential solution is for health care systems to increase their focus on overuse and to balance it with the priority of targeting underuse. This is no small task; data show that physicians improve more readily on quality indicators aimed at underuse rather than overuse [56]. Institutions should counter these tendencies by incentivizing physicians to be equally focused on safely

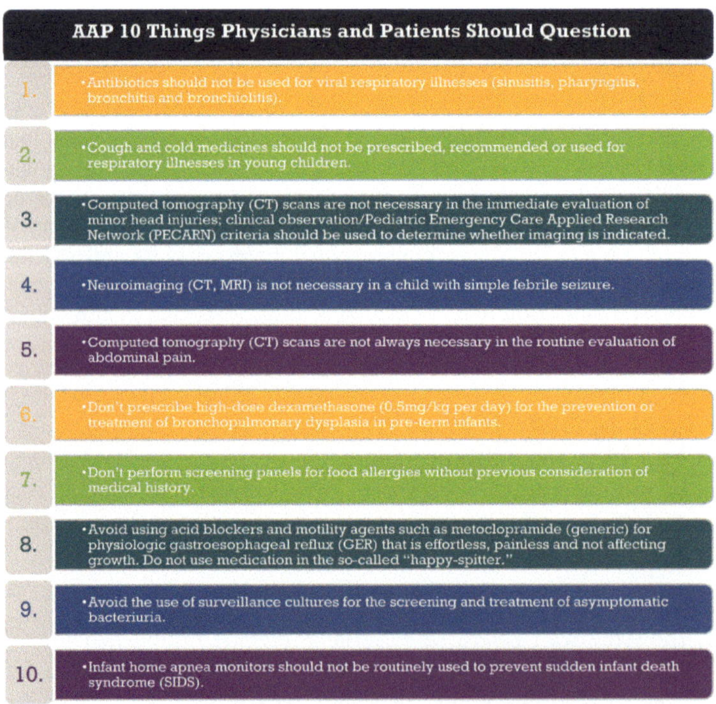

Fig. 4. American Academy of Pediatrics (AAP): 10 things physicians and patients should question. *Adapted from* Choosing Wisely, American Academy of Pediatrics, "Ten Things Physicians and Patients Should Question". Released February 21, 2013 (1–5) and March 17, 2014 (6–10); #1, 3, 9 updated July 13, 2016; #1, 2, 4, 5 and 10 updated June 12, 2018. https://www.choosingwisely.org/wp-content/uploads/2015/02/AAP-Choosing-Wisely-List.pdf. Accessed November 30, 2020.

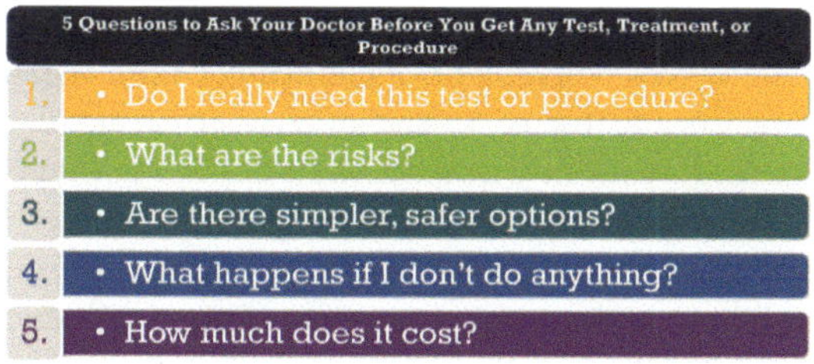

Fig. 5. Five questions to ask a doctor before getting any test, treatment, or procedure. *Adapted from* Choosing Wisely, "Five Questions to Ask Your Doctor Before You Get Any Test, Treatment, or Procedure". Accessed on November 30, 2020. https://www.choosingwisely.org/wp-content/uploads/2018/03/5-Questions-Poster_8.5x11-Eng.pdf.

doing less. Attempts to increase cost visibility for practitioners, such as displaying a dollar amount or otherwise denoting particularly expensive testing or treatment, have been implemented in order to encourage practitioners to avoid unnecessary tests and treatments. The data on these interventions are mixed, but there is some evidence that this transparency does help guide physician decision-making and may encourage physicians not to order unnecessary testing and treatment [57].

There should be increased research on the impacts of overuse, both as measured directly and as inferred by measuring variability that otherwise cannot be explained. Major medical journals should endeavor to prioritize publication not only of positive studies but also negative studies–those demonstrating a lack of benefit of a given test or treatment.

Patient-provider communication

Improvement in physician communication may be another important way to reduce overuse. Engaging and empowering patients to understand the benefits–and importantly, the limitations–of testing and treatment can help to limit unnecessary interventions. Few patients undergoing cancer screening report being fully informed by their physicians about the risks of overdiagnosis and overtreatment, and they would choose to opt out of a screening test if there were a high risk of false-positive results and a low likelihood of benefit [58]. The quality of the patient-provider relationship has a powerful impact in preventing overuse: increased continuity of care in Medicare patients has been found to reduce instances of overused procedures [59]. A training program for family medicine physicians in shared decision-making led to a reduction in antibiotic overuse for upper respiratory infections [60]. In a study of oncology patients, Zafar and colleagues [61] found that most patients want to discuss costs with their physicians and that having cost conversations with patients led to a reduction in costs of care.

Medical student and trainee education

Finally, curricula on overdiagnosis and overtreatment should be incorporated into medical education. Physicians often demonstrate a poor understanding of the risks of overdiagnosis in screening tests [58]; medical educators should ensure that learners have a working understanding of the risk of overdiagnosis. Case-based learning should focus on not only uncovering the rare zebras but also developing an understanding of what the most likely diagnosis is in a given scenario. At the University of Colorado, the internal medicine residency program implemented the Do No Harm Project, in which trainees studied cases illustrating harm from medical overuse [62]. Only by increasing awareness from the earliest stages of training and education can it be hoped to develop a workforce that avoids overuse.

SUMMARY

Overuse, overdiagnosis, and overtreatment contribute to the already high and rising costs of healthcare. More importantly, unnecessary testing and treatment can be causes of harm to patients. There are many pressures on physicians and patients to do more when less is best, including complex cultural factors and top-down pressures from health care systems as well as perceived pressures from patients as health care consumers. When providers develop strong relationships with patients, engage in shared decision-making, and take time to fully educate them about risks and benefits, however, patients often prefer to avoid excessive testing and treatment. Health care systems should educate practitioners about the risks and consequences of overuse and should implement quality practices related to reducing overuse with the same emphasis as problems related to underuse. Finally, providers should be aware of the cognitive biases that contribute to the tendency to overtest and overtreat and should be educated about overuse starting in medical school and residency training. Over time, with increased awareness, providers can move toward a culture of safely doing less.

DISCLOSURE

Audrey D. Kamzan and Elayna Ng have no commercial or financial conflicts of interest and have not received funding for this work.

References

[1] Skinner J. Causes and consequences of geographic variation in health care. In: McGuire TG, Pauly M, Barros PP, editors. Handbook of health economics, Vol. 2 2012 North Holland: Amsterdam.
[2] Cooper Z, Craig SV, Gaynor M, et al. The price ain't right? hospital prices and health spending on the privately insured. Q J Econ 2019;134(1):51–107.
[3] Fisher ES, Wennberg DE, Stukel TA, et al. The implications of regional variations in Medicare spending. Part 1: The content, quality, and accessibility of care. Ann Intern Med 2003;138(4):273–87.
[4] Institute of Medicine. To err is human: building a safer health system. Washington, DC: The National Academies Press; 2000; https://doi.org/10.17226/9728.
[5] Landrigan CP, Parry GJ, Bones CB, et al. Temporal trends in rates of patient harm resulting from medical care. N Engl J Med 2010;363:2124–34.
[6] Miller MR, Takata G, Stucky ER, et al. Policy statement - principles of pediatric patient safety: reducing harm due to medical care. Pediatrics 2011;127(6):1199–210.
[7] Allen DB, Lou MM, Mullen B. A meta-analysis of the effect of oral and inhaled corticosteroids on growth. J Allergy Clin Immunol 1994;93(6):967–76.

[8] Lancet T. Time to be serious about children's health care. Lancet 2001;358(9280):431.
[9] Gillis J, Loughlan P. Not just small adults: the metaphors of paediatrics. Arch Dis Child 2007;92(11):946–7.
[10] Santell JP, Hicks R. Medication errors involving pediatric patients. Jt Comm J Qual Patient Saf 2005;31(6):348–53.
[11] OECD 2014, health expenditure. Available at: https://stats.oecd.org/. Accessed November 20 2020.
[12] OECD 2014, health status. Available at: https://stats.oecd.org/. Accessed November 20 2020.
[13] Berwick DM, Hackbarth AD. Eliminating waste in US health care. JAMA 2012;307(14): 1513–6.
[14] Shrank WH, Rogstad TL, Parekh N. Waste in the US Health Care System: estimated costs and potential for savings. JAMA 2019;322(15):1501–9.
[15] Chassin MR, Galvin RW, Donaldson MS. The urgent need to improve health care quality: Institute of Medicine National Roundtable on Health Care Quality. J Am Med Assoc 1998;280(11):1000–5.
[16] Brownlee S, Chalkidou K, Doust J, et al. Evidence for overuse of medical services around the world. Lancet 2017;390(10090):156–68.
[17] Lee CN, Hultman CS, Sepucha K. Do patients and providers agree about the most important facts and goals for breast reconstruction decisions? Ann Plast Surg 2010;64:563–6.
[18] Mulley AG, Trimble C, Elwyn G. Stop the silent misdiagnosis: patients' preferences matter. BMJ 2012;345:e6572.
[19] Handy LK, Bryan M, Gerber JS, et al. Variability in antibiotic prescribing for community-acquired pneumonia. Pediatrics 2017;139(4):e20162331.
[20] Brownlee S, Hurley V. Elective heart procedures in California: a close-up of geographic variation. California Healthcare Foundation; 2014. Available at: http://www.chcf.org/~/media/MEDIA%20LIBRARY%20Files/PDF/PDF%20V/PDF%20VariationCloseUpHeartProcedures2014.pdf. Accessed November 28, 2016.
[21] Brodersen J, Schwartz LM, Heneghan C, et al. Overdiagnosis: what it is and what it isn't. BMJ 2018;23(1):1–3.
[22] Wolraich ML, Hagan JF, Allan C, et al. Clinical practice guideline for the diagnosis, evaluation, and treatment of attention-deficit/hyperactivity disorder in children and adolescents. Pediatrics 2019;144(4):e20192528.
[23] Sherman J, Rasmussen C, Baydala L. The impact of teacher factors on achievement and behavioural outcomes of children with Attention Deficit/Hyperactivity Disorder (ADHD): a review of the literature. Educ Res 2008;50(4):347–60.
[24] Morrow RL, Garland EJ, Wright JM, et al. Influence of relative age on diagnosis and treatment of attention-deficit/hyperactivity disorder in children. CMAJ 2012;184(7):755–62.
[25] Visser SN, Danielson ML, Wolraich ML, et al. Vital signs: national and state-specific patterns of attention deficit/hyperactivity disorder treatment among insured children aged 2-5 years - United States, 2008-2014. MMWR Morb Mortal Wkly Rep 2016;65(17):443–50.
[26] Kuzniewicz MW, Escobar GJ, Newman TB. Impact of universal bilirubin screening on severe hyperbilirubinemia and phototherapy use. Pediatrics 2009;124(4):1031–9.
[27] Usatin D, Liljestrand P, Kuzniewicz MW, et al. Effect of neonatal jaundice and phototherapy on the frequency of first-year outpatient visits. Pediatrics 2010;125(4):729–34.
[28] Tilburt JC, Wynia MK, Sheeler RD, et al. Views of US physicians about controlling health care costs. JAMA 2013;310(4):380–8.
[29] Schleifer D, Rothman DJ. "The ultimate decision is yours": exploring patients' attitudes about the overuse of medical interventions. PLoS One 2012;7(12):e52552.
[30] Carman KL, Maurer M, Yegian JM, et al. Evidence that consumers are skeptical about evidence-based health care. Health Aff 2010;29(7):1400–6.

[31] Korenstein D, Chimonas S, Barrow B, et al. Development of a conceptual map of negative consequences for patients of overuse of medical tests and treatments. JAMA Intern Med 2018;178(10):1401–7.
[32] Schpero WL, Morden NE, Sequist TD, et al. Datawatch: for selected services, blacks and hispanics more likely to receive low-value care than whites. Health Aff 2017;36(6): 1065–9.
[33] Schilling FH, Spix C, Berthold F, et al. Neuroblastoma screening at one year of age. N Engl J Med 2002;346(14):1047–53.
[34] Woods WG, Tuchman M, Robison LL, et al. A population-based study of the usefulness of screening for neuroblastoma. Lancet 1996;348(9043):1682–7.
[35] Sankila R. Lessons learned from neuroblastoma screening. *Evaluation and monitoring of screening programs*. Luxembourg, Luxembourg: Office for Official Publications of the European Communities; 2001. p. 233–42.
[36] Ioka A, Inoue M, Yoneda A, et al. Effects of the cessation of mass screening for neuroblastoma at 6 months of age: a population-based study in Osaka, Japan. J Epidemiol 2016;26(4):179–84.
[37] Farnan JM, Johnson JK, Meltzer DO, et al. Resident uncertainty in clinical decision making and impact on patient care: a qualitative study. Qual Saf Health Care 2008;17(2):122–6.
[38] Borg MA. Prolonged perioperative surgical prophylaxis within european hospitals: an exercise in uncertainty avoidance? J Antimicrob Chemother 2014;69(4):1142–4.
[39] Cutler D, Skinner JS, Stern AD, et al. Physician beliefs and patient preferences: a new look at regional variation in health care spending. Am Econ J Econ Policy 2019;11(1):192–221.
[40] Kahneman D, Tversky A. Prospect theory: an analysis of decision under risk. Econometrica 1979;47(2):263.
[41] Kessler D, McClellan M. Do doctors practice defensive medicine? Q J Econ 1996;111(2): 353–90.
[42] Wallace E, Lowry J, Smith SM, et al. The epidemiology of malpractice claims in primary care: a systematic review. BMJ Open 2013;3(7):e002929.
[43] Clemens J, Gottlieb JD. Do physicians' financial incentives affect medical treatment and patient health? Am Econ Rev 2014;104(4):1320–49.
[44] Mangione-Smith R, DeCristofaro AH, Setodji CM, et al. The quality of ambulatory care delivered to children in the United States. N Engl J Med 2007;357(15):1515–23.
[45] Fanari Z, Abraham N, Kolm P, et al. Aggressive measures to decrease "door to balloon" time and incidence of unnecessary cardiac catheterization: potential risks and role of quality improvement. Mayo Clin Proc 2015;90(12):1614–22.
[46] Natale JAE, Joseph JG, Rogers AJ, et al. Cranial computed tomography use among children with minor blunt head trauma: association with race/ethnicity. Arch Pediatr Adolesc Med 2012;166(8):732–7.
[47] Rolfe A, Burton C. Reassurance after diagnostic testing with a low pretest probability of serious disease: systematic review and meta-analysis. JAMA Intern Med 2013;173(6): 407–16.
[48] Sah S, Elias P, Ariely D. Investigation momentum: the relentless pursuit to resolve uncertainty. JAMA Intern Med 2013;173(10):932–3.
[49] Fanelli D. Negative results are disappearing from most disciplines and countries. Scientometrics 2012;90(3):891–904.
[50] Moynihan RN, Cooke GPE, Doust JA, et al. Expanding disease definitions in guidelines and expert panel ties to industry: a cross-sectional study of common conditions in the United States. PLoS Med 2013;10(8):e1001500.
[51] History. Available at: https://www.choosingwisely.org/our-mission/history/. Accessed November 28, 2020.
[52] Wolfson D, Santa J, Slass L. Engaging physicians and consumers in conversations about treatment overuse and waste: a short history of the choosing wisely campaign. Acad Med 2014;89(7):990–5.

[53] Facts and Figures. Available at: https://www.choosingwisely.org/our-mission/facts-and-figures/. Accessed November 30, 2020.
[54] American Academy of Pediatrics | Choosing Wisely. Ten things physicians and patients should question. 2018. Available at: https://www.choosingwisely.org/societies/american-academy-of-pediatrics. Accessed November 30, 2020.
[55] Additional Materials for Patients. 5 questions to ask your doctor before you get any test, treatment or procedure. Available at: https://www.choosingwisely.org/getting-started/resource-library/additional-materials-for-patients/. Accessed November 30, 2020.
[56] Kale MS, Bishop TF, Federman AD, et al. Trends in the overuse of ambulatory health care services in the United States. JAMA Intern Med 2013;173(2):142–8.
[57] Goetz C, Rotman SR, Hartoularos G, et al. The effect of charge display on cost of care and physician practice behaviors: a systematic review. J Gen Intern Med 2015;30(6):835–42.
[58] Wegwarth O, Gigerenzer G. Overdiagnosis and overtreatment: evaluation of what physicians tell their patients about screening harms. JAMA Intern Med 2013;173(22):2086–7.
[59] Romano MJ, Segal JB, Pollack CE. The association between continuity of care and the overuse of medical procedures. JAMA Intern Med 2015;175(7):1148–54.
[60] Légaré F, Labrecque M, Cauchon M, et al. Training family physicians in shared decision-making to reduce the overuse of antibiotics in acute respiratory infections: a cluster randomized trial. CMAJ 2012;184(13):E726.
[61] Zafar SY, Chino F, Ubel PA, et al. The utility of cost discussions between patients with cancer and oncologists. Am J Manag Care 2015;21(9):607–15.
[62] The Do No Harm Project | Division of General Internal Medicine | University of Colorado Denver. Available at: https://medschool.cuanschutz.edu/general-internal-medicine/education/do-no-harm-project. Accessed November 30, 2020.

Advances in Pediatrics 68 (2021) 37–53

ADVANCES IN PEDIATRICS

Antibiotic Stewardship in Pediatrics

Kurlen S.E. Payton, MD[a,*], Marissa A. Brunetti, MD[b]

[a]Department of Pediatrics, Division of Neonatology, Cedars-Sinai Medical Center, 8700 Beverly Boulevard, NT Suite 4221, Los Angeles, CA 90048, USA; [b]University of Pennsylvania Perelman School of Medicine, Children's Hospital of Philadelphia, 3401 Civic Center Boulevard Suite 8NE51, Philadelphia, PA 19104, USA

Keywords

• Antibiotic • Antimicrobial • Stewardship • Pediatrics
• Neonatal intensive care unit • Pediatric intensive care unit

Key points

- Unnecessary antibiotic use occurs in most areas of pediatrics. Antibiotic exposure in early life is linked to short- and long-term adverse effects that can impact health across the lifespan.
- Antibiotics disrupt normal microbiome development, are linked to later development of several diseases, are implicated in more rapid development of antibiotic resistance, and increase costs while decreasing the value of health care.
- Antibiotic stewardship has been shown to effectively decrease antibiotic use, prescription errors, and cost.
- Coordinated antibiotic stewardship efforts are a requirement for hospitals and ambulatory care settings.
- Pediatric antibiotic stewardship resources and support for individuals, hospitals, and health systems are readily available to help guide antibiotic stewardship efforts.

INTRODUCTION

The discovery and development of antimicrobials is one of the most important advances in modern medicine. Antimicrobial use targeting life-threatening infections has saved countless lives and continues to be a mainstay of successful medical management. However, antibiotics and other antimicrobials have notable short- and long-term adverse effects that have become more evident

*Corresponding author. *E-mail address:* kurlen.payton@cshs.org

https://doi.org/10.1016/j.yapd.2021.05.002

with time. Striking a balance between the obvious benefits of antimicrobials and the unintended consequences is now possible because the adverse effects are becoming more clearly defined. Antibiotic stewardship (AS) seeks to navigate this balance by prioritizing appropriate antibiotic use.

For the purposes of this review, we consider AS as any coordinated effort to decrease the negative impact of antibiotic exposure. This review summarizes the current knowledge regarding antimicrobial overuse, specific challenges, and stewardship strategies encountered in distinct areas of pediatrics. We use the term *antibiotic* to refer to all antimicrobials as it relates to stewardship. Pediatric oncology deserves special attention and is not included in this review.

The scope of the problem of antimicrobial overuse and the potential solutions vary greatly by context. Thus, this review is organized as follows:

- Consequences of unnecessary antibiotic use
- Newborns and neonates
  - Newborn nursery
  - Neonatal intensive care unit (NICU)
- Infant, children, and adolescents
  - Outpatient and emergency departments
  - Pediatric intensive care unit (PICU)

CONSEQUENCES OF ANTIBIOTIC OVERUSE

Antibiotic exposure early in life is linked to several short- and long-term adverse effects. Antibiotics disrupt normal microbiome development and diversity, they are linked to later development of several diseases, they are implicated in more rapid development of antibiotic resistance, and they increase costs while decreasing the value of health care by overuse of resources.

Microbiome

Microbiome disruption is an important mediator of many consequences of antibiotics use [1]. Newborn infants are frequently impacted by antibiotic exposure altering the microbiome even before birth [2]. The newborn period and infancy are critical times for the development of the microbiome and seems to be extremely sensitive to antibiotic exposure that occurs at this time [1,3].

Link to later disease

Antenatal antibiotic exposure has been linked to neurodevelopmental deficits, childhood infections, obesity, febrile seizures, and epilepsy. Other diseases linked to early antibiotic exposure include asthma, allergic rhinitis, celiac disease, type 2 diabetes, inflammatory bowel disease, attention deficit hyperactivity disorder, and learning disabilities [4–9].

Antibiotic resistance and economic impact

All antibiotic use inherently encourages resistance to antibiotics and antibiotic resistance is increasing [10]. Antibiotic resistance is associated with increased morbidity, mortality, length of stay, and hospital costs [11–13]. Redundant antibiotic treatment in US hospitals was shown to be a frequent and avoidable example of health care waste with an estimated cost of $12 million over a 3-year period from 2008 to 2011 [14].

Antibiotic overuse begins as a pediatric issue, but ultimately impacts health across the lifespan. Safely decreasing antibiotic use, decreasing errors, and decreasing antimicrobial resistance are all feasible goals of stewardship efforts [15].

ANTIBIOTIC STEWARDSHIP STRATEGIES AND ANTIBIOTIC STEWARDSHIP PROGRAMS

There is less evidence and relatively less guidance on AS in pediatrics relative to adult medicine, but a wide range of strategies have evolved from AS efforts and studies. Pediatric-specific AS and antibiotic stewardship programs (ASPs) are needed to meet the unique needs of AS efforts in pediatrics. Children's hospitals with ASPs have been shown to be more effective at reducing antibiotic use than those without ASPs [16]. Several publications and resources provide guidance for clinicians developing ASPs within pediatrics [17,18].

Professional societies and government agencies have called for mandatory implementation of stewardship efforts to improve health care [19,20]. The Joint Commission mandates antimicrobial stewardship activities for both hospitals and ambulatory care settings [21]. The Centers for Disease Control and Prevention's released core elements of hospital AS in 2014 to help hospitals implement ASPs (Table 1). Evidence-based AS strategies with grade of recommendation and quality of evidence are summarized in Table 2.

NEONATES

Forty percent of mothers receive antibiotics before delivery [22] and antibiotics account for 80% of maternal medications [23]. Most studies have focused on the benefits of maternal antibiotics and have overlooked the potential consequences [22,24,25]. There are notable short- and long-term effects on newborns and infants linked to maternal antibiotic administration [2]. There is overuse and large variation in rates of antibiotic use in neonates [26,27].

There are many efforts and collaborations among institutions and government agencies aimed at understanding the scope of neonatal antibiotic exposure, benchmarking, and development of strategies to minimize harm related to antibiotics in this population [28].

Unique challenges in the newborn nursery

The presumably well newborn infant presents a challenge to AS because the appropriate expectation of wellness in most babies is contrasted with the potential for rapid deterioration and the high risk of morbidity and mortality associated with early-onset sepsis (EOS). The ever-present phrase, "well-baby nursery" implies that this is a place for newborns without illness. Historically, newborn nurseries have not been equipped to provide rigorous and continuous monitoring with the expectation of identifying newborns with sepsis. These contrasting factors have contributed to what is now accepted as the overuse

Table 1
Centers for Disease Control and Prevention core elements of hospital AS programs

Core element	Description
Hospital leadership commitment	Support for time and resources Regularly scheduled interaction for reporting to senior hospital leadership
Accountability	Clear leader of program accountable for management and results
Pharmacy expertise	Ideally, a pharmacist represented in a leadership role
Action	Priority interventions include prospective audit and feedback, preauthorization, and local treatment recommendations
Tracking	Monitor use/prescribing, impact of interventions, and outcomes
Reporting	Regularly report use and resistance information to staff and leadership
Education	Recommends case-based education through prospective audit and feedback and preauthorization

Adapted from Core Elements of Hospital AS Programs. Atlanta, GA: US Department of Health and Human Services, CDC; 2019, https://www.cdc.gov/antibiotic-use/core-elements/hospital.html.

of antibiotics for newborn infants in the nursery environment. Previous guidelines recommended blood culture and empiric antibiotics for a newborn infant with a history of antenatal sepsis risk factors, such as maternal chorioamnionitis [29]. Screening laboratory tests with poor positive predictive values have been

Table 2
Evidence based pediatric AS strategies

Strategy	Grade of recommendation/evidence quality
Preauthorization and prospective audit and feedback	Strong/moderate
Targeting interventions to decrease *Clostridium difficile* infections	Strong/moderate
Targeting reduction of treatment to shortest effective duration	Strong/moderate
Use oral antibiotics as able	Strong/moderate
Educational interventions	Weak/low
Local guidelines should be developed and used with dissemination and implementation strategy	Weak/low
Target specific diseases	Weak/low
Prescriber-oriented interventions	Weak/low
Computer decision support	Weak/moderate
Cycling antibiotics	Weak/low

Data from Barlam TF, Cosgrove SE, Abbo LM, et al. Implementing an Antibiotic Stewardship Program: Guidelines by the Infectious Diseases Society of America and the Society for Healthcare Epidemiology of America. *Clinical Infectious Diseases*. 2016;62(10):e51-e77.

used to screen for sepsis. These laboratory tests are frequently abnormal and can lead to a prolonged courses of antibiotic treatment in newborns without signs of sepsis [30]. Historically, these newborns have been treated with antibiotics even in the absence of any clinical signs of illness leading to treatment of risk factors alone, without targeting their current diagnosis. More recent guidelines offer approaches with less antibiotic use [31,32].

Full-term and late preterm infants in the neonatal intensive care unit

Most newborns admitted to NICUs are full term and late preterm infants. Thus, this target of AS efforts is of high value. Current guidelines recommend judicious antibiotic use in this relatively low-risk population of full-term and late preterm infants [31]. Table 3 summarizes recommendations for evaluation and management of EOS for infants $35^{0/7}$ weeks of gestation or older. These recommendations are relevant for newborns being managed in the nursery and NICU.

Table 3
Summary of strategies and pearls to consider for evaluation and management of EOS

Local guidelines [31]	Hospitals caring for newborns should develop local documented EOS evaluation and management guidelines
Risk stratification strategies [31]	Categorical risk factor assessment Multivariate risk assessment (eg, neonatal sepsis calculator) Clinical condition based assessment (eg, serial clinical/physical examinations)
Laboratory testing	
Blood culture [31]	The diagnostic gold standard Effectively detects low level bacteremia[a] (minimum volume of 1 mL) Time to positivity not effected by intrapartum antibiotics
WBC [31]	Commonly used to evaluate EOS Low usefulness in settings with low EOS rates Traditionally used WBC indices (WBC count, ANC, I/T ratio) do not perform well in identifying culture proven EOS Antibiotics should not be continued for abnormal WBC indices alone
C-reactive protein and procalcitonin	Low positive predictive value [33]; good negative predictive value with serial measurements [34]; frequently elevated in healthy newborns and trends up during first 48 h in healthy newborns [35,36]; should not be used in well appearing newborns; abnormal values should not dictate whether to administer antibiotics [31]

Abbreviations: ANC, absolute neutrophil count; I/T, immature to total; WBC, white blood cell count.
[a]Detects at level of 1 to 10 bacteremia colony forming units per milliliter.

Challenges managing preterm infants in the neonatal intensive care unit

Preterm infants present one of the most difficult AS challenges. They can be the most vulnerable and also the most susceptible to the adverse effects of antibiotics [37].

The risk of EOS increases with decreasing gestational age [38]. Preterm infants have very little reserve and tolerance for delays in treatment of sepsis and mortality rates are notably higher than for term and late preterm infants. Additionally, almost all preterm infants present at birth with some degree of respiratory illness requiring support. These clinical signs are not easily distinguished from clinical signs of sepsis. This creates a dilemma leading to nearly all preterm infants being treated with empiric antibiotics after birth and a general acceptance of this as an appropriate practice. Sentinel events and deaths owing to sepsis understandably challenge the justification for reducing antibiotic exposure in this unique population.

Adverse effects of antibiotics in preterm infants

The evidence supporting a link between antibiotic exposure and short- and long-term adverse effects is most extensive in the preterm infant, with multiple studies linking exposure with morbidity and mortality. Prolonged antibiotic exposure in preterm infants is linked to death and necrotizing enterocolitis in multiple studies, even with attempts to control for confounders [39–44].

Culture-negative sepsis

Culture-negative sepsis is a diagnosis of exclusion given to an infant when the care provider is convinced that sepsis is present despite a negative blood culture. This factor is one of the primary drivers of unwarranted antibiotic use in EOS management among neonatologists [45]. Provider perception of culture-negative sepsis leads to notable variation in antibiotic management in the evaluation of EOS and late-onset sepsis in NICUs [46]. Frequent maternal treatment with antibiotics, perceived low sensitivity of blood cultures, and persistent clinical signs beyond 48 hours after blood culture results are commonly reported reasons for concern regarding culture negative sepsis. Infants in NICUs are commonly treated with prolonged courses of antibiotics for culture-negative sepsis with no clear source of infection. An alternative perspective for culture negative sepsis proposes that culture-negative sepsis is not plausible and not a common cause of illness in infants being evaluated for sepsis. Current blood culture technology is extremely sensitive and able to detect bacteria with very low colony counts. One could reasonably expect that concentrations of organisms high enough to cause sepsis should be high enough to be captured in contemporary culture medium, if adequate blood volume was obtained [47]. Despite these facts, neonatologists are impacted by past cases of infants becoming ill and there is a high risk of mortality with any delay in the administration of antibiotics. Sentinel events make it difficult for providers to change practice and limit antibiotics for fear of missing cases of sepsis. These dilemmas are notable barriers to antimicrobial stewardship in the NICU.

Discussions and consideration of prescriber perspectives of culture-negative sepsis may be an integral part of stewardship efforts.

Antibiotic stewardship strategies in the nursery and neonatal intensive care unit

Contemporary strategies focused on decreasing antibiotic use in the well newborn nursery setting and NICU are becoming more accepted and quality improvement studies are showing how to safely implement these strategies in various contexts.

Sepsis calculator

The neonatal EOS calculator has been shown to decrease antibiotic use, laboratory testing use, and NICU admissions in a diverse group of newborn care settings. The calculator has provided a long-needed objective sepsis risk stratification method for newborn infants. The calculator was developed by using a large cohort of neonates to create a 2-part risk model [48–50]. Systematic reviews and meta-analyses comparing the outcomes related to the neonatal EOS calculator show consistent decreased in antibiotic use without evidence of harm related to mortality or missed cases [51,52].

It is vital to acknowledge that the neonatal EOS calculator does not effectively identify all newborns who will have EOS [49,53], but it seems to be as effective as traditional methods of care. The neonatal EOS calculator is endorsed by the American Academy of Pediatrics' most recent EOS guidelines clinical report as an objective method of multivariate risk stratification [31]. The calculator is a feasible option for many nurseries and NICUs aiming to safely reduce antibiotic exposure in newborns.

Serial physical and clinical examinations

Using the physical examination as a screening tool is accepted as a method of management for select newborns being evaluated for EOS [31]. This approach capitalizes on the fact that well-appearing newborn infants, even with history of risk factors such as maternal infection, are unlikely to have sepsis. This method significantly decreases antibiotic exposure and blood draws for screening laboratory tests without evidence of harm [54,55]. Frymoyer and colleagues [55] showed sustained improvements with this approach 5 years after implementation.

Biomarkers for evaluating sepsis in the nursery and neonatal intensive care unit

Using biomarkers to aid in sepsis evaluations in infants in nurseries and NICUs is a widespread practice, but has significant limitations (see Table 3). C-reactive protein is the most commonly used and studied biomarker in neonates, with procalcitonin being the second most commonly used. In theory, these biomarkers are intended to help to identify and/or rule out sepsis for infants being evaluated. Serial C-reactive protein and procalcitonin tests have a good negative predictive value, but a poor positive predictive value for sepsis [33]. Studies show mixed results related to impact on antibiotic use, because limitations in performance of biomarkers can actually lead to inappropriate antibiotic use

[56,57]. Thirty percent of NICU prescribers chose to start antibiotics in a well-appearing newborn with an elevated C-reactive protein in a vignette study of individual provider antibiotic use variation in EOS [46]. The American Academy of Pediatrics recommendations published after this study now recommend against using biomarkers for well-appearing infants and advise that serial abnormal C-reactive protein and/or procalcitonin values should not dictate whether or not to administer antibiotics in neonates without a culture-confirmed infection.

Using biomarkers for EOS is particularly problematic because events related to normal and complicated deliveries cause predictable increases in C-reactive protein. Increases in C-reactive protein are directly correlated with the stress of delivery. Vaginal deliveries and a longer duration of labor result in predictably higher C-reactive proteins than cesarean deliveries in healthy newborns. Healthy newborns also consistently show increasing C-reactive proteins and procalcitonin during the first 48 hours after delivery [35,36]. C-reactive protein does not benefit diagnosis or antibiotic use decisions during initial evaluation of late onset sepsis infection in preterm infants in NICUs [58,59].

Blood cultures in this NICU population are reliable indicators of sepsis and rarely become positive after 24 hours [60]. Thus, appropriately drawn blood cultures may effectively eliminate the need for the use of biomarkers that require serial values over time. Ultimately, the impact of using biomarkers lies in the prescriber's interpretation of the results as well as their perspective of culture-negative sepsis. In summary, the currently available biomarkers used for the evaluation of sepsis in the NICU population may not necessarily aid diagnostic evaluations and may encourage unnecessary antibiotic use.

Guidelines and stewardship implementation for early onset sepsis in preterm infants

The 2018 American Academy of Pediatrics Clinical Report is the first national guideline with recommendations for EOS management in preterm infants [38]. These guidelines suggest that identifying low-risk preterm infants may be the most feasible method of safely decreasing unnecessary antibiotic exposure in this vulnerable group of infants.

In contrast with the past practice of default empiric antibiotic treatment of all these infants, the guidelines recommend considering the "risk/benefit ratio of low risk infants" to guide whether or not empiric antibiotics are given for the initial management of suspected EOS. This approach was shown to be feasible in a retrospective single-site study with decreased antibiotic exposure of 48.8% and 65.3% during the first 7 days in very low birth weight and extremely low birth weight infants, respectively [29].

In summary, the rationale and urgency for AS in nurseries and NICUs is clear. Changing long-standing prescribing preferences and behavior can be challenging. The specific strategies that will lead to more appropriate antibiotic use are not well-defined. Multiple studies have documented safe decreases in antibiotic use in several contexts of neonatal care. Clinicians providing care for newborns in the nursery and NICU have ample examples of strategies to implement effective AS processes to optimize appropriate antibiotic use.

PEDIATRIC INTENSIVE CARE UNIT

AS in the PICU encompasses infant, school-aged, and adolescent patients with general medical and surgical disease in the PICU and patients with medical and surgical cardiac disease in the cardiac intensive care unit (CICU). AS is a balance between decreasing the likelihood of antimicrobial resistance and recognition with rapid administration of antibiotics in those with possible sepsis. The point prevalence of severe sepsis in the PICU population has been reported as 7.7% in North America and 8.2% globally with an in-hospital mortality rate of 25% [61]. The incidence of sepsis in the CICU is unknown. Using the Society of Thoracic Surgeons Congenital Heart Surgery Database, Barker and colleagues [62] found that 2.6% of patients with congenital heart disease in North America had sepsis, but their study population was limited to patients status post surgery for congenital heart disease. Because patients with acquired heart disease and those being managed preoperatively are also at significant risk for sepsis, this rate underestimates the true incidence. Both previously healthy and medically complex children may present critically ill with community-acquired infections, such as bacterial meningitis and pneumonia, leading to sepsis. And because critically ill patients are managed with support devices such as central lines, endotracheal tubes, and foley catheters, they are at risk for hospital-acquired infections, such as central line–associated blood stream infections, during the ICU stay. The American College of Critical Care Medicine's clinical practice guidelines for the management of pediatric sepsis call for the rapid administration of "broad-spectrum antibiotics within 60 minutes" from the recognition of possible sepsis [63]. Given these facts, PICUs have been found to have very high rates of antibiotic use, making AS more challenging. In a study of antibiotic use across PICUs, CICUs, and NICUs, patients in the PICU and CICU had double the days of antibiotic treatment when compared with NICU patients (697 days of treatment per 1000 patient-days vs 324.5 days of treatment per 1000 patient-days) [64]. In addition, once a PICU patient is on antibiotics, the lack of clear diagnosis may make a critical care team reluctant to stop antibiotics. In a study analyzing antibiotic use across all services at Mayo Children's Hospital, Levy and colleagues [65] found that the PICU had the highest rates of vancomycin and cefepime use with failure to discontinue or de-escalate when appropriate for nonsurgical pediatric patients.

Tenets of antibiotic stewardship in the pediatric intensive care unit

AS in the PICU includes the following basic tenets:

1. Stopping antibiotic administration if cultures are negative after 48 hours.
2. Narrowing antibiotic coverage when cultures are positive based on culture sensitivity results to avoid the use of unnecessary broad-spectrum antibiotics.

3. Stopping antibiotics when specimen results are consistent with bacterial colonization rather than infection.
4. Working closely with infectious disease specialists.

There have been several studies regarding antibiotic use and AS in the PICU. Lee and associates [66] created and implemented guidelines for empiric antibiotic treatment of common community-acquired and hospital-acquired infections in pediatric hospital ICUs, which included the NICU, PICU, and CICU. The goal was to decrease broad-spectrum antibiotic use and cost. Days of treatment with broad-spectrum antibiotics decreased by 33% and cost decreased by 62% after guideline implementation. Unit-specific decreases in days of treatment with broad-spectrum antibiotics ranged from 61% to 99%. There were no changes in ICU mortality after guideline implementation. Aizawa and colleagues [67] implemented having infectious disease specialists on ICU rounds every day, infectious disease consultations for any aspect of infectious disease management, and AS interventions such as restricting certain broad-spectrum antibiotics. They found a significant decrease in days of treatment with anti-pseudomonal agents but not non–anti-pseudomonal agents after implementation of these interventions. The number of extracorporeal membrane oxygenation runs, ICU length of stay, infection-related deaths, and PICU readmissions were all unchanged after the implementation of their interventions. Adams and colleagues [68] published a quality improvement project in which an antibiotic time out was done on PICU rounds after 48 to 72 hours of treatment with vancomycin, meropenem, or zosyn to decrease days of treatment. The time out significantly reduced treatment days for vancomycin and meropenem. Zosyn days of treatment were lower, but did not reach significance. Days of treatment were also significantly less for all other antibiotics after time out implementation. Overall direct costs for the 3 study antibiotics were decreased by 39%. There were no adverse effects to patients reported.

Biomarkers for antibiotic stewardship in the pediatric intensive care unit

There have been adult and pediatric studies on using inflammatory markers to aid in the de-escalation of antibiotic therapy in patients unlikely to have bacterial infection. Downes and colleagues [69] studied 8 biomarkers in pediatric patients with presumed sepsis admitted to the PICU. They found that C-reactive protein combined with procalcitonin or serum amyloid A measured at presentation had a sufficient negative predictive value and specificity to identify patients with low risk of bacterial infection. They then conducted a follow-up study where a protocol was implemented using a C-reactive protein of less than 4 mg/dL and procalcitonin of less than 1 ng/mL at presentation and no signs of bacterial infection by 48 hours to guide broad-spectrum antibiotic discontinuation [70]. The aim was to decrease excess antibiotic administration. A multivariable analysis did not show a decrease in excess antibiotic administration, which was attributed to a low number of patients qualifying as low risk with low C-reactive protein and procalcitonin values at presentation. The usefulness of biomarkers as an effective AS tool in the PICU population is unclear.

The practice at the Children's Hospital of Philadelphia is to start broad-spectrum antibiotics at the onset of an episode of suspected sepsis ideally after obtaining blood cultures and cultures of any relevant support devices, such as an endotracheal tube, or any possible source based on history and physical examination, such as lumbar puncture for suspected meningitis. If cultures are negative at 48 hours, antibiotics are stopped. If cultures are positive, we narrow antibiotic coverage at 48 hours. Any desire to continue broad-spectrum antibiotics beyond 48 hours or to use restricted antibiotics (such as linezolid) requires an infectious disease consultation. An order to continue broad-spectrum antibiotics beyond 48 hours is stopped by pharmacy review of the order entry system before filling.

OUTPATIENT ANTIBIOTIC USE

Outpatient antibiotic use has attracted less attention relative to inpatient settings, but contributes to a significant proportion of all prescribed antibiotics. Outpatient antibiotics make up the majority of antibiotic expenditures [71]. Several studies have documented antibiotic overuse and variation in outpatient settings [72–76]. Practice guidelines are frequently not followed in pediatric ambulatory care settings [77]. In 2010 and 2011, a randomly assigned national survey sampling pediatrics office visits found that 30% of outpatient antibiotic prescriptions were inappropriate [73]. There is relatively little evidence guiding AS in outpatient settings, but studies show effective results from stewardship interventions [78].

Emergency department

Pediatric emergency departments are in need of AS, but there is little guidance and few studies informing AS in this setting [79,80]. Most pediatric emergency visits occur in nonpediatric emergency departments and emergency department care in children presents unique challenges for AS, with many of the barriers seen in other ambulatory or office settings. Eighty-five percent of emergency department visits for children were noted to occur in nonpediatric emergency departments and 32% of antibiotic prescriptions in the emergency department were found to be inappropriate. Nonpediatric physicians were more likely to prescribe antibiotics inappropriately relative to pediatric physicians in emergency departments [81]. Effective antibiotic strategies in emergency departments may require unique solutions targeting pediatric and nonpediatric providers.

Factors contributing to antibiotic overuse in outpatient settings

There are unique challenges and barriers to AS in outpatient settings. Describing and understanding these factors is essential. Specific factors identified as drivers of inappropriate antibiotic use in outpatient settings include [82]:

- Patient satisfaction and parental pressure
- Time constraints
- Diagnostic uncertainty
- Externalized responsibility

Outpatient antibiotic stewardship interventions

There are relatively few studies informing outpatient pediatric AS. Most studies identified targets of interventions. Few studies have tested the effectiveness of interventions [83]. Broad-spectrum antibiotics are overused in outpatient settings and retrospective studies have shown no benefit over narrow spectrum treatment. One notable study investigated effectiveness of an intervention related to broad-spectrum antibiotic use. Gerber and colleagues [78,84] showed decreased broad-spectrum antibiotic use with a single 1-hour, on-site, clinical education session coupled with audit and feedback of prescribing for bacterial and viral upper respiratory tract infections. As is the case with many AS interventions, the improvements were not sustained when assessed after the active phase of the interventions [85].

Kilgore and Smith reviewed current literature and adapted the Centers for Disease Control and Prevention core elements to summarize potentially effective outpatient stewardship strategies (Table 4).

Table 4
Potentially effective outpatient stewardship strategies to optimize sustainable guideline-based prescribing

Strategy	Description
Mentorship	Build and maintain relationship with a leader in outpatient AS to help direct AS activities
Provider education	Target all stakeholders and not just prescribers Target pediatric and nonpediatric providers Active based learning, instead of lecture
Family education	Target parent and patient education with appropriate educational materials to engage them in their own care
Watchful waiting	Pragmatic purposeful delay in prescribing with contingency plan to actively engage families as opposed to sending the message of "nonmanagement"
Metric reporting	Support audit and feedback of metrics to empower and engage providers in efforts
Recognition of barriers	Be aware of special populations that may have geographic, cultural, or other reasons impeding stewardship

Data from Kilgore JT, Smith MJ. Outpatient Pediatric Antibiotic Use: a Systematic Review. *Current Infectious Disease Reports*. 2019;21(4).

SUMMARY

Antibiotic stewardship is required to preserve the effectiveness and benefit of life-saving antimicrobials. These life-saving medications also play a role in contributing to short- and long-term adverse effects. Pediatrics is arguably best situated to greatly impact lives by targeting efforts to more effectively define appropriate antimicrobial use and to implement strategies to safely decrease unnecessary antimicrobial use. AS and ASPs have been shown to safely decrease antibiotic use in various contexts. This decrease can enhance quality of care, medication errors, and health care costs. Creative consideration of innovative antibiotic stewardship strategies is required to prevent the adverse consequences of overuse of antimicrobials in pediatrics.

CLINICS CARE POINTS

- Hospitals caring for newborns should develop local EOS evaluation and management guidelines and perform surveillance after implementation.
- An abnormal complete blood count indices and elevated biomarkers such as C-reactive protein and procalcitonin have poor correlation with true infection in for early and late onset sepsis.
- The usefulness of biomarkers as a stewardship tool is unclear in the NICU and PICU populations.
- Antibiotics should be discontinued at 36 to 48 hours in most cases in which cultures are negative without a site-specific source of infection.
- The antibiotic regimen should be narrowed when cultures are positive based on culture sensitivity results to avoid the use of unnecessary broad-spectrum antibiotics.
- Antibiotics should be discontinued when the evaluation is consistent with bacterial colonization rather than infection.
- Preauthorization and prospective audit and feedback, target interventions to decrease *Clostridium difficile* infections, targeting a decrease in treatment to the shortest effective duration, and use oral antibiotics are all strongly recommended strategies with a moderate quality of evidence.

References

[1] Tanaka M, Nakayama J. Development of the gut microbiota in infancy and its impact on health in later life. Allergol Int 2017;66(4):515–22.

[2] Dierikx TH, Visser DH, Benninga MA, et al. The influence of prenatal and intrapartum antibiotics on intestinal microbiota colonisation in infants: a systematic review. J Infect 2020;81(2):190–204.

[3] Underwood MA, Mukhopadhyay S, Lakshminrusimha S, et al. Neonatal intestinal dysbiosis. J Perinatology 2020;40(11):1597–608.

[4] Aversa Z, Atkinson EJ, Schafer MJ, et al. Association of infant antibiotic exposure with childhood health outcomes. Mayo Clinic Proc 2020;96(1):66–77.

[5] Renz H, Skevaki C. Early life microbial exposures and allergy risks: opportunities for prevention. Nat Rev Immunol 2020;21(3):177–91.
[6] Ng SC, Bernstein CN, Vatn MH, et al. Geographical variability and environmental risk factors in inflammatory bowel disease. Gut 2013;62(4):630–49.
[7] Del Fiol FS, Balcão VM, Barberato-Fillho S, et al. Obesity: a new adverse effect of antibiotics? Front Pharmacol 2018;9(1408):1408.
[8] Miller JE, Pedersen LH, Vestergaard M, et al. Maternal use of antibiotics and the risk of childhood febrile seizures: a Danish population-based cohort. PLoS One 2013;8(4):e61148.
[9] Mikkelsen KH, Knop FK, Frost M, et al. Use of antibiotics and risk of type 2 diabetes: a population-based case-control study. J Clin Endocrinol Metab 2015;100(10):3633–40.
[10] Bell BG, Schellevis F, Stobberingh E, et al. A systematic review and meta-analysis of the effects of antibiotic consumption on antibiotic resistance. BMC Infect Dis 2014;14:13.
[11] Laxminarayan R, Duse A, Wattal C, et al. Antibiotic resistance—the need for global solutions. Lancet Infect Dis 2013;13(12):1057–98.
[12] Smith R, Coast J. The true cost of antimicrobial resistance. BMJ 2013;346:f1493.
[13] Maragakis LL, Perencevich EN, Cosgrove SE. Clinical and economic burden of antimicrobial resistance. Expert Rev Anti Infect Ther 2008;6(5):751–63.
[14] Schultz L, Lowe TJ, Srinivasan A, et al. Economic impact of redundant antimicrobial therapy in US hospitals. Infect Control Hosp Epidemiol 2014;35(10):1229–35.
[15] Donà D, Barbieri E, Daverio M, et al. Implementation and impact of pediatric antimicrobial stewardship programs: a systematic scoping review. Antimicrob Resist Infect Control 2020;9(1):3.
[16] Hersh AL, De Lurgio SA, Thurm C, et al. Antimicrobial stewardship programs in freestanding children's hospitals. Pediatrics 2015;135(1):33.
[17] Klatte JM. Pediatric antimicrobial stewardship programs: current perspectives. Pediatr Health Med Ther 2020;11:245–55.
[18] Barlam TF, Cosgrove SE, Abbo LM, et al. Implementing an antibiotic stewardship program: guidelines by the Infectious Diseases Society of America and the Society for Healthcare Epidemiology of America. Clin Infect Dis 2016;62(10):e51–77.
[19] Quick Safety Issue 16: national action plan: use antibiotics wisely. 2015. Available at: https://www.jointcommission.org/resources/news-and-multimedia/newsletters/newsletters/quick-safety/quick-safety–issue-16-national-action-plan-use-antibiotics-wisely/. Accessed November 28, 2020.
[20] Fishman N. Policy Statement on Antimicrobial Stewardship by the Society for Healthcare Epidemiology of America (SHEA), the Infectious Diseases Society of America (IDSA), and the Pediatric Infectious Diseases Society (PIDS). Infect Control Hosp Epidemiol 2015;33(4):322–7.
[21] R3 report issue 23: antimicrobial stewardship in ambulatory health care. The Joint Commission; 2019. Available at: https://www.jointcommission.org/standards/r3-report/r3-report-issue-23-antimicrobial-stewardship-in-ambulatory-health-care/. Accessed November 1, 2020.
[22] de Tejada B. Antibiotic use and misuse during pregnancy and delivery: benefits and risks. Int J Environ Res Public Health 2014;11(8):7993–8009.
[23] Bookstaver PB, Bland CM, Griffin B, et al. A review of antibiotic use in pregnancy. Pharmacotherapy 2015;35(11):1052–62.
[24] Ledger WJ, Blaser MJ. Are we using too many antibiotics during pregnancy? BJOG 2013;120(12):1450–2.
[25] Kuperman AA, Koren O. Antibiotic use during pregnancy: how bad is it? BMC Med 2016;14(1):91.
[26] Schulman J, Dimand RJ, Lee HC, et al. Neonatal intensive care unit antibiotic use. Pediatrics 2015;135(5):826–33.
[27] Schulman J, Benitz WE, Profit J, et al. Newborn antibiotic exposures and association with proven bloodstream infection. Pediatrics 2019;144(5):e20191105.

[28] O'Leary EN, van Santen KL, Edwards EM, et al. Using NHSN's antimicrobial use option to monitor and improve antibiotic stewardship in neonates. Hosp Pediatr 2019;9(5):340–7.
[29] Polin RA. Management of neonates with suspected or proven early-onset bacterial sepsis. Pediatrics 2012;129(5):1006–15.
[30] Ayrapetyan MCD, Lakshminrusimha S, Bhandari V, et al. Infants born to mothers with clinical chorioamnionitis: a cross-sectional survey on the use of early-onset sepsis risk calculator and prolonged use of antibiotics. Am J Perinatol 2018;36(4):428–33.
[31] Puopolo KM, Benitz WE, Zaoutis TE. Management of neonates born at ≥35 0/7 weeks' gestation with suspected or proven early-onset bacterial sepsis. Pediatrics 2018;142(6): e20182894.
[32] Benitz WE, Wynn JL, Polin RA. Reappraisal of guidelines for management of neonates with suspected early-onset sepsis. J Pediatr 2015;166(4):1070–4.
[33] Eschborn S, Weitkamp J-H. Procalcitonin versus C-reactive protein: review of kinetics and performance for diagnosis of neonatal sepsis. J Perinatology 2019;39(7):893–903.
[34] Benitz WE, Han MY, Madan A, et al. Serial serum C-reactive protein levels in the diagnosis of neonatal infection. Pediatrics 1998;102(4):e41.
[35] Perrone S, Lotti F, Longini M, et al. C-reactive protein in healthy term newborns during the first 48 hours of life. *Arch Dis Child Fetal Neonatal Ed* 2018;103(2):F163–6.
[36] Mjelle AB, Guthe HJT, Reigstad H, et al. Serum concentrations of C-reactive protein in healthy term-born Norwegian infants 48 - 72 hours after birth. Acta Paediatr 2018;108(5):849–54.
[37] Sola A. Abuse of antibiotics in perinatology: negative impact for health and the economy. NeoReviews 2020;21(8):e559.
[38] Puopolo KM, Benitz WE, Zaoutis TE. Management of neonates born at ≤34 6/7 weeks' gestation with suspected or proven early-onset bacterial sepsis. Pediatrics 2018;142(6): e20182896.
[39] Ting JY, Roberts A, Sherlock R, et al. Duration of initial empirical antibiotic therapy and outcomes in very low birth weight infants. Pediatrics 2019;143(3):e20182286.
[40] Ting JY, Synnes A, Roberts A, et al. Association between antibiotic use and neonatal mortality and morbidities in very low-birth-weight infants without culture-proven sepsis or necrotizing enterocolitis. JAMA Pediatr 2016;170(12):1181.
[41] Cotten CM. Adverse consequences of neonatal antibiotic exposure. Curr Opin Pediatr 2016;28(2):141–9.
[42] Cotten CM, Taylor S, Stoll B, et al. Prolonged duration of initial empirical antibiotic treatment is associated with increased rates of necrotizing enterocolitis and death for extremely low birth weight infants. Pediatrics 2009;123(1):58–66.
[43] Kuppala VS, Meinzen-Derr J, Morrow AL, et al. Prolonged initial empirical antibiotic treatment is associated with adverse outcomes in premature infants. J Pediatr 2011;159(5): 720–5.
[44] Alexander VN, Northrup V, Bizzarro MJ. Antibiotic exposure in the newborn intensive care unit and the risk of necrotizing enterocolitis. J Pediatr 2011;159(3):392–7.
[45] Klingenberg C, Kornelisse RF, Buonocore G, et al. Culture-negative early-onset neonatal sepsis — at the crossroad between efficient sepsis care and antimicrobial stewardship. Front Pediatr 2018;6:285.
[46] Payton KSE, Wirtschafter D, Bennett MV, et al. Vignettes identify antibiotic use variation in suspected early onset sepsis. Hosp Pediatr 2021 [in press].
[47] Cantey JB, Baird SD. Ending the culture of culture-negative sepsis in the neonatal ICU. Pediatrics 2017;140(4):e20170044.
[48] Kerste M, Corver J, Sonnevelt MC, et al. Application of sepsis calculator in newborns with suspected infection. J Matern Fetal Neonatal Med 2016;29(23):3860–5.
[49] Kuzniewicz MW, Puopolo KM, Fischer A, et al. A quantitative, risk-based approach to the management of neonatal early-onset sepsis. JAMA Pediatr 2017;171(4):365–71.

[50] Kuzniewicz MW, Walsh EM, Li S, et al. Development and implementation of an early-onset sepsis calculator to guide antibiotic management in late preterm and term neonates. Joint Comm J Qual Patient Saf/Joint Comm Resour 2016;42(5):232–9.

[51] Achten NB, Klingenberg C, Benitz WE, et al. Association of use of the neonatal early-onset sepsis calculator with reduction in antibiotic therapy and safety: a systematic review and meta-analysis. JAMA Pediatr 2019;173(11):1032–40.

[52] Deshmukh M, Mehta S, Patole S. Sepsis calculator for neonatal early onset sepsis – a systematic review and meta-analysis. J Matern Fetal Neonatal Med 2019;34(11):1832–40.

[53] Benitz WE, Long SS. The holy grail of ascertainment of early-onset neonatal sepsis. J Pediatr 2019;213:10–2.

[54] Berardi A, Buffagni AM, Rossi C, et al. Serial physical examinations, a simple and reliable tool for managing neonates at risk for early-onset sepsis. World J Clin Pediatr 2016;5(4):358.

[55] Frymoyer A, Joshi NS, Allan JM, et al. Sustainability of a Clinical Examination-Based Approach for Ascertainment of Early-Onset Sepsis in Late Preterm and Term Neonates. *J Pediatr* 2020;225:263–8.

[56] Stocker M, van Herk W, el Helou S, et al. Procalcitonin-guided decision making for duration of antibiotic therapy in neonates with suspected early-onset sepsis: a multicentre, randomised controlled trial (NeoPIns). Lancet 2017;390(10097):871–81.

[57] Mukherjee A, Davidson L, Anguvaa L, et al. NICE neonatal early onset sepsis guidance: greater consistency, but more investigations, and greater length of stay. Arch Dis Child - Fetal Neonatal Edition 2015;100(3):F248–9.

[58] Brown JVE, Meader N, Wright K, et al. Assessment of C-reactive protein diagnostic test accuracy for late-onset infection in newborn infants. JAMA Pediatr 2020;174(3):260.

[59] Brown JVE, Meader N, Cleminson J, et al. C-reactive protein for diagnosing late-onset infection in newborn infants. *Cochrane Database Syst Rev* 2019;1(1):CD012126.

[60] Marks L, de Waal K, Ferguson JK. Time to positive blood culture in early onset neonatal sepsis: a retrospective clinical study and review of the literature. J Paediatr Child Health 2020;56(9):1371–5.

[61] Weiss SL, Fitzgerald JC, Pappachan J, et al. Global epidemiology of pediatric severe sepsis: the sepsis prevalence, outcomes, and therapies study. Am J Respir Crit Care Med 2015;191(10):1147–57.

[62] Barker GM, O'Brien SM, Welke KF, et al. Major infection after pediatric cardiac surgery: a risk estimation model. Ann Thorac Surg 2010;89(3):843–50.

[63] Davis AL, Carcillo JA, Aneja RK, et al. American College of Critical Care Medicine clinical practice parameters for hemodynamic support of pediatric and neonatal septic shock. Crit Care Med 2017;45(6):1061–93.

[64] Balkhy HH, El-Saed A, AlShehri A, et al. Antimicrobial consumption in three pediatric and neonatal intensive care units in Saudi Arabia: 33-month surveillance study. Ann Clin Microbiol Antimicrob 2019;18(1):20.

[65] Levy ER, Swami S, Dubois SG, et al. Rates and appropriateness of antimicrobial prescribing at an academic children's hospital, 2007–2010. Infect Control Hosp Epidemiol 2015;33(4):346–53.

[66] Lee KR, Bagga B, Arnold SR. Reduction of broad-spectrum antimicrobial use in a tertiary children's hospital post antimicrobial stewardship program guideline implementation*. Pediatr Crit Care Med 2016;17(3).

[67] Aizawa Y, Suwa J, Higuchi H, et al. Antimicrobial stewardship program in a pediatric intensive care unit. J Pediatr Infect Dis Soc 2018;7(3):e156–9.

[68] Adams SM, Ngo L, Morphew T, et al. Does an antimicrobial time-out impact the duration of therapy of antimicrobials in the PICU?*. Pediatr Crit Care Med 2019;20(6).

[69] Downes KJ, Weiss SL, Gerber JS, et al. A pragmatic biomarker-driven algorithm to guide antibiotic use in the pediatric intensive care unit: the Optimizing Antibiotic Strategies in Sepsis (OASIS) Study. J Pediatr Infect Dis Soc 2017;6(2):134–41.

[70] Downes K, Schriver E, Russo M, et al. Implementation of a pragmatic biomarker-driven algorithm to guide antibiotic use in the pediatric intensive care unit: the Optimizing Antibiotic Strategies in Sepsis (OASIS) II Study. Open Forum Infect Dis 2017;4(Suppl 1):S504.
[71] Suda KJ, Hicks LA, Roberts RM, et al. Antibiotic expenditures by medication class, and healthcare setting in the United States, 2010–2015. Clin Infect Dis 2018;66(2):185–90.
[72] Gerber JS, Prasad PA, Russell Localio A, et al. Variation in antibiotic prescribing across a pediatric primary care network. J Pediatr Infect Dis Soc 2014;4(4):297–304.
[73] Fleming-Dutra KE, Hersh AL, Shapiro DJ, et al. Prevalence of inappropriate antibiotic prescriptions among US ambulatory care visits, 2010-2011. JAMA 2016;315(17):1864.
[74] Fierro JL, Prasad PA, Localio AR, et al. Variability in the diagnosis and treatment of group A Streptococcal pharyngitis by primary care pediatricians. Infect Control Hosp Epidemiol 2014;35(S3):S79–85.
[75] Handy LK, Bryan M, Gerber JS, et al. Variability in antibiotic prescribing for community-acquired pneumonia. Pediatrics 2017;139(4):e20162331.
[76] Hicks LA, Bartoces MG, Roberts RM, et al. US outpatient antibiotic prescribing variation according to geography, patient population, and provider specialty in 2011. Clin Infect Dis 2015;60(9):1308–16.
[77] Islam S, Mannix MK, Breuer RK, et al. Guideline adherence and antibiotic utilization by community pediatricians, private urgent care centers, and a pediatric emergency department. Clin Pediatr (Phila) 2020;59(1):21–30.
[78] Gerber JS, Prasad PA, Fiks AG, et al. Effect of an outpatient antimicrobial stewardship intervention on broad-spectrum antibiotic prescribing by primary care pediatricians: a randomized trial. JAMA 2013;309(22):2345–52.
[79] Mistry RD, Newland JG, Gerber JS, et al. Current state of antimicrobial stewardship in children's hospital emergency departments. Infect Control Hosp Epidemiol 2017;38(4):469–75.
[80] Yadav K, Meeker D, Mistry RD, et al. A multifaceted intervention improves prescribing for acute respiratory infection for adults and children in emergency department and urgent care settings. Acad Emerg Med 2019;26(7):719–31.
[81] Poole NM, Shapiro DJ, Fleming-Dutra KE, et al. Antibiotic prescribing for children in United States emergency departments: 2009–2014. Pediatrics 2019;143(2):e20181056.
[82] Zetts RM, Stoesz A, Smith BA, et al. Outpatient antibiotic use and the need for increased antibiotic stewardship efforts. Pediatrics 2018;141(6):e20174124.
[83] Kilgore JT, Smith MJ. Outpatient pediatric antibiotic use: a systematic review. Curr Infect Dis Rep 2019;21(4).
[84] Gerber JS, Ross RK, Bryan M, et al. Association of broad- vs narrow-spectrum antibiotics with treatment failure, adverse events, and quality of life in children with acute respiratory tract infections. JAMA 2017;318(23):2325.
[85] Gerber JS, Prasad PA, Fiks AG, et al. Durability of benefits of an outpatient antimicrobial stewardship intervention after discontinuation of audit and feedback. JAMA 2014;312(23):2569.

Advances in Pediatrics 68 (2021) 55–69

ADVANCES IN PEDIATRICS

Balancing Autonomy and Protection in Pediatric Treatment and Research

Tiffany Chenneville, PhD[a,*], Kemesha Gabbidon, PhD[a], Stefanie Hornschuh, MSc[b], Janan Dietrich, PhD[b,c]

[a]Department of Psychology, University of South Florida, 140 7th Avenue South, DAV 117, St. Petersburg, FL 33701, USA; [b]Perinatal HIV Research Unit, Faculty of Health Sciences, University of Witwatersrand, New Nurses Home, Diepkloof, Soweto 1864, Johannesburg, Gauteng, South Africa; [c]Health Systems Research Unit, South African Medical Research Council, Cape Town, South Africa

Keywords

• Pediatric health care • Pediatric research • Children • Adolescents • Autonomy • Protection • Ethics

Key points

- Competing discourses—children as vulnerable versus children as autonomous—exist and influence views about how much to involve children and adolescents in pediatric treatment and research.
- Legal and ethical issues around informed consent, privacy, and confidentiality frame discussions about the protection–autonomy balance in pediatric health care and research settings.
- Health equity and access as well as developmental, family, and cultural factors must be considered when examining the protection versus autonomy dilemma among minor children and adolescents.
- Fisher's goodness-of-fit ethics and Chenneville's protection–autonomy model provide frameworks for thinking through how best to involve minors in pediatric treatment or research.
- Pediatric health care providers and scientists are encouraged to consider best practices for informed consent/assent and privacy/confidentiality when treating or conducting research with children.

*Corresponding author. *E-mail address:* chennevi@usf.edu

https://doi.org/10.1016/j.yapd.2021.05.009

INTRODUCTION

In a policy statement issued by the American Academy of Pediatrics, the Committee on Pediatric Workforce described the demand for primary care pediatricians and pediatric specialists to meet needs of the increasing numbers of children with significant and chronic health care needs [1]. As demands for pediatric health care increase, so do demands for pediatric research. As Connor and colleagues [2] explained, research is needed to guide health care decisions for children. Basing health care decisions on research conducted solely with adults is insufficient at best and unethical at worst. As pediatric health care and, consequently, research demands continue to increase, it is important for health care providers and scientists to consider the delicate balance between protection and autonomy when working with minor children. In this article, we explore some of the overarching issues related to finding such balance, present relevant ethical decision-making models, and offer recommendations and future directions for pediatric health care providers and scientists.

CHILD PROTECTION VERSUS CHILD AUTONOMY

Competing views complicate decisions about how much or how little to involve children in pediatric treatment and research. On one end of the continuum, minor children are viewed as vulnerable and in need of protection. On the other end, minor children, particularly adolescents, are viewed as autonomous agents whose participation and involvement in decisions regarding treatment and research is critical (Fig. 1). As Carter [3] noted, these discourses–child as vulnerable versus child as autonomous–are at odds with one another. Legally, the former view prevails with a few exceptions. For example, the mature minor doctrine in the United States allows adolescent patients, even those who are not emancipated from their parents, to make certain health care decisions without parental permission or even parental knowledge. The ability of adolescents to test and obtain treatment for sexually transmitted infections (STIs), including HIV, without parental consent or knowledge in many states in the United States provides one example of the application of the mature minor doctrine. Meanwhile, institutional review boards (IRBs) in the United States and institutional

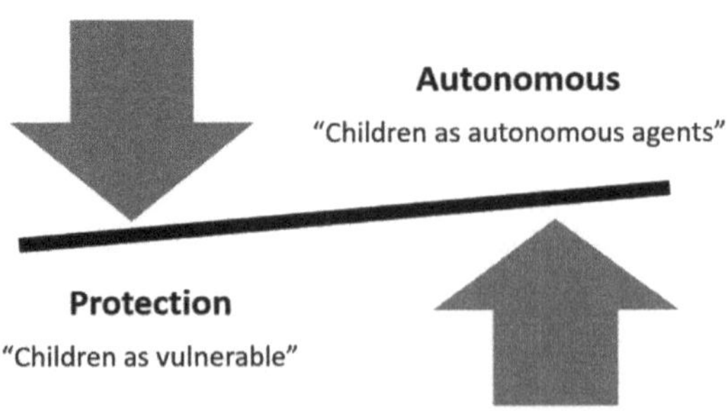

Fig. 1. The child protection–autonomy continuum.

or research ethics committees in other parts of the world sometimes grant waivers of parental permission for research that poses a minimal risk.

Wilhelms and Reyna [4] posit that mature minor status should be treated as an exception rather than a rule. Although they acknowledge the developmental models and theories that suggest cognitive abilities are similar between adolescents and adults, they argue that adolescents have limited gist intuition, which refers to understanding the essence of something and is different from verbatim analysis. Wilhelms and Reyna [4] stress the importance of gist intuition for medical decision-making. Other factors may also affect risk taking and decision-making among adolescents, including emotional maturity, impulsivity, poor self-control, and sensation seeking. Regardless of the application of the mature minor doctrine on health care decision-making, Iltis [5] contends that the doctrine should not be expanded to research settings, instead favoring greater parental involvement in decisions regarding adolescents' participation in research.

Despite arguments in favor of protection, child or minor assent requirements acknowledge the importance of child participation in treatment and research [6]. Also, the fact that research has demonstrated that minor adolescents often possess the capacity to make decisions about medical treatment similar to that of adults serves as an argument in favor of granting adolescents the autonomy to make decisions about their treatment or participation in research, particularly when doing so presents a minimal risk [7]. In response to arguments about the limited maturity of adolescents and the impact of maturity on decision-making, Steinberg [7] argues that adolescents demonstrate maturity equivalent to that of adults in situations where emotional arousal and peer influence are minimized, as is the case for many decisions about pediatric treatment and minimal risk research.

LEGAL AND ETHICAL CONSIDERATIONS

Informed consent

Informed consent is a core aspect of research and treatment endeavors. In pediatric treatment and research settings, informed consent is not only crucial, but required. The basis of informed consent are the principles of respect for persons and autonomy of the individual as outlined in the Nuremberg Code, the Declaration of Helsinki, and the Belmont Report [8–10]. For research conducted in the United States, the Common Rule, a federal policy for the Protection of Human Subjects, details the requirement for informed consent from all research participants unless a waiver of consent is granted by an IRB [11]. In the case of minors, informed consent or parental permission must be obtained from parents or caregivers, and minor assent must be obtained from children ages 7 and older (until adult age or age of majority, which is 18 years in most jurisdictions) except under certain specified circumstances (e.g., when a child has been emancipated from his or her parents or legal guardians). Child assent is a minor's affirmative agreement to participate in treatment or research and is not simply a failure to object to assent.

Informed consent of parents and child or minor assent involve several elements all of which are necessary:

- Full disclosure from the clinician or researcher,
- Voluntary agreement from the patient, client, or participant and/or their parent,
- Comprehension of the information to which the person is consenting or assenting, and
- Documentation.

There are times in which a minor, especially an adolescent, may be able to provide informed consent to clinical services and treatment. For example, as noted elsewhere in this article, in many states in the United States and also other parts of the world, minor adolescents are legally permitted to consent to testing for HIV or other STIs, although the exact age varies across jurisdictions and countries (e.g., 12 years in some places, 13 or 14 years in others). However, regulations do not allow these same adolescent minors to assent to research without parental permission unless a waiver of parental permission has been granted by the IRB. This factor may negatively affect recruitment for research involving sensitive topics (e.g., sexual behavior), especially for adolescents who identify as lesbian, gay, bisexual, transgender, or queer (LGBTQ) [12]. Pediatric researchers and clinicians have advocated for a more nuanced approach to adolescent assent without parental permission for minimal risk treatment and research including the use of decision-making models that aim to better balance protection with respect for autonomy [13,14].

Although pediatric settings are designed to provide care for children and adolescents, there are times in which providing care to parents (or legal guardians) may arise. For example, providing mental health services to parents may be important for addressing the needs of the child (e.g., in cases where parental depression or anxiety is interfering with disease management for a child's condition). Also, in some settings, there are family clinics as opposed to pediatric or adult clinics. These situations and settings may pose unique ethical dilemmas. Andrews [15] shares best practices for obtaining informed consent for parents who receive services within the pediatric setting. These include [15]:

- Always obtaining informed consent when initiating parent-centered services, regardless of any previous consent obtained from either the parent or assent from the child;
- Clearly outlining the limitations of confidentiality by describing what information will be documented and where it will be recorded, who will have access to these records, and what information will be shared with the child care team; and
- Clarifying the nature of all relationships between the clinician, parent, child and others.

Similarly, parent–child dyadic research may pose unique challenges associated with informed consent. Specifically, parental coercion of the minor child may be an issue in parent–child dyadic research, particularly when incentives are favorable to parents [16]. Wittenborn and colleagues [17] recommend obtaining assent without the parent(s) present in the room and verifying assent with probing questions designed to ensure the child is assenting of his or her own volition.

Privacy and confidentiality

Privacy and confidentiality are both legal and ethical constructs relevant to pediatric research and practice [18]. Confidentiality is an agreement about the protection of private information and a determination of who has access to that information. As posed by Chenneville [19], when reflecting on the privacy and confidentiality obligations of clinicians in a pediatric setting, to whom is the right to privacy owed? Is it the parent, the minor child, or both? This concern will likely intensify as children age into adolescence, during which time their need for autonomy increases. Pediatric clinicians and researchers are then tasked with balancing the adolescent's right to privacy with the parent's right to information about their minor child. With the increased need for autonomy, adolescents may wish to withhold information about their identity, medical health, and health behaviors (e.g., sexual health and behaviors, STI status, LGBTQ identity) from their parents (or legal guardians). Clinicians' and researchers' decisions must be framed within the legal and ethical requirements of their profession and government. For example, in the United States, some states require parental (or legal guardian) consent or notification to provide HIV screening and/or treatment to the adolescent minor, whereas others do not. Considering these difficulties, the Society for Adolescent Medicine recommends that ensuring the confidentiality of the adolescent's privacy should be commensurate with the adolescent's maturity level and autonomy rights [20].

For certain health conditions, confidentiality may be further complicated by competing legal and ethical demands. For example, unique to adolescents living with HIV or other STIs, there may also be instances in which providers will need to weigh their ethical and legal duty to maintain confidentiality against their ethical and legal duty to protect third parties from harm. This situation may likely occur if the adolescent patient living with an STI, including HIV, discloses engaging in sexual behavior with someone unaware of their HIV status. The cross-section of these duties has resulted in a practical quandary for mental health professionals in the United States, whose duty to protect third parties from potential harm resulted from the well-known case, *Tarasoff v. Regents of the University of California* [21]. There remains significant controversy around if and how much information should be disclosed to a third party in these circumstances [22]. Although the American Psychological Association advocates for strict confidentiality to preserve the therapeutic relationship wherein HIV disclosure can be explored as a part of treatment, public health and medical professionals may support limited disclosure (e.g., compliance with partner notification services) [19,23]. These differences in professional ethical standards further complicate decision-making within pediatric integrated care or research settings [24].

Although most practice and research literature has focused on balancing the autonomy of minor children and adolescents with their parent's right to information, as noted elsewhere in this article, there are circumstances in which pediatric providers may provide care to parents or legal guardians [15]. In this situation, and except for emergency care, clinicians must determine and outline their ethical responsibilities regarding privacy and confidentiality clearly [15]. Practitioners should monitor accidental breaches of confidentiality, including how confidential information is learned and discussed, and are advised to minimize disclosure of parent's information to the child's health care team [15]. Precautions around recordkeeping and documentation and who and under what circumstances they would have access to this information should be considered. If clinicians are not able to protect parents' confidentiality or to decrease the harm resulting from these multiple relationships, then they should refer rather than provide services [15]. Similarly, privacy and confidentiality may pose unique ethical considerations in parent–child dyadic research. Specifically, inadvertent confidentiality breaches resulting from the way in which data are collected, analyzed, or disseminated may occur, which speaks to a need for caution when designing such studies [25]. Decisions about whether to collect data jointly or separately are important and should consider concerns about privacy. Gabbidon and colleagues [16] provide a thorough discussion of the pros and cons of joint versus separate data collection methods in parent–child dyadic research, as well as ways to minimize inadvertent breaches to confidentiality when collecting data remotely (e.g., online, via email, telephonically, virtually) and when disseminating findings.

DEVELOPMENTAL CONSIDERATIONS

Developmental factors are important to consider when trying to adequately balance protection and autonomy for minors in both accessing medical treatment and participating in research. Even though age is one of the most widely used parameters for establishing developmental competence and maturity, there may be differences around the developmental competencies of children the same age owing to varying factors, and these need to be taken into consideration [26]. Developmental and cognitive disabilities or chronic medical illnesses (e.g., HIV) may also have an impact on the ability to make informed decisions and affect children and adolescents' capacity to assent to treatment and research [27]. It has been recommended that decisional capacity be assessed before a child provides assent to medical treatment or participation in a study [13,28]. Grisso and Appelbaum [29] describe decisional capacity as a construct composed of 4 essential components: understanding, appreciation, reasoning and the ability to express a choice.

For children and minor adolescents to be able to provide informed assent, it is imperative that they have the ability to comprehend and feel prepared enough to process and engage with the information presented to them. The literature suggests that by the age of 14 years, adolescents approach comprehension levels similar to adults [30]. Children under the age of 10 years are usually not giving informed consent and those older than 10 years of age do not possess the legal status to consent to treatment or research without parental or guardian permission until reaching the age of maturity (i.e., age 18 in many countries). However, it is still important to directly involve them in all aspects of the decision-making process. In fact, children as young as 6 to 7 years of age have been shown to have the capacity to understand research aspects and take some form of responsibilities for their own wellbeing [30]. Therefore, access to developmentally appropriate information about their treatment and research participation is vital. This process can have many short- and long-term benefits for treatment and research aspects, including improved adherence to health care regimens in the case of treatment and procedures, and protocols in the case of research.

FAMILY CONSIDERATIONS

Parents or guardians/caregivers are considered the best proxy for advocating for the needs of their child and protecting their rights and health [31]. They are legally responsible for treatment and research decisions, except in cases where parental waivers have been granted. Nevertheless, decision-making around treatment and research should be managed through an interdisciplinary team and collaboratively between the family, child, and health practitioner or investigator [32]. Family dynamics and the strength and vulnerabilities of the parent providing informed consent need to be taken into consideration during the decision-making process. This also includes the parent–child and parent–parent (in those instances where both parties are involved) relationships [31]. This process might become more complex in situations where the parents are divorced or separated and informed consent might need to be obtained from both parties before initiating treatment or research procedures. However, in general, it is only required to obtain permission from 1 parent when the treatment or research procedures are considered minimal risk, whereas permission from both parties is required for procedures posing a greater than minimal risk to the child. During the informed consent process, health practitioners and investigators have the dual role of not only supporting the parent's decision-making responsibilities in their child's best interest, but to also support the child's developing autonomy [31].

Support by family members, close peers, and community members has been shown to help facilitate adherence to treatment and study participation. This includes being reminded about medication intake, appointment reminders, emotional support and efforts for health promotion needs [33–36]. Open and ongoing parent–child and also physician/investigator–child–parent communication and the fostering thereof may have benefits for treatment and research participation and decision-making. Similarly, parenting styles and approaches can influence the child's own decision-making autonomy, with authoritative parenting approaches facilitating the best balance around this [37,38].

CULTURAL CONSIDERATIONS

Across the world, cultural diversity is becoming increasingly important in addressing public health outcomes among youth. Participation in research and adherence to study procedures and/or medical treatment may be affected negatively if cultural factors are not considered. In many parts of the world, cultural practices and norms form the basis for decision-making of minors in treatment and research. Cultural norms can be protective of children, especially those who are particularly vulnerable as a result of their living situation (e.g., children who are orphaned or who, for other reasons, are living with legal or nonlegal guardians). For instance, in some countries with high rates of HIV, many children are orphans as a result of HIV. More research among minors living with chronic illnesses or infectious diseases such as HIV is taking place in low- and middle-income settings. Therefore, the protection of children from potential exploitation is a key factor when attempting to balance the risks and benefits of involving children and adolescents in research [39]. In many places, access to communities for research–even if low risk–requires the approval of community leaders or gatekeepers, so this factor must also be considered.

In many countries, legislation governs the ability of minors to self-consent (or assent without parental permission), even adolescent minors who may possess the requisite decisional capacity. Further, cultural norms will influence the extent to which minors perceive their caregivers as having the authority to make decisions about their health including decisions about whether to participate in research. Therefore, in some cultures, even when minors possess decisional capacity and are permitted to self-consent, they will still seek guidance from key adults for decision-making. Further, minors may regard community leaders and other adults as a source of decision-making in pediatric treatment and research. In these instances, longer term outcomes, such as adherence to treatment and research protocols, may be affected without the support of key adults. The involvement of key adults also may help to promote continuity of care. For example, a study involving youth living with HIV in Zimbabwe found that continuity of care improved when maternal and paternal family members of orphans were consulted during the consenting process [39]. A family-centered approach to decision-making has been documented in Botswana [40]. Clinical researchers can mitigate potential conflict and tension by learning about the cultural norms in a particular community through formative research, stakeholder engagements, and employing local researchers. Cultural competence will facilitate bridging the gap between public health priorities and the cultural background of young people [41]. Cultural awareness and sensitivity also is important with regard to data collection methods. For example, there may be cultural taboos associated with providing hair samples or bodily fluids for the purpose of research.

HEALTH EQUITY AND ACCESS CONSIDERATIONS

Equity and access are important factors to consider when thinking about pediatric treatment and research. The social determinants of health framework explains the ways in which factors such as food insecurity, unstable housing, exposure to physical and sexual violence, and poor access to services affect health. Across the world, health access is often structured around the majority population with few considerations for marginalized groups who face systemic discrimination based on race, ethnicity, sexual orientation, gender identity, and other intersecting identities. The ethical principle of justice demands that children and adolescents have equal access to health care, yet this is not the case in many places, including the United States. The principle of justice also applies to pediatric research. Within the context of research, justice speaks to the need for equal access to the benefits and burdens of research. In certain instances, youth (e.g., youth living with a chronic health condition) may be overlooked for research owing to physical access, limited financial resources, or the potential for intimate partner violence. Further, participation may be limited as a result of not having consent from a legal guardian or fear of disclosing these risk factors.

The principles of justice and beneficence can be addressed through the health system by ensuring that health care professionals have an awareness of their own biases through sensitivity training and through addressing structural barriers. Additionally, parental or caregiver waivers of consent could be considered on a case-by-case basis to ensure that key populations are not excluded from care and research, especially situations deemed low risk [31]. To decrease health inequities, it is important for minors and their caregivers to explicitly know that their decision regarding participation in research would not affect their continuity of care. This factor would ensure that minors' decisional capacity would not be biased or coerced to ensure that research objectives can be met. Last, in certain countries like the United States, if a child does not wish to participate in research that would benefit them–such as if previous treatments were unsuccessful–then the parent may consent for the child's participation [31]. In this case, health inequities may be decreased but the minor's participation and/or compliance may be affected.

RELEVANT ETHICAL MODELS

Goodness-of-fit ethical framework

The goodness-of-fit ethical framework emphasizes the value of empirical research on informed consent that outlines important considerations for potential participant strengths and vulnerabilities; this research may inform best practices while addressing the unique needs of the research context [31]. The vulnerability of minor youth is fluid and can be created or worsened by the social, cultural, or political context in which research is implemented or care is provided [31]. Participant characteristics relevant to minors include their decisional capacity, the parent's (or legal guardian's) understanding of clinical or research-related information, and the personal and cultural norms and values that shape decision making [31]. Framed around HIV, the goodness-of-fit ethical framework as outlined by Fisher and colleagues [31] provides best practices for informed consent, confidentiality, and disclosure.

The protection–autonomy model

The protection–autonomy model is a conceptual framework that incorporates the protection–autonomy continuum, which emphasizes an assessment of the decisional capacity of youth to consent to medical treatment or research [13]. Historically, this has been viewed through the lens of protectionists versus autonomists; however, making decisions about youth's ability to consent is far more nuanced. In this model, researchers and clinicians are encouraged to assess the decisional capacity of minors to consent to treatment or research rather than relying on the parents (or legal guardians) or health professionals as the authority figure(s). The application of this model and the associated results gathered from determining decisional capacity will inform the level of protective or autonomous action that is endorsed. For example, when decisional capacity is low, more protective action from parents and health care providers would be needed. However, when decisional capacity is high, more emphasis on respecting the autonomy of the child may be ideal. Chenneville and colleagues [13] ask professionals to recognize that protection and autonomy are not mutually exclusive, but rather considerations for the child's developmental stage and emotional, cognitive, and medical needs must be addressed.

RECOMMENDATIONS FOR BALANCING AUTONOMY AND PROTECTION IN PEDIATRIC TREATMENT AND RESEARCH

We offer recommendations for balancing protection and autonomy in pediatric treatment and research. They take into account arguments on both ends of the protection–autonomy continuum, ethical and legal issues, and considerations related to development, family, culture, and health equity as well as relevant ethical models (Fig. 2). Specifically, best practices for obtaining informed consent and assent and best practices for protecting confidentiality and disclosures in pediatric treatment and research are outlined.

Best practices for informed consent and assent

Consistent with recommendations summarized by Fisher and colleagues, health care providers and scientists are encouraged to create informed consent/assent procedures keeping in mind [31,42,43]:

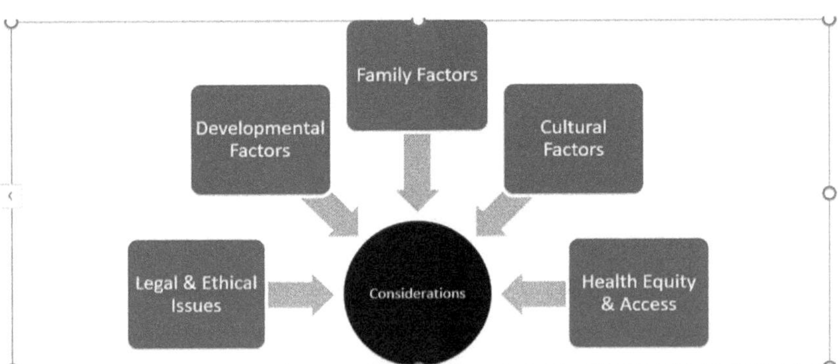

Fig. 2. Important considerations for balancing autonomy and protection in pediatric treatment and research.

- The developmental and health-related factors that shape a child's ability to provide a voluntary, informed, and rational choice
- The parent's (or legal guardian's) comprehension of the child's health and their health-related literacy
- The cultural and familial norms around decision-making, and any specific considerations relevant to the research and clinical context

In the case of adolescents, minors, and consistent with Chenneville and colleagues's recommendations, it also is important to assess decisional capacity, given research that has shown that youth's decisional capacity at age 14 is comparable with that of adults, barring any neuropsychological impairments [13,44]. Decisional capacity notwithstanding, the cognitive and emotional challenges of youth living with a chronic illness will need to be considered and used to tailor fit their informed assent needs. Tailoring of the informed consent procedures for parents (or legal guardians) may also be necessary and should include consideration for the parent's educational background, health literacy, and knowledge of the medical aspects of their child's illness. Applying an HIV-specific example, Fisher and colleagues [31] outline the importance of considering the cultural and familial norms around decision-making and how this would inform the consent process. Although researchers and clinicians may hope to support the child's developing autonomy by emphasizing their informed assent in deciding to participate in treatment or research, Fisher and colleagues [31,45] warn against elevating the child's autonomy over the parent's responsibility to decide what is best. When the benefits of autonomy outweigh the risks, then the mature minor doctrine should be considered (e.g., STI testing and treatment). Similarly, for minimal risk research, particularly research on sensitive topics wherein parental permission requirements might prevent adolescent participation, scientists should consider seeking waivers of parental permission although some IRBs will not grant such waivers.

Best practices for protecting confidentiality and disclosures

Also consistent with recommendations summarized by Fisher and colleagues [31], best practices suggest that health care providers and scientists:

- Establish confidentiality limits before beginning research or practice,
- Outline the legal and ethical obligations of the health care provider or researcher,
- Decide how to respond to parent's request for information on their child, and
- Be prepared to breach confidentiality if the child poses a risk to themselves or others.

Before initiating treatment or research, professionals should consider the emotional and cognitive needs of the child, the goals of the treatment or research being implemented, and the role of the parent (or legal guardian). With regard to outlining legal and ethical obligations, the goodness-of-fit ethical framework supports professionals in being specific about the types of information that would be shared versus kept confidential. This determination should be made early in the process to manage ethical dilemmas that may arise from multiple relationships between health care providers and patients/clients or scientists and research participants. Before initiating treatment, health care providers in conjunction with the family should develop a confidentiality and disclosure policy that is aligned with the relevant cultural and familial norms around decision-making [31]. Attention should be given to parental views and concerns and should be revisited to ensure best practices. There may be times (e.g., if a child's behavior poses a risk to themselves or others) in which disclosure of the minor child's health information or behaviors may need to be disclosed to parents (or legal guardians). Fisher and colleagues [31] outline 4 guiding principles to aid professionals in deciding if and how much information should be disclosed. First, professionals are encouraged to assess and address the risk behaviors of the youth. Second, professionals should consider options if the minor client is unable or unwilling to reduce risk behaviors. Third, professionals should prepare the client for disclosure by being responsive to their concerns and needs. Finally, professionals should emphasize and respond to parents' feelings in a positive way, outlining ways in which they can support the child.

SUMMARY

Given the increasing numbers of children with significant and chronic health care needs, the demand for specialized pediatric health care and research in this population is high. When working with children and adolescents, it is important to balance autonomy and protection. Although an increased focus on minors' rights may thwart needed protections, an overemphasis on the vulnerability of minors may impede autonomy rights, particularly for adolescents who are transitioning into early adulthood. As we have described, there are important legal and ethical issues as well as factors related to development, family, culture, and health equity that health care providers and scientists should acknowledge when engaging in treatment or research with children and adolescents. Taking into account relevant ethical models, health care providers and scientists are encouraged to consider best practices around informed consent/assent and confidentiality/disclosures. Going forward, additional research is needed to further examine the cognitive, social, emotional, and cultural factors that influence medical decision-making among adolescents in an effort to develop evidence-based policies and procedures that achieve the important balance between protection and autonomy in pediatric health care and research settings. Among other examples, longitudinal research that allows for an examination of the outcomes of decisions related to pediatric treatment over time, including an analysis of differential outcomes based on who is making the decision–parent or child–is needed. It also is important to educate pediatric health care providers, scientists, and IRBs (or independent ethics committees or research ethics committees) about these issues.

CLINICS CARE POINTS

- Pediatric health care providers and scientists are encouraged to familiarize themselves with competing discourses related to how much to involve children and adolescents in pediatric treatment and research, and to examine their own position along the continuum of viewing children as vulnerable on one end to viewing children as autonomous on the other end.
- Pediatric health care providers and scientists are encouraged to familiarize themselves with the ways in which legal and ethical issues around informed consent, privacy, and confidentiality frame discussions about the protection–autonomy balance in pediatric health care and research settings.
- Pediatric health care providers and scientists are encouraged to consider issues related to health equity and access as well as developmental, family, and cultural factors when examining the protection versus autonomy dilemma among minor children and adolescents.
- Pediatric health care providers and scientists are encouraged to use Fisher's goodness-of-fit ethics and/or Chenneville's protection–autonomy model as frameworks for thinking through how best to involve minor children and adolescents in pediatric treatment or research.
- Pediatric health care providers and scientists are encouraged to consider best practices for informed consent and assent as well as privacy and confidentiality when treating or conducting research with children.

DISCLOSURE

Authors acknowledge partial support through University of South Florida Nexus Initiative (UNI) Award. Dr Hornschuh was supported by the Consortium for Advanced Research Training in Africa (CARTA). CARTA is jointly led by the African Population and Health Research Center and the University of the Witwatersrand and funded by the Carnegie Corporation of New York (Grant No-B 8606.R02), Sida (Grant No:54100029), the DELTAS Africa Initiative (Grant No: 107768/Z/15/Z). The work reported herein for JJD was made possible through partial funding by the South African Medical Research Council (SAMRC) through its Division of Research Capacity Development under the SAMRC Postdoctoral Programme from funding received from the South African National Treasury as well as the CIPHER GROWING THE LEADERS OF TOMORROW grant from the International AIDS Society.

References

[1] Basco WT, Rimsza ME, Committee on Pediatric W, American Academy of Pediatrics. Pediatrician workforce policy statement. Pediatrics 2013;132(2):390–7.
[2] Connor EM, Smoyer WE, Davis JM, et al. Meeting the demand for pediatric clinical trials. Sci Transl Med 2014;6(227):227fs211.
[3] Carter B. Tick box for child? The ethical positioning of children as vulnerable, researchers as barbarians and reviewers as overly cautious. Int J Nurs Stud 2009;46(6):858–64.

[4] Wilhelms EA, Reyna VF. Fuzzy trace theory and medical decisions by minors: differences in reasoning between adolescents and adults. Great Britain: Oxford University Press; 2013. p. 268.
[5] Iltis AS. Parents, adolescents, and consent for research participation. J Med Philos 2013;38(3):332–46.
[6] Committee on Bioethics. Informed consent in decision-making in pediatric practice. Pediatrics 2016;138(2):e20161484.
[7] Steinberg L. Does recent research on adolescent brain development inform the mature minor doctrine? J Med Philos 2013;38(3):256–67.
[8] Code N, 1949. The Nuremberg Code. *Trials of war criminals before the Nuremberg military tribunals under control council law,* 10, 1949. p. 181–2.
[9] World Medical Association General A. World Medical Association Declaration of Helsinki: ethical principles for medical research involving human subjects. J Int Bioethique 2004;15(1):124–9.
[10] US Department of Health and Human Services, 1979. The belmont report.
[11] US Department of Health and Human Services, 1991. The Common Rule, Title 45 (Public Welfare), Code of Federal Regulations, Part 46 (Protection of Human Subjects).
[12] Mustanski B, Fisher CB. HIV rates are increasing in gay/bisexual teens: IRB barriers to research must be resolved to bend the curve. Am J Prev Med 2016;51(2):249–52.
[13] Chenneville T, Sibille K, Bendell-Estroff D. Decisional capacity among minors with HIV: a model for balancing autonomy rights with the need for protection. Great Britain: Taylor & Francis; 2010. p. 83.
[14] Chenneville T, Gabbidon K, Drake H, et al. Considerations and recommendations for balancing protection and autonomy in the context of adolescent HIV research. Translational Issues Psychol Sci 2020;6(3):196–206.
[15] Andrews JH. Ethically uncharted territory: providing psychological services to parents in pediatric settings. Ethics Behav 2020;31(2):77–90.
[16] Gabbidon K, Chenneville, T., & Rote, W. Methodological and ethical considerations for parent-child dyadic research. (under review).
[17] Wittenborn AK, Dolbin-MacNab ML, Keiley MK. Dyadic research in marriage and family therapy: methodological considerations. J Marital Fam Ther 2013;39(1):5–16.
[18] Nagy TF. Essential ethics for psychologists. [electronic resource]: a primer for understanding and mastering core issues. 1st ed. Washington, DC: American Psychological Association; 2011.
[19] Chenneville T. Pediatric/adolescent HIV: legal and ethical issues. In: HIV/AIDS in rural communities. Switzerland: Springer; 2017. p. 73–88.
[20] Ford C, English A, Sigman G. Confidential health care for adolescents: position paper for the society for adolescent medicine. J Adolesc Health 2004;35(2):160–7.
[21] Tarasoff V. Regents of the University of California, 17 Cal.3d 425, 551 P.2d 334 1976 1974.
[22] Chenneville T, Gabbidon K. HIV, confidentiality, and duty to protect: considerations for psychotherapists in the age of treatment as prevention. Psychotherapy (Chic) 2020;57(1): 7–14.
[23] Association AP. Legal liability related to confidentiality and the prevention of HIV transmission. 1991. Available at: http://www.apa.org/about/policy/confidentiality.aspx. Accessed November 28, 2020.
[24] Chenneville T, Gabbidon K. Application of the APA ethics code for psychologists working in integrated care settings: potential conflicts and resolutions. Ethics Behav 2020;30(4): 264–74.
[25] Ummel D, Achille M. Transplant trajectory and relational experience within living kidney dyads. Qual Health Res 2016;26(2):194–203.

[26] Grootens-Wiegers P, Hein IM, van den Broek JM, et al. Medical decision-making in children and adolescents: developmental and neuroscientific aspects. BMC Pediatr 2017;17(1): 120.
[27] Kuther TL. Medical decision-making and minors: issues of consent and assent. Adolescence 2003;38(150):343–58.
[28] Dunn LB, Nowrangi MA, Palmer BW, et al. Assessing decisional capacity for clinical research or treatment: a review of instruments. Am J Psychiatry 2006;163(8):1323–34.
[29] Grisso T, Appelbaum PS. Assessing competence to consent to treatment: a guide for physicians and other health professionals. USA: Oxford University Press; 1998.
[30] Field MJ, Behrman RE, editors. Ethical conduct of clinical research involving children. 2004 Washington (DC): National Academy of Sciences.
[31] Fisher CB, Arbeit MR, Chenneville T. Goodness-of-fit ethics for practice and research involving children and adolescents with HIV. In: A clinical guide to pediatric HIV. Switzerland: Springer; 2016. p. 229–58.
[32] Harrison C, Society CP, Committee B. Treatment decisions regarding infants, children and adolescents. Paediatr Child Health 2004;9(2):99–114.
[33] Mutwa PR, Van Nuil JI, Asiimwe-Kateera B, et al. Living situation affects adherence to combination antiretroviral therapy in HIV-infected adolescents in Rwanda: a qualitative study. PLoS One 2013;8(4):e60073.
[34] Obirikorang C, Selleh PK, Abledu JK, et al. Predictors of adherence to antiretroviral therapy among HIV/AIDS patients in the upper west region of Ghana. ISRN AIDS 2013;2013: 873939.
[35] Taddeo D, Egedy M, Frappier JY. Adherence to treatment in adolescents. Paediatr Child Health 2008;13(1):19–24.
[36] Scott K, Campbell C, Madanhire C, et al. In what ways do communities support optimal antiretroviral treatment in Zimbabwe? Health Promot Int 2014;29(4):645–54.
[37] Hein IM, De Vries MC, Troost PW, et al. Informed consent instead of assent is appropriate in children from the age of twelve: policy implications of new findings on children's competence to consent to clinical research. BMC Med Ethics 2015;16(1):76.
[38] Partridge BC. Adolescent psychological development, parenting styles, and pediatric decision making. J Med Philos 2010;35(5):518–25.
[39] Bwakura-Dangarembizi M, Musesengwa R, Nathoo KJ, et al. Ethical and legal constraints to children's participation in research in Zimbabwe: experiences from the multicenter pediatric HIV ARROW trial. BMC Med Ethics 2012;13:17.
[40] Shaibu S. Ethical and cultural considerations in informed consent in Botswana. Nurs Ethics 2007;14(4):503–9.
[41] Gray B. Culture, cultural competence and the cross-cultural consultation. J Paediatr Child Health 2018;54(4):343–5.
[42] Fisher CB. A goodness-of-fit ethic for child assent to nonbeneficial research. Am J Bioeth 2003;3(4):27–8.
[43] Fisher CB. Adolescent and parent perspectives on ethical issues in youth drug use and suicide survey research. Ethics Behav 2003;13(4):303–32.
[44] Behrman RE, Field MJ, Institute of Medicine (U.S.). Committee on clinical research involving children. *Ethical conduct of clinical research involving children.* Washington, D.C.: National Academies Press; 2004.
[45] Young AJ, Kim L, Shu L, et al. Agency and communication challenges in discussions of informed consent in pediatric cancer research. Qual Health Res 2010;20(5):628–43.

Advances in Pediatrics 68 (2021) 71–88

ADVANCES IN PEDIATRICS

Addressing Parental Adverse Childhood Experiences in the Pediatric Setting

Rupal C. Gupta, MD[a,b,c,*], Kimberly A. Randell, MD, MSc[b,c,d], M. Denise Dowd, MD, MPH[b,c,d]

[a]Division of General Academic Pediatrics, Children's Mercy Kansas City, 2401 Gillham Road, Kansas City, MO 64109, USA; [b]University of Missouri–Kansas City School of Medicine, Kansas City, MO, USA; [c]University of Kansas School of Medicine, Kansas City, KS, USA; [d]Division of Emergency Medicine, Children's Mercy Kansas City, 2401 Gillham Road, Kansas City, MO 64109, USA

Keywords

• Parent trauma • Adverse childhood experiences • Toxic stress • Childhood trauma • Parenting • Resilience

Key points

- A parent's own adverse childhood experiences (ACEs) may have an impact on the future health and well-being of their children.
- All parents can benefit from universal education on the impact of childhood trauma on parenting and the benefits of positive parenting techniques.
- Using a strengths-based approach when working with parents who have been affected by ACEs allows parents to build on resilience factors.

INTRODUCTION

A 27-year-old mother of an asthmatic 8-year-old struggles with anxiety and depression and feels overwhelmed with her parental responsibilities. Her child has been hospitalized 3 times in the past year with severe asthma exacerbations. A 30-year-old father responds to his 4-year-old's challenging behaviors with anger and harsh verbal discipline. He wants his child prescribed something to "calm him down." From comments made by these parents the provider

*Corresponding author. Division of General Academic Pediatrics, Children's Mercy Kansas City, 2401 Gillham Road, Kansas City, MO 64109, USA. *E-mail address:* rcgupta@cmh.edu

https://doi.org/10.1016/j.yapd.2021.05.003

understands that each of them had what they both refer to as a "tough" upbringing. The provider ponders the relationship between those parental experiences and the children's health and development challenges.

Adverse childhood experiences (ACEs) are part of the contemporary pediatric lexicon. The term describes traumatic experiences, occurring prior to the age of 18 years, which are strongly associated in a dose-response manner with lifelong negative physical and mental health consequences [1], including cardiovascular disease [2], liver disease [3], depression [4], substance abuse [5,6], and suicidality [7]. Multiple studies consistently have reproduced these findings, and related associations have been expanded to include poor educational, social-emotional, and employment outcomes [1,8]. ACEs are common, with one-half to two-thirds of the adult population experiencing at least 1 ACE [9,10]. ACEs occur at all income levels but there is a direct linear relationship between high ACE score ($\geq$4) and lower incomes [11,12]. The ACEs in Felitti and colleagues' [1] original work included psychological, physical, or sexual abuse; violence against the mother; and living with household members with substance use disorder, mental illness, suicidality, or history of imprisonment. More recently, researchers have proposed expanding ACEs criteria to include witnessing violence, experiencing discrimination, lacking a safe neighborhood, being bullied, and living in foster care [13].

Although the conventional term, *parental ACEs*, is used in this article, the authors recognize that many children live with a nonparent primary caregiver. Thus, readers are asked to keep in mind that the concepts and recommendations discussed may be applied to any of a child's caregivers.

PARENTAL ADVERSE CHILDHOOD EXPERIENCES AND CHILD HEALTH OUTCOMES

More recent work expands the understanding of the impact of ACEs to include the negative impact of parental ACEs on child health broadly across multiple domains. A population-based study of Philadelphia parent-child dyads found that for each point increase in parental expanded ACE score, the odds of poor overall child health increased by 19% and asthma by 17% [14]. Maternal ACEs also predict impaired birthweight and missed child preventive care [15,16]. Multiple studies demonstrate a dose-response relationship between parental ACE score and risk for child developmental delay, with 1 study finding maternal ACE score of 3 or greater associated with 2.2-times greater likelihood of suspected child developmental delay and an increasing number of developmental domains affected [17–19]. Maternal ACEs also are associated with reduced child Ages and Stages Questionnaire: Social-Emotional Score [15]. Additionally, a dose-response relationship is seen with parental ACEs and child hyperactivity, emotional disturbance, and aggressive behavior [20,21]. Available studies primarily examine maternal data; much less is known about the impact of paternal ACEs but it is likely that they affect children's health similarly [16,20].

EARLY EXPERIENCES AND THE IMPACT OF PARENTAL ADVERSE CHILDHOOD EXPERIENCES ON PARENTING BEHAVIORS

Causal mechanisms for the relationship between parental ACEs and child health outcomes are not yet fully understood, but evidence to date suggests that multiple pathways are contributory. Chief among these is the impact of parental ACEs on parenting behaviors [22]. The early years are a critical developmental period because experiences during this time embed themselves in the brain circuitry and provide scaffolding for behavior, emotionality, and physiology across the life span [23]. Safe, stable, nurturing relationships and growth through positive experiences form the roots of resilience, defined by Masten [24] as the dynamic process of positive adaption to, or in spite of, significant adversity. Forkey's [25] THREADS mnemonic initially was developed to identify factors critical to child resilience: thinking and learning brain, hope, regulation or self-control, efficacy, attachment, developmental skill mastery, and social connectedness. An adaptation of this mnemonic can aid in understanding the impact of the presence or absence of parental ACEs on parent resilience and parenting behaviors (Table 1).

A child's capacity for resilient adaptation across the life course develops within the context of their relationships with primary caregivers. Individuals who experienced a positive family emotional climate, positive attachment with their parents, and less authoritarian parenting during their childhood are more likely to show warm, sensitive, stimulating maternal behavior in adulthood [26]. In the absence of a nurturing parental relationship, however, adults may develop a heightened stress response and altered capacity to respond effectively to life's stressors, such as raising their own children.

The biological mechanism by which ACEs impair parenting is hypothesized to be multifold, correlating with the known impact of ACEs on child brain development. Parental emotionality and nurturing behavior are dependent on autonomic nervous system and hypothalamic-pituitary-adrenal (HPA) axis functioning, and ACEs have a negative impact on both [27]. Sustained activation of the stress response system in response to ACEs results in cell hypertrophy and proliferation as well as brain remodeling in the amygdala, hippocampus, and prefrontal cortex [28]. These architectural shifts impair the development of critical areas related to memory, learning, decision-making, and stress response [28,29]. They also increase parental risk of depression, posttraumatic stress disorder (PTSD), anxiety, and poor emotional regulation, which may decrease parental availability to respond to a child's needs [15,30,31].

INTERGENERATIONAL TRANSMISSION OF ADVERSE CHILDHOOD EXPERIENCES

Parental ACEs may have a further impact on child health through intergenerational transmission of ACEs. One hypothesized pathway for this transmission is epigenetic modification. Epigenetics refers to molecular-level changes in gene

Table 1
Potential impact of parental adverse childhood experiences on the THREADS of resilience and parenting

THREADS of childhood [25]	Relevance to parenting	How adverse childhood experiences may disrupt THREADS, impairing parental resiliency
Thinking and learning brain	Parenting is a skill that can be developed, with opportunity for continued growth and cognitive development.	Reflexive behaviors and actions of brain may take over to manage small and large threats; parents may have increased short-/long-term response to stimuli and increased reactivity to harsh environmental cues [27].
Hope	Belief, faith, and optimism in a future for oneself can motivate positive parenting behavior	Parents may have abandoned hope to deal with present challenges, experience negative emotions more strongly, and have impaired coping [77].
Regulation and self-control	Executive function, including working memory, problem-solving, inhibition control, and attention control, are critical to responsive parenting.	Parent may react impulsively to unpredictable events. This carries high risk of unhealthy behaviors (eg, smoking during pregnancy, alcohol, marijuana, and illicit drug use), which impair ability to parent positively [6,36].
Efficacy	Parent has knowledge that they can have an impact on their environment or situation.	Parent may not be able to maintain efficacy when reacting to situations rather than being in control of them. Mental illness, if present, and additional stressors and adversities, such as poverty, can compound already heightened parenting stress [23,78].
Attachment and attunement	Parent has secure attachment, marked by responsiveness and concern for their child [79].	Attachment may be impaired. Depression, PTSD, or anxiety, if present, can lead to a parent having reduced emotional responsiveness to child's needs and intrusive behavior toward children [80,81].

(*continued on next page*)

Table 1
(continued)

THREADS of childhood [25]	Relevance to parenting	How adverse childhood experiences may disrupt THREADS, impairing parental resiliency
Developmental skill mastery Distance and self-care	Parent succeeds in building life skills alongside nurturing skills. Parent realizes self-worth without relying on child for sense of personal accomplishment.	In having to deal with the present threat, parents may lose ability to focus on future goals, nurturing their child, or both.
Social connectedness (home-based, school-based, and community-based)	Parent can achieve resilience and effective parenting behaviors within a network of positive, supportive social relationships.	Parent may have lost social connectedness due to past or present trauma.

expression that occur as a result of environmental factors, such as toxins, and social-emotional factors, such as manner of care and nurturing [32]. ACEs have been found in human and animal studies to increase methylation of DNA in the promoter region of several genes, including the glucocorticoid receptor gene, functionally reducing expression of those genes and leading to dysfunction of the HPA axis [27]. It is understood that some epigenetic changes are inherited [33], and thus potentially affect the stress response and behaviors of future generations, but the inevitability of transmission and extent of impact are not known. Pregnant women with high ACEs have a greater risk of fetal demise [34], giving birth to a preterm infant [35], and high-risk health behaviors during their pregnancy [36]. Research into the epigenetic mechanisms around ACEs and parenting abilities still is in its infancy, with further work needed to evaluate how the epigenetics of ACEs may have an impact on other hormones and neurotransmitters, including dopamine, oxytocin, and other neuropeptides thought to be involved in nurturing.

These gaps notwithstanding, it is clear that parental ACEs may directly beget children's ACEs. Children of parents with a high ACE score are themselves more likely to experience childhood adversity [37], in part because ACE-related adult health outcomes, such as mental illness and substance use disorder, may themselves be ACEs for their children. The conditions contributing to childhood adversity may continue to be present in adulthood, thus setting up potential for exposure of the next generation to the ACEs of poverty and violence. Additionally, parents who have experienced childhood adversity and poor modeling by their parents are more likely to take on suboptimal attitudes and parenting beliefs [38,39]. Mothers who experienced child physical abuse have been found to be 1.5 times more likely to use corporal punishment than those who had not been abused [39]. Fathers who experienced ACEs were more likely to be perpetrators of violence against their partners [40].

FRAMEWORK FOR ADDRESSING PARENTAL ADVERSE CHILDHOOD EXPERIENCES IN PEDIATRIC CARE SETTINGS

Trauma-informed care and healing-centered engagement provide a general framework for addressing parental ACEs. A trauma-informed approach to parental ACEs recognizes the high prevalence of ACEs, that any parent may have experienced childhood adversity, and that these experiences will influence parenting practices, the stresses of parenting, and interactions with the pediatric health care team [41]. Central to trauma-informed care is a shift from the question of "What is wrong with you?" to the question of "What happened to you?" Healing-centered engagement adds the question, "What is right with you?" in recognition that all individuals, including those with a history of trauma, have strengths [42]. Further, healing-centered engagement views healing as a collective experience, stresses culture as central to well-being, and empowers individuals to play an active role in their healing [42]. Health care teams must keep in mind that although trauma has a significant impact, these experiences do not fully define any individual. Practicing healing-centered engagement can enable pediatricians to work with families from a perspective that focuses just as strongly on strengths and possibility as it does on trauma and its negative impacts. Above all, this approach frames ACEs as history and not destiny. It emphasizes resilience and success despite exposure to adversities.

RECOGNITION OF PARENTAL ADVERSE CHILDHOOD EXPERIENCES IN CLINICAL SETTINGS

A trauma-informed perspective enables pediatricians to recognize parent behaviors that may be a consequence of ACEs. Table 2 depicts an adaptation of the mnemonic FRAYED, based on the understanding that trauma may fray the fabric of healthy human development [25]. As defined by Forkey, elements of FRAYED childhood include Fits, Frets, and Fear, Regulation disorders, Attachment problems, Yawning and Yelling, Educational and developmental delays, Defeat and Dissociation [25]. Initially developed to aid in identification of child symptoms related to trauma, the mnemonic also may be applied to parents. Considering how ACEs can fray the THREADS of parental resilience (see Table 2) may aid pediatric health providers in identifying manifestations of parental ACEs. Some behavioral consequences of parental ACEs may be a downstream consequence of multiple impacts of ACEs (eg, decreased engagement may be due to attunement challenges, substance use disorder, and/or depression). Although issues other than parental ACEs (eg, current psychosocial stressors) may trigger these parental behaviors, pediatricians must consider that these behaviors may be indicative of past trauma. When these behaviors occur, pediatricians can use this as an opportunity to explore what may be driving the behavior and model safe and nurturing responses (Box 1).

Table 2
Possible manifestations when parental resilience is FRAYED

Elements of FRAYED parenting [25]	How parents may present in the pediatric setting
Fear, fighting, and fretting	• Interaction with the health care setting may trigger an emotional response related to past trauma • Missed or delayed appointments • Difficulty following through with treatment plans • Easy frustration with the health care team or child behaviors
Regulation disorders	• Difficulty controlling emotions and temper • Quickness to anger • Disrespectful or demanding interactions
Attunement challenges	• Difficulty perceiving child needs and responding appropriately • Challenges in supporting their child during painful medical procedures • Challenges recognizing urgency of a child's medical needs in relationship to more immediate needs
Alcohol and substance abuse	• Past or current substance abuse may o Have an impact on engagement with health care system, such as aversion to medical procedures o Decrease ability to parent effectively
Yelling	• Harsh, punitive parenting • Harsh interactions with child and/or health care team
Exhaustion	• Decreased engagement with the child's health care team • Difficulty following through with treatment plans
Defeat/detachment	• Depression and/or hopelessness • Lack of attachment with their child • Decreased engagement with the child's health care team

THE CHALLENGES OF SCREENING

Research on incorporating ACEs screening, including parental ACE screening, as a routine component of health care, is in its infancy, and no gold standard screening tool exists. Many experts have cautioned against universal ACE screening for both patients and their caregivers [43–46]. Concerns about adoption of ACEs screening include lack of standardized screening tools or criteria. It also is unclear at this point what should be assessed, that is, individual ACEs and/or an ACE score. Currently available ACE screening tools do not capture duration, frequency, or magnitude of trauma. Moreover, providing resource information and service referral based solely on ACE score may overlook parents experiencing ongoing negative impacts of fewer ACEs. An algorithmic approach to parental ACEs based on ACE score also may limit appreciation of resilience factors and strengths and alienate or stigmatize parents without necessarily empowering them to address their past. ACE questionnaires also are population health tools and do not predict outcomes at the individual level [47].

Conversely, other investigators advocate for universal ACE screening as a means to identify risk and guide treatment and resource allocation [48].

Box 1: Examples of statements and questions a provider can use to start a conversation with a parent when THREADS may be FRAYED

In our practice we work to recognize that families may have trauma in the past, and that there are strengths that everyone can use and build on. Would you be open to discussing the strengths you rely on to be an effective parent?

Many families find it challenging to [make it to every appointment, get every medication dose, and so forth]. What are some things that make this challenging for your family?

(In response to a parent's frustration with a young child's behavior in the moment) It is so hard for kids to be cooped up in these small rooms, and for parents, too. Can we get your child [a snack, something to color, a book to look at]?

You are frustrated with [how the school is handling a situation, your child's behavior, and so forth.]. You are worried about your child, and the process is not what you expected [pause for parent response].

Being a parent is hard and can feel exhausting. Our own experiences as children might make parenting harder. How do you think your experiences while you were growing up might have an impact on how you parent?

I notice you are [checking the time or checking your phone]. I know the rest of your life does not slow down just because you are here for your child's appointment [pause for parent response].

- Follow-up statement: Tell me about your priorities today and how we can best meet your needs today.

What can we do to help you comfort your child today when we complete your child's [visit, immunizations, or blood testing]? What might help your child feel more comfortable during the procedure?

Some practices have implemented traditional ACEs screening tools with parents. Gillespie and colleagues [49] introduced universal parental ACE screening in their private, primary care practice with evidence of feasibility, including acceptability among parents and providers. Components of this written screening include a framing statement that normalizes the screening, screening for ACE score, and assessment for resilience factors. Providers were given guidance for addressing positive screens, including verbal prompts from the American Academy of Pediatrics resource, Connected Kids, to facilitate provider-parent discussions, developmental promotion activity handouts, and social services resource lists for parents [49]. Although the intervention has shown acceptability among parents and providers, the impact of this screening on parenting behaviors and child health outcomes is not yet known.

Screening for parental ACEs, if pursued, works best if conducted within the context of a nurturing clinician-family relationship, with acknowledgment and identification of resilience factors as well as provision of concrete resources [46]. Pediatricians also must keep in mind the need to address current psychosocial issues, including intimate partner violence, mental health issues, and substance use disorder, which have immediate consequences to the child and available interventions [46]. Identification of current psychosocial stressors for which there are evidence-based interventions (eg, cognitive behavioral therapy for relapse prevention [50]) should not be eschewed in favor of parental ACEs screening [50].

IMPLICATIONS FOR PRACTICE

Pediatric health care providers have multiple options to support parents affected by ACEs. These may be viewed as a 2-pronged approach, with universal interventions provided to all families and targeted interventions provided when risk and negative impacts are identified. The goal of both levels of intervention is to mitigate the potential impact of parental ACEs on child health and well-being and to strengthen parent and family resilience factors.

Recognizing the sensitive nature of such disclosures, documentation of parental ACEs in a child's medical record should be limited. This ensures confidentiality of a disclosure of experiences that other caregivers with access to the child's chart may not know or that the parent would not wish the child to learn should the child eventually access the chart. A caregiver who entrusts a particular member of the care team with this disclosure may not desire that it be known or accessible to the full team [51]. Templated documentation denoting that the impact of parental ACEs was discussed and that appropriate resources were provided may be useful.

When past trauma or ongoing stressors are identified during a trusted provider-parent discussion, the disclosure should not be addressed as a diagnostic item to be scored. Rather, it is an opportunity to validate the challenges created by trauma, recognize the caregiver's resilience, and discuss how the caregiver sees their ACEs having an impact on their parenting and their child. Health care teams must recognize parents as the experts on their lives and empower parents to make informed choices on their own terms about use of available resources [25,52].

Pediatric providers should always put the child's safety at the forefront. If parent behaviors put the child's health at risk, referral to child protective services may be necessary as mandated by state law or to facilitate connection to more intensive services. Any such referrals should be carried out with transparency and with the provider showing consistent and reliable support to the parent.

UNIVERSAL INTERVENTIONS

At baseline, pediatricians and other health care team members can provide consistent, trusting relationships with both parent and child, modeling compassionate availability. Each encounter with a member of the health care team, from a phone call to making an appointment to the provider visit, is an opportunity to nurture the relationships that are key for disclosure and discussion of parental ACEs [25,53]. Furthermore, social support and trusting relationships in parents' lives may reduce intergenerational transmission of trauma and improve child health [54,55]. Just as importantly, members of the health care team can model safe, stable, and nurturing relationships through their interactions with one another.

Emerging evidence supports universal education to address psychosocial issues [56–58]. This approach is in line with the research finding that parents desire to learn more about ACEs and resilience [49]. For example, Vu and colleagues [51] found that key stakeholders, including adult patients, recommended conversations addressing psychosocial adversity rather than screening questionnaires. For parental ACEs, universal education may include conversations about the prevalence of ACEs, their impact on parent well-being, parenting practices, child well-being, and resilience factors. Providers also may suggest additional resources for parenting and to address consequences of parental ACEs [59]. Universal education creates opportunity for caregivers to learn about the impact of parental ACEs and resources without a required disclosure and to access those resources at the time and place of their choosing. This approach signals to caregivers that the provider is open to conversations about trauma, while also minimizing pressure toward disclosure that may result from a screening approach. The Connected Parents, Connected Kids pocket card (Fig. 1) is a universal education intervention that uses the CUES framework [60]. CUES uses healing-centered engagement to empower parents to utilize resources for themselves and to serve as a resource for their community.

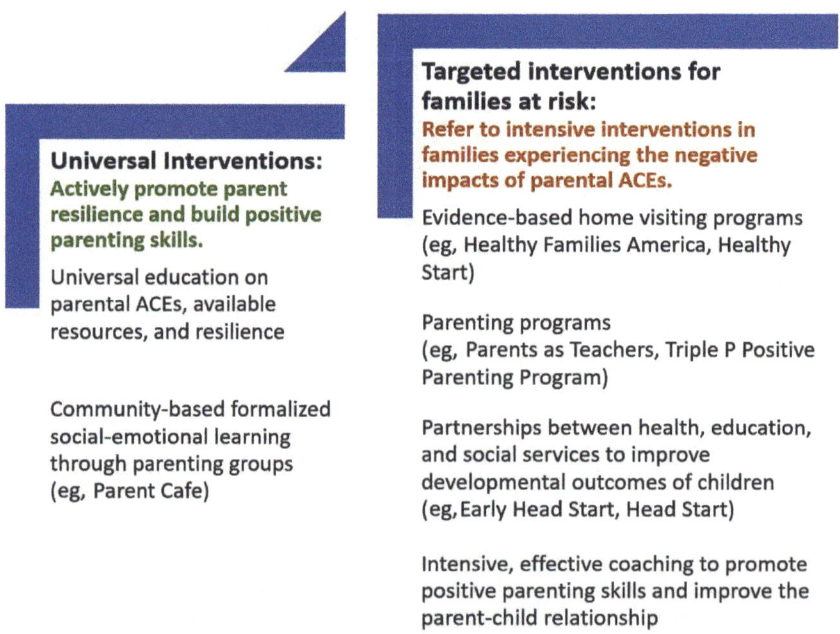

Fig. 1. Stepwise approach to addressing parental ACEs in pediatric health care settings. The interventions listed are examples; the list is not exhaustive.

Two pocket cards are provided to caregivers, using a script that includes (1) confidentiality, (2) universal education and empowerment, and (3) support (Box 2).

Interventions promoting parenting skills can benefit all parents but perhaps especially those with a history of ACEs who themselves did not experience positive parenting practices as children. Pediatricians can model positive parenting behaviors in their interactions with their patients, such as calling out good (or good enough) behavior and ignoring undesired behaviors. Programs, such as Reach Out and Read and the Incredible Years, also offer opportunities to model parenting skills, among a host of additional evidence-based interventions that have been introduced in the primary setting [61–64]. As part of routine anticipatory guidance, pediatricians can provide practical tips and concrete examples, such as scripts, for approaches to common parenting challenges. Additionally, they can normalize the frustrations of

Box 2: Using CUES and the CONNECTED PARENTS, CONNECTED KIDS card to support parents[a]

Confidentiality

- Share limits of confidentiality.
- Assure the caregiver that the challenges shared with the provider will be kept confidential and will not go into the child's record unless by caregiver request or if the provider has concerns about a child's safety.

Universal education and empowerment

- Give caregivers 2 pocket cards. Open the card and encourage the caregivers to take a look.
- Make sure the caregivers know that their provider is a safe person to talk to.
- Explain to parents that 2 cards are given to all parents/caregivers. Tell caregivers, "These cards talk about how our past experiences may affect how we act as parents. They also share some ways to take care of yourself and your kids. You can look through the card and share one with a friend or family member. On the back of the card are resources to call or text, and you can always talk to me about how parenting is going."

Support

- Know how to support someone who discloses their ACEs. Disclosure is not the goal of universal education, but it will happen.
- Offer parenting strategies and a care plan that take a history of ACEs into consideration.
- "Thank you for sharing your challenge me. I'm sorry this happened. A lot of parents have experienced things like this. There are resources that can help [share resources]. We can help make the connection to any of these if you would like."

[a]*Data from* Beyond Screenings: Easy Steps to Support Survivors in Health Settings Infographic. Available at: https://store.futureswithoutviolence.org/index.php/product/cues-poster/. Accessed 25 November, 2020.

parenting and offer strategies for coping during these moments. BehaviorChecker.org is a free, evidence-based online resource that provides parents a structured approach to help address challenging behaviors in their children [65]. Promotion of mindfulness practices that aid in self-regulation also may be of benefit; there are multiple mindfulness apps to which parents may be directed. Parents also can be directed to resources, such as Small Moments Big Impact, a free, pediatrician-developed app for parents of infants ages birth through 6 months that supports infant-parent relationships and addresses the challenges of early parenting [66].

TARGETED PREVENTION STRATEGIES FOR HIGH-RISK FAMILIES

More intensive and focused interventions are needed for families identified as higher risk for or acutely experiencing negative effects of parental ACEs. Multidisciplinary team-based approaches have been found effective in addressing parental ACEs and may be particularly useful in implementation of targeted interventions for families at risk. For example, family navigators on the primary care team can connect families to services, help parents develop problem-solving skills and address parenting stress, and provide emotional support [67]. Some pediatric practices have mental health providers embedded within their practice [68]. Some institutions have piloted 2-generational programs that bridge the psychosocial, economic, and health sectors to assist parents affected by ACEs and their children, but further study is required to evaluate effects and scalability of these innovative models [69,70]. These approaches may counteract barriers families face when seeking services (eg, difficulty obtaining timely appointments, transportation barriers, and reluctance to engage with mental health providers) [71].

High-risk parents showing evidence of FRAYED THREADS may benefit from intensive community-based social support services and parenting programs. Pediatricians should maintain an updated list of such services in their community and be equipped to facilitate referral to these services. There are multiple evidence-based interventions, including community programs, that may help build resilience capacity in families with parents who have experienced ACEs. Fig. 1 provides examples of such interventions. These interventions were not designed solely for parents with histories of ACEs. This list is not exhaustive; a wide array of additional programming is being developed in primary care settings. Providers also can reference Web sites, such as Aunt Bertha (findhelp.org) and The Children's Advocacy Project of America (CAP4Kids.org), to find services available in their localities [64,72–74].

Families may be reluctant to engage with a social services professional. This barrier may be addressed by using a warm hand-off approach when feasible, with a health care team member directly connecting the family and resource provider. Additionally, practices can consider implementing a closed-loop referral system to facilitate enrollment of families in such services.

RESOURCES

Box 3 provides summarized points that can assist pediatricians to address parental ACEs routinely. Resources that can aid pediatric health care teams in promoting patient and family resilience after trauma include the American Academy of Pediatrics Trauma Toolbox for Primary Care and Pediatric Approach to Trauma, Treatment and Resilience Project. Furthermore, Bair-Merritt and colleagues [75] developed measurable standards for addressing

Box 3: Pearls and pitfalls of addressing parental adverse childhood experiences in pediatric health care settings

Take a strengths-based approach:

- Focus on positive aspects of child-parent relationships/interactions.
- Emphasize that ACEs are history and not destiny.
- Acknowledge the parent's resilience.

Engage with the parent as a true partner:

- Respect the parent's expertise in their lived experience.
- Allow the parent to guide the discussion and establish boundaries.
- Respect the parent's choice for next steps.

Keep the child at the forefront of the relationship with the parent.

Keep in mind that trauma not always is the answer and may be accompanied by other issues. Trust parental report and do not jump to conclusions that the parent's current situation or past history is the cause of the child's health issues.

Be mindful of what is important to the parent as well as the provider relationship with the parent. It may put off a parent to raise issues around FRAYED THREADS at the wrong time or in the context of a new parent-provider relationship.

Do not ignore current factors, such as intimate partner violence, parental substance use disorder, and parental mental health concerns.

Be aware how the clinical setting may create or have undue barriers to care. Consider how the practice can improve its processes or offer additional needed services to increase parental success in navigating the setting, such as offering walk-in visits, telephone services, closed-loop referral, or other services to improve engagement.

Create an environment that promotes open discussion about family challenges:

- Display information on resources for psychosocial needs.
- Implement universal education on parental ACEs and resilience.

Be aware of how implicit biases may impact the provider's relationship with families and management of child health issues. Strive to provide equitable treatment.

Attending to self-care is critical.

- Be aware of and maintain personal boundaries.
- Develop and maintain a self-care plan.
- Discuss with parents how they take care of themselves and what they think they can try.

psychosocial adversity within the patient-centered medical home that provide practical and detailed actions, many of which may be translated to pediatric care provided in nonprimary care settings.

SUMMARY

> All adults were once children.
>
> —Dr Bob Block

The existing evidence on the impact of parental ACEs on child health and development is significant and growing. The implications for the policy and practice of pediatric health care are numerous and present an abundance of opportunities to improve child well-being. Certainly, the gap between what is known and what is done is immense, and providers have far to go to incorporate evidence into routine practice. Pediatrician and child mental health experts have called for a 2-generation model of child health care, which has at its center the parent-child relationship [76]. As more is learned about early childhood adversity, its impact on health outcomes across the life span, and its cross-generational effect, the more the potential of pediatrics is revealed.

Acknowledgments

The authors are grateful to the following individuals for their assistance with this manuscript: Elizabeth Miller, MD, PhD, for her review and feedback on Box 2, and to Tanuj Gupta, MD, MBA, Jeffrey Colvin, MD, JD, and Paul Ramírez, PhD, for their support and review at various stages of the project.

Disclosure

Funding: Dr K.A. Randell is supported by the Eunice Kennedy Shriver National Institute of Child Health & Human Development of the National Institutes of Health under Award Number K23HD098299. The content is solely the responsibility of the authors and does not necessarily represent the official views of the National Institutes of Health.

References

[1] Felitti VJ, Anda RF, Nordenberg D, et al. Relationship of childhood abuse and household dysfunction to many of the leading causes of death in adults. The Adverse Childhood Experiences (ACE) Study. Am J Prev Med 1998;14(4):245–58.
[2] Pierce JB, Kershaw KN, Kiefe CI, et al. Association of childhood psychosocial environment with 30-year cardiovascular disease incidence and mortality in middle age. J Am Heart Assoc 2020;9(9):e015326.
[3] Dong M, Dube SR, Felitti VJ, et al. Adverse childhood experiences and self-reported liver disease: new insights into the causal pathway. Arch Intern Med 2003;163(16):1949–56.
[4] Ege MA, Messias E, Thapa PB, et al. Adverse childhood experiences and geriatric depression: results from the 2010 BRFSS. Am J Geriatr Psychiatry 2015;23(1):110–4.
[5] Dube SR, Anda RF, Felitti VJ, et al. Growing up with parental alcohol abuse: exposure to childhood abuse, neglect, and household dysfunction. Child Abuse Negl 2001;25(12):1627–40.

[6] Dube SR, Felitti VJ, Dong M, et al. Childhood abuse, neglect, and household dysfunction and the risk of illicit drug use: the adverse childhood experiences study. Pediatrics 2003;111(3):564–72.
[7] Merrick MT, Ports KA, Ford DC, et al. Unpacking the impact of adverse childhood experiences on adult mental health. Child Abuse Negl 2017;69:10–9.
[8] Robles A, Gjelsvik A, Hirway P, et al. Adverse Childhood Experiences and Protective Factors With School Engagement. Pediatrics 2019;144(2):e20182945.
[9] Centers for Disease Control and Prevention. Adverse childhood experiences reported by adults — five states, 2009. MMWR Morb Mortal Wkly Rep 2010;59(49):1609–13.
[10] Gilbert LK, Breiding MJ, Merrick MT, et al. Childhood adversity and adult chronic disease: an update from ten states and the District of Columbia, 2010. Am J Prev Med 2015;48(3): 345–9.
[11] Halfon N, Larson K, Son J, et al. Income inequality and the differential effect of adverse childhood experiences in US children. Acad Pediatr 2017;17(7s):S70–8.
[12] Anda RF, Felitti VJ, Bremner JD, et al. The enduring effects of abuse and related adverse experiences in childhood. A convergence of evidence from neurobiology and epidemiology. Eur Arch Psychiatry Clin Neurosci 2006;256(3):174–86.
[13] Cronholm PF, Forke CM, Wade R, et al. Adverse childhood experiences: expanding the concept of adversity. Am J Prev Med 2015;49(3):354–61.
[14] Lê-Scherban F, Wang X, Boyle-Steed KH, et al. Intergenerational associations of parent adverse childhood experiences and child health outcomes. Pediatrics 2018;141(6): e20174274.
[15] McDonnell CG, Valentino K. Intergenerational effects of childhood trauma: evaluating pathways among maternal ACEs, perinatal depressive symptoms, and infant outcomes. Child Maltreat 2016;21(4):317–26.
[16] Eismann EA, Folger AT, Stephenson NB, et al. Parental adverse childhood experiences and pediatric healthcare use by 2 years of age. J Pediatr 2019;211:146–51.
[17] Folger AT, Eismann EA, Stephenson NB, et al. Parental adverse childhood experiences and offspring development at 2 years of age. Pediatrics 2018;141(4):e20172826.
[18] Sun J, Patel F, Rose-Jacobs R, et al. Mothers' adverse childhood experiences and their young children's development. Am J Prev Med 2017;53(6):882–91.
[19] Racine N, Plamondon A, Madigan S, et al. Maternal adverse childhood experiences and infant development. Pediatrics 2018;141(4):e20172495.
[20] Schickedanz A, Halfon N, Sastry N, et al. Parents' adverse childhood experiences and their children's behavioral health problems. Pediatrics 2018;142(2):e20180023.
[21] Yoon Y, Cederbaum JA, Mennen FE, et al. Linkage between teen mother's childhood adversity and externalizing behaviors in their children at age 11: Three aspects of parenting. Child Abuse Negl 2019;88:326–36.
[22] Coe JL, Huffhines L, Contente CA, et al. Intergenerational effects of maternal childhood experiences on maternal parenting and infant developmental progress. J Dev Behav Pediatr 2020;41(8):619–27.
[23] Hertzman C, Boyce T. How experience gets under the skin to create gradients in developmental health. Annu Rev Public Health 2010;31:329–47.
[24] Masten AS. Ordinary magic: resilience processes in development. Am Psychol 2001;56(3):227–38.
[25] Forkey H. Putting your trauma lens on. Pediatr Ann 2019;48(7):e269–73.
[26] Belsky J, Jaffee SR, Sligo J, et al. Intergenerational transmission of warm-sensitive-stimulating parenting: a prospective study of mothers and fathers of 3-year-olds. Child Dev 2005;76(2): 384–96.
[27] Lomanowska AM, Boivin M, Hertzman C, et al. Parenting begets parenting: a neurobiological perspective on early adversity and the transmission of parenting styles across generations. Neuroscience 2017;342:120–39.

[28] McEwen BS. Early life influences on life-long patterns of behavior and health. Ment Retard Dev Disabil Res Rev 2003;9(3):149–54.
[29] National Scientific Council on the Developing Child. Excessive Stress Disrupts the Architecture of the Developing Brain: Working Paper 3. Updated Edition. 2014. Available at: http://www.developingchild.harvard.edu. Accessed November 15, 2020.
[30] Spertus IL, Yehuda R, Wong CM, et al. Childhood emotional abuse and neglect as predictors of psychological and physical symptoms in women presenting to a primary care practice. Child Abuse Negl 2003;27(11):1247–58.
[31] Smith AL, Cross D, Winkler J, et al. Emotional dysregulation and negative affect mediate the relationship between maternal history of child maltreatment and maternal child abuse potential. J Fam Violence 2014;29(5):483–94.
[32] McEwen BS. Understanding the potency of stressful early life experiences on brain and body function. Metabolism 2008;57(Suppl 2):S11–5.
[33] Verhoeven KJ, vonHoldt BM, Sork VL. Epigenetics in ecology and evolution: what we know and what we need to know. Mol Ecol 2016;25(8):1631–8.
[34] Hillis SD, Anda RF, Dube SR, et al. The association between adverse childhood experiences and adolescent pregnancy, long-term psychosocial consequences, and fetal death. Pediatrics 2004;113(2):320–7.
[35] Christiaens I, Hegadoren K, Olson DM. Adverse childhood experiences are associated with spontaneous preterm birth: a case-control study. BMC Med 2015;13:124.
[36] Chung EK, Nurmohamed L, Mathew L, et al. Risky health behaviors among mothers-to-be: the impact of adverse childhood experiences. Acad Pediatr 2010;10(4):245–51.
[37] Randell KA, O'Malley D, Dowd MD. Association of parental adverse childhood experiences and current child adversity. JAMA Pediatr 2015;169(8):786–7.
[38] O'Dougherty Wright M, Fopma-Loy J, Oberle K. In their own words: the experience of mothering as a survivor of childhood sexual abuse. Dev Psychopathol 2012;24(2):537–52.
[39] Chung EK, Mathew L, Rothkopf AC, et al. Parenting attitudes and infant spanking: the influence of childhood experiences. Pediatrics 2009;124(2):e278–86.
[40] Fonseka RW, Minnis AM, Gomez AM. Impact of adverse childhood experiences on intimate partner violence perpetration among Sri Lankan men. PLoS One 2015;10(8):e0136321.
[41] Menschner C, Maul A. Issue brief: key ingredients for successful trauma-informed care implementation. Advancing Trauma-Informed Care, Center for Health Care Strategies, Inc, Robert Wood Johnson Foundation; 2016. Available at: https://www.samhsa.gov/sites/default/files/programs_campaigns/childrens_mental_health/atc-whitepaper-040616.pdf. Accessed June 6, 2021.
[42] Ginwright S. The future of healing: Shifting from trauma informed care to healing centered engagement. 2018. Available at: https://medium.com/@ginwright/the-future-of-healing-shifting-from-trauma-informed-care-to-healing-centered-engagement-634f557ce69c. Accessed November 20, 2020.
[43] Finkelhor D. Screening for adverse childhood experiences (ACEs): Cautions and suggestions. Child Abuse Negl 2018;85:174–9.
[44] Dube SR. Continuing conversations about adverse childhood experiences (ACEs) screening: a public health perspective. Child Abuse Negl 2018;85:180–4.
[45] McLennan JD, MacMillan HL, Afifi TO, et al. Routine ACEs screening is NOT recommended. Paediatr Child Health 2019;24(4):272–3.
[46] Bair-Merritt MH, Zuckerman B. Exploring parents' adversities in pediatric primary care. JAMA Pediatr 2016;170(4):313–4.
[47] Baldwin JR, Caspi A, Meehan AJ, et al. Population vs individual prediction of poor health from results of adverse childhood experiences screening. JAMA Pediatr 2021;175(4):385–93.
[48] Stevens JE. To prevent childhood trauma, pediatricians screen children and their parents...and sometimes, just parents...for childhood trauma. Aces Connection. 2014. Available at: https://www.acesconnection.com/blog/to-prevent-childhood-trauma-pediatricians-

screen-children-and-their-parents-and-sometimes-just-parents-for-aces. Accessed November 23, 2020.
[49] Gillespie RJ, Folger AT. Feasibility of assessing parental ACEs in pediatric primary care: implications for practice-based implementation. J Child Adolesc Trauma 2017;10(3): 249–56.
[50] Wells EA, Kristman-Valente AN, Peavy KM, et al. Social workers and delivery of evidence-based psychosocial treatments for substance use disorders. Soc Work Public Health 2013;28(3–4):279–301.
[51] Vu C, Rothman E, Kistin CJ, et al. Adapting the patient-centered medical home to address psychosocial adversity: results of a qualitative study. Acad Pediatr 2017;17(7):S115–22.
[52] Svendsen S, Griffin J, Forkey H. Using the attachment relationship and positive parenting principles to build childhood resilience. Adv Pediatr 2020;67:15–28.
[53] Brown JD, King MA, Wissow LS. The central role of relationships with trauma-informed integrated care for children and youth. Acad Pediatr 2017;17(7):S94–101.
[54] Schofield TJ, Lee RD, Merrick MT. Safe, stable, nurturing relationships as a moderator of intergenerational continuity of child maltreatment: a meta-analysis. J Adolesc Health 2013;53(4 Suppl):S32–8.
[55] Appleton AA, Kiley K, Holdsworth EA, et al. Social support during pregnancy modifies the association between maternal adverse childhood experiences and infant birth size. Matern Child Health J 2019;23(3):408–15.
[56] Miller E, Goldstein S, McCauley HL, et al. A school health center intervention for abusive adolescent relationships: a cluster RCT. Pediatrics 2015;135(1):76–85.
[57] Miller E, Jones KA, McCauley HL, et al. Cluster randomized trial of a college health center sexual violence intervention. Am J Prev Med 2020;59(1):98–108.
[58] Tancredi DJ, Silverman JG, Decker MR, et al. Cluster randomized controlled trial protocol: addressing reproductive coercion in health settings (ARCHES). BMC Womens Health 2015;15:57.
[59] Purewal SK, Bucci M, Gutiérrez Wang L, et al. Screening for adverse childhood experiences (ACEs) in an integrated pediatric care model. Zero Three 2016;37(1):10–7.
[60] Beyond Screenings: Easy Steps to Support Survivors in Health Settings Infographic. Available at: https://store.futureswithoutviolence.org/index.php/product/cues-poster/. Accessed 25 November, 2020.
[61] Zuckerman B, Needlman R. 30 Years of reach out and read: need for a developmental perspective. Pediatrics 2020;145(6):e20191958.
[62] Perrin EC, Sheldrick RC, McMenamy JM, et al. Improving parenting skills for families of young children in pediatric settings: a randomized clinical trial. JAMA Pediatr 2014;168(1):16–24.
[63] Woods-Jaeger B, Thompson JE, Foye-Fletcher A, et al. Parent engagement in an integrated care parenting intervention to prevent toxic stress. Clin Pract Pediatr Psychol 2020;8(3): 298.
[64] Smith JD, Cruden GH, Rojas LM, et al. Parenting interventions in pediatric primary care: a systematic review. Pediatrics 2020;146(1):e20193548.
[65] Raised with Love and Limits Foundation. Behavior checker. 2020. Available at: http://www.behaviorchecker.org. Accessed November 23, 2020.
[66] WGBH Educational Foundation and Boston Medical Center. Small moments, big impact. 2020. Available at: http://smallmomentsbigimpact.com. Accessed November 23, 2020.
[67] Godoy L, Hodgkinson S, Robertson HA, et al. Increasing mental health engagement from primary care: the potential role of family navigation. Pediatrics 2019;143(4):e20182418.
[68] Chakawa A, Belzer LT, Perez-Crawford T, et al. Which model fits? Evaluating models of integrated behavioral health care in addressing unmet behavioral health needs among underserved sociodemographic groups. Evid Based Pract Child Adolesc Ment Health 2020;5(3): 251–70.

[69] Babcock E, Ruiz De Luzuriaga N. Families disrupting the cycle of poverty: coaching with an intergenerational lens. Boston: Economic Mobility Pathways; 2016. Available at: http://s3.amazonaws.com/empath-website/pdf/EMPath-Families_Disrupting_the_Cycle_of_-Poverty-Intergen-7-12-16.pdf. Accessed November 17, 2020.
[70] Ivanova MY, Dewey L, Swift P, et al. Health promotion in primary care pediatrics: initial results of a randomized clinical trial of the vermont family based approach. Child Adolesc Psychiatr Clin N Am 2019;28(2):237–46.
[71] Wissow LS, van Ginneken N, Chandna J, et al. Integrating children's mental health into primary care. Pediatr Clin North Am 2016;63(1):97–113.
[72] Dunne L, Craig N, Connolly P, et al. Community-based early childhood programmes for improving developmental outcomes for children: a systematic review and meta-analysis. Campbell Collaboration; 2016. Available at: https://campbellcollaboration.org/media/k2/attachments/ECG-Dunne_Title.pdf.s.
[73] Aunt Bertha (findhelp.org). Available at: https://findhelp.org. Accessed 26 November, 2020.
[74] The children's advocacy project of America. Available at: https://cap4kids.org. Accessed 26 November, 2020.
[75] Bair-Merritt MH, Mandal M, Garg A, et al. Addressing psychosocial adversity within the patient-centered medical home: expert-created measurable standards. J Prim Prev 2015;36(4):213–25.
[76] Zuckerman B. Two-generation pediatric care: a modest proposal. Pediatrics 2016;137(1):e20153447.
[77] Shah AN, Beck AF, Sucharew HJ, et al. Parental adverse childhood experiences and resilience on coping after discharge. Pediatrics 2018;141(4):e20172127.
[78] Hugill M, Berry K, Fletcher I. The association between historical childhood sexual abuse and later parenting stress: a systematic review. Arch Womens Ment Health 2017;20(2):257–71.
[79] Numan M. Hypothalamic neural circuits regulating maternal responsiveness toward infants. Behav Cogn Neurosci Rev 2006;5(4):163–90.
[80] Moehler E, Biringen Z, Poustka L. Emotional availability in a sample of mothers with a history of abuse. Am J Orthopsychiatry 2007;77(4):624–8.
[81] Tronick E, Reck C. Infants of depressed mothers. Harv Rev Psychiatry 2009;17(2):147–56.

Advances in Pediatrics 68 (2021) 89–102

ADVANCES IN PEDIATRICS

Caring for Medically Complex Children in the Outpatient Setting

Michelle A. Blanco, MD*, Carol M. Lilly, MD, MPH, Brooke C. Bavinger, MD, Sara Garcia, MD, Michelle P. Hojnicki, DO

Department of Pediatrics, Division of General Pediatrics, University of South Florida Morsani College of Medicine, 2 Tampa General Circle, Tampa, FL 33606, USA

Keywords

• Children with medical complexity • Complex care • Chronic care • Outpatient care • Pediatric health care transitions

Key points

- Outpatient pediatric care for children with medical complexity is a rapidly growing field.
- Early identification of children with medical complexity is key for improving their long-term outcomes.
- The extraordinary costs, resources, time, and coordination needed to appropriately care for medically complex children pose significant challenges to families and providers.
- The development of pediatric complex care clinics can provide options for overcoming some of the challenges facing this population.

INTRODUCTION

Advances in neonatal, pediatric, and surgical care have led to the survival of a greater number of children with special health care needs who are cared for at home [1]. In the United States, approximately 1 in 25 children are considered children with medical complexity (CMC), and this population is expected to double in the next decade [2]. Due to the growing need for comprehensive care for these children, expanding and improving outpatient pediatric complex

*Corresponding author. *E-mail address:* mblanco@usf.edu

https://doi.org/10.1016/j.yapd.2021.05.012

care services is necessary. This article reviews strategies and tools for identifying CMC and their degree of complexity, discusses different outpatient complex clinic models, identifies and evaluates challenges of delivering and managing complex care in the outpatient setting, describes current options for patient and family support, and discusses important transitions of care throughout these children's lives.

IDENTIFYING COMPLEX PATIENTS

The Maternal and Child Health Bureau defines children with special health care needs as children at "increased risk of chronic physical, developmental, behavioral, or emotional conditions" who "require health care and related services of a type or amount beyond that required by children generally" [3]. Although this population constitutes a small proportion of the medical pediatric community (13%–18%) [3], it is important given its high level of unmet health care needs, substandard quality of care received, poor health outcomes, and high health care costs [4]. CMC, a subgroup within the population of children with special health care needs, are recognized as those with the most medical fragility and highest health care resource use. They typically have multiple chronic conditions, functional limitations, and often rely on adaptive technology [5].

The definition of medical complexity often differs when describing individuals versus populations. Even when evaluating an individual patient, identifying at what point the patient should be diagnosed as medically complex and to what degree the complexity should be categorized can often seem to be a subjective distinction and moving target. As such, approaches to detecting and recognizing medical complexity are inconsistent and unreliable [6]. Cohen and colleagues [3] proposed the characterization of chronic medical conditions of childhood into 4 broad domains: needs, chronic conditions, functional limitations, and health care use. The needs domain encompasses substantial service needs identified by families (medical care, specialized therapy, and educational needs), that significantly affect the family, such as time expenditure on direct care, care coordination, frequent medical visits, and financial burden [3]. The chronic conditions domain refers to CMC having 1 or more diagnosed or unknown chronic medical conditions that are severe and/or associated with high morbidity/mortality. CMC have functional limitations that may be categorized as impairment, activity limitation, or participation restriction as defined by the World Health Organization's International Classification and Functioning, Disability and Health framework [6]. The functional limitation domain describes CMC as having limitations that are typically severe, often requiring the assistance of technology, such as tracheostomy tubes, gastrostomy tubes, supplemental oxygen, or a wheelchair [3,6]. The health care use domain projects that CMC will have high health care resource use; for example, ongoing or frequent involvement of multiple subspecialty services/providers, multiple surgeries, and/or frequent or prolonged hospitalizations [3].

- Family-identified needs
  - Financial burden
  - Transportation challenges
  - Specialized educational needs
  - Time-intensive care and appointments
- Chronic conditions
  - Typically categorized as severe
  - Associated with high morbidity/mortality
- Functional limitations
  - Interferes with activities of daily living or participation
  - Often requires adaptive technology: tracheostomy tubes, gastrostomy tubes, orthopedic braces, walkers, wheelchairs, and so forth
- Health care use
  - High resource use
  - Multiple subspecialists
  - Various surgeries or procedures
  - Frequent or prolonged hospitalizations

Scoring of complexity

Given the difficulty in defining CMC at an individual and population level, multiple classification systems have emerged. Feudtner and colleagues [4] describe 4 different examples of classification systems developed for the identification of health problems experienced by CMC.

- Complex chronic conditions (CCC): CCCs in childhood are strongly associated with high morbidity, mortality, functional limitations, high health-resource use, and pursuit of complex care clinical programs. Tables of CCC categories with their analogous International Classification of Diseases (ICD) 9 and ICD-10 diagnoses and procedures codes are available to the public. However, these listings do not differentiate all CMC because they do not contain all chronic conditions of childhood, such as asthma, attention-deficit/hyperactivity disorder, obesity, or depression [4].
- Patient Medical Complexity Algorithm: The Patient Medical Complexity Algorithm was developed by Seattle Children's Hospital Center of Excellence on Quality of Care Measures for Children with Complex Needs as a diagnosis classification system for CMC. It is a pediatric-specific, open-source system that uses ICD-9 codes to classify CMC complexity into 1 of 3 categories: (1) complex, chronic disease; (2) noncomplex, chronic disease; (3) nonchronic disease. Although this system allows the classification of CMC, developers recommend at least 2 years of patient data be available for effective classification [4].
- Chronic Condition Indicators (CCI): The CCI is an open-source system developed by the Agency for Healthcare Research and Quality. It is designed to categorize 14,000 ICD-9 and 68,000 ICD-10 diagnosis codes into chronic versus nonchronic conditions. The system arranges the chronic conditions into 18 major clinical groups (eg, group 1, Infectious and Parasitic Disease; group 2, Neoplasms, and so forth). The number of clinical groups in which a child has a chronic condition correlates with their degree of health-resource use.

However, the utility of this system for CMC is limited because multiple organ systems may be in 1 clinical category, making the patient seem less complex. It is also important to note that the CCI system is not specific to children [4].

- Clinical Risk Groups (CRGs): CRGs were developed by 3M Health Information Systems to categorize pediatric diagnoses into hierarchical, severity-adjusted groups. These groups range from healthy children without a chronic condition (CRG group 1, Acute Condition) to high morbidity/mortality-associated catastrophic chronic conditions in unhealthy children (CRG group 9, "Catastrophic Condition") [6]. The advantage of CRGs include their ability to differentiate children with minor, moderate, dominant, and catastrophic chronic conditions. CRGs also distinguish children with single versus 2 to 3 chronic conditions and allows a diagnosis to be incorporated into multiple CRG groups. However, it is recommended to have at least 3 years of health care data to accurately categorize children into a CRG, which limits the use of this tool for infants and toddlers [4].

Benefits of identifying complex patients

The recognition and identification of CMC has received attention in the clinical setting for many reasons, including the more than 400% increase in the proportion of children with a chronic condition since the 1960s [7]. Vestal and colleagues [8] reported that this trend may be explained by increased survival rates for infants born prematurely, improvements in treatment options for acute illnesses in fields such as intensive care and oncology, and other advances in medicine and technology that reduce mortalities. Although CMC have the highest health care needs and resource use, and are the most medically fragile population of children, they have high levels of unmet health care needs, receive substandard quality of care, and have poor health outcomes. About one-third of overall health care spending for children is accounted for by approximately 1% of children, of whom most are CMC [6]. In addition, this 1% also accounts for an increasing percentage of pediatric hospitalizations and recurrent admissions. Therefore, it is important to identify CMC early so their quality of care and quality of life can be improved by providing them and their families the necessary resources and support. In addition, early identification of CMC allows the assessment of temporal trends in their morbidity and mortality, which can be used to provide counseling and identify ways to improve outcomes. Collecting data on patterns of health care use in this population may also provide the information needed to better advocate for resources for these children.

COMPLEX CARE CLINIC MODELS

Several clinical care models have been used to accommodate the needs of CMC. No single model has yet to be established as the gold standard of care, likely because clinic needs differ depending on location, population, and scope of practice. However, the overall goal of clinics for CMC remains the same: to maximize family support, facilitate coordination of care and communication with subspecialists, assist in transitions of care, and minimize emergency room visits and hospital admissions [2]. The challenges to providing care to CMC in the outpatient setting that have pushed providers to search for alternative care options include high care costs, insufficient reimbursement, time constraints, inadequate knowledge of more rare or complex disorders, and insufficient staff and resources [5]. Most complex care clinics have multidisciplinary teams to help provide the comprehensive care that these children require. Team members often include physicians, nurses, nutritionists, care coordinators, social workers, and mental health specialists [2]. Three of the more popular models of care for CMC include the medical home model, consultative model, and episode-based model [5]. Although these models aim to accommodate a variety of CMC with different diagnoses, they are not typically created to address children with mental and behavioral health issues, a population frequently left with inadequate support and resources.

Medical home model

The medical home model is primary care centered, and the care team is led by the primary care physician (PCP) who provides well, acute, and chronic care. As in any general pediatric office, growth and development are monitored, preventive care such as vaccinations is given, and care for acute illness is provided. However, the PCP also takes the lead in managing chronic and complex issues by coordinating communication between subspecialists, overseeing and reconciling medications and adaptive technology, and being the primary liaison with home health providers and inpatient teams. Longer appointment times allow providers to deliver this comprehensive care. Emergency care plans, after-hours services, and acute sick visits are regularly provided and are useful in reducing emergency room visits and hospital admissions [6]. Advantages of this model often include proximity to a patient's home, continuity of care, and familiarity with community resources. Some clinics even offer care for siblings to reduce the travel burden on families [9]. Certain complex clinics are affiliated with larger hospital systems for seamless integration with specialists and inpatient services. Teams may have general pediatricians who rotate between the outpatient and inpatient settings, enabling them to offer an even higher degree of continuity.

Consultative model

The consultative model of complex care involves comanagement between the community pediatrician and a complex team that is typically affiliated with a tertiary care center. It allows patients to stay with their community pediatricians and established medical homes. The complex team in this model does not offer routine health care, but instead serves as a bridge between the PCP and subspecialists. Patients can continue their preventive and acute care with their PCPs, who are often closer to home, but then have periodic visits with the complex team to address chronic issues and coordinate subspecialty care and adaptive technology. For some patients, a condition-specific complex clinic, such as those specializing in Down syndrome, can be beneficial. Condition-specific philanthropy, research, and resources are sometimes easier to champion and access [10]. Clear and consistent communication between the PCP and complex team in this consultative model is key to avoiding unclear patient ownership and overlooked medical issues [9].

Episode-based model

The episode-based model of complex care revolves around discrete care episodes that are limited in time and location, usually during a period surrounding critical illness or a significant transitional phase of care. An example is a rehabilitation clinic that cares for a patient after traumatic injury. A multidisciplinary team familiar with managing complex medical issues manages care until transition to the care of the PCP. Another example of episode-based care is transitional care homes that provide a safe period for family education between hospitalization and home. With guidance, parents can become comfortable managing new medical equipment, feeding routines, and medication administration before completing the transition home [5] (Table 1).

CHALLENGES OF DELIVERING AND MANAGING COMPLEX CARE

CMC face numerous barriers to inclusive, efficacious, and safe health care services and environments. A survey of pediatricians revealed the top 3 barriers to be time, reimbursement, and lack of support services [11]. Even within complex clinics that are specifically structured to care for CMC, these obstacles remain a challenge.

Finances

Inadequate health insurance negatively affects health outcomes, access to primary and specialty care, and therapeutic interventions [6,12]. Although policies have been proposed to address gaps in insurance coverage, families still often struggle to get coverage for all specialty medications, imaging, equipment, and therapy. Health care providers also struggle to obtain adequate reimbursement for the extraordinarily time-intensive services CMC require.

The impact of lost parental employment or decreased work hours remains a significant burden for families of CMC. Parents must dedicate an enormous amount of time to attending medical appointments, coordinating their children's care, and providing direct health care to their children as their primary care givers. Many parents with CMC have to terminate employment in order

Table 1
Summary of complex care clinic models

	Preventive care	Acute care	Complex care
Medical Home Model	✓	✓	✓
Consultative Model	—	—	✓
Episode-based Model	—	✓ For a discrete episode	✓ For a discrete episode

to have the time to care for their children, and often report financial difficulties [13]. Social security benefits for children with disabilities, home health services, and medical daycares are some of the resources that can offer families of CMC financial and medical support.

Geographic access

Transportation remains a significant access barrier for CMC. Specialty and care coordination services needed for CMC are often located in central hubs requiring long-distance travel for care. For families without cars whose children are on Medicaid insurance, Medicaid taxis can often be reserved but typically require at least a 48 hours advanced notice, which can be challenging when trying to address acute medical issues. Some CMC, such as children on ventilators, are so medically fragile that they require transportation by ambulance to all appointments to ensure their safety. Given the obstacles to transporting CMC, complex clinics located at tertiary centers often try to coordinate multiple specialty appointments for the same day, at the same location, to help minimize travel burden for families.

Infrastructure and care coordination

The current health infrastructure within the United States is based on an episodic illness model of care. CMC comprise 1% of children but account for one-third of health care spending for children [14]. CMC benefit from a so-called medical neighborhood focused on (1) integration and coordination of services and community resources, (2) long-term care planning, and (3) engagement of families in shared decision making [6]. Although there are many examples of health maintenance and disease management guidelines, most health spending involves hospitalizations and emergency care [13,14]. Fee-for-service systems do not cover ambulatory costs such as [6]:

- 24/7 access
- Care coordination
- Care plan development
- Family psychosocial assessments
- Reconciliation of medications
- Oversight of home health care plans

Medical complexity itself might be a primary determinant of unmet needs, even when accounting for other inequities, including financial, racial, or English-as-second-language barriers in the family [6]. Programs intended to improve care access and comprehensive coordination are inconsistently funded and have proved difficult to sustain. Avritscher and colleagues [15] reported several benefits to providing a medical home in a trial that compared children receiving traditional versus comprehensive care. Program success was linked to several key practice activities, including 24/7 phone access; follow-up after emergency room visits; acute, primary, and specialty care within the same venue; low patient-to-provider ratios; and extensive consultation between team members [15]. These strategies improved outcomes and addressed medication management, laboratory and radiology monitoring, and care planning. Notably, a key barrier to comprehensive care sustainability was a lack of reimbursement.

Workforce readiness

Several studies have addressed comfort levels of medical providers related to meeting complex needs within a primary care practice. Agrawal and colleagues [11] reviewed pediatricians' perceptions of barriers, noting that they reported feeling unprepared to address individualized education program planning for school, respite care, or management of invasive technologies. Bogetz and colleagues [16] sorted training focus into 3 domains: learner attitudes, motivation, and concrete experiences to support skills acquisition. The investigators noted that recruitment efforts are hampered by a lack of infrastructure within pediatric programs. Half of the respondents reported that their institutions had no infrastructure for complex care education [16]. Few formal curricula are available to address CMC.

PATIENT AND FAMILY SUPPORT

Family members of CMC usually assume a significant responsibility for providing medical care for their children. These families often report physical, emotion, social, and financial burdens [17]. A report from the National Survey of Children with Special Health Care Needs found that a significant percentage of families provide greater than 21 hours per week on health care at home and approximately 11 hours per week on coordination of care. The survey found that approximately 25% of parents decrease their work duties or leave their jobs to care for their children [18].

Home health care

Because of the complex and time-intensive care CMC require, the American Academy of Pediatrics recommends that pediatric home health care be available and accessible to families [19]. Home health can involve a large array of professional services, including nurses, physical and occupational therapists, speech therapists, respiratory therapists, psychologists, dieticians, and social workers. Some locations have programs that enable this team of professionals to support children from their own homes or in a medical day care setting. Home nursing can be provided as a daily continuous in-home service versus intermittent brief skilled visits. Private daily skilled nursing is important for children who require intensive care, such as those with significant physical impairments, on respiratory support, or receiving tube feedings. Periodic skilled nursing visits are helpful for assisting with discrete tasks such as intermittent infusions or central line care. Home nursing can help deliver patient-centered and family-centered care and decrease avoidable medical appointments, emergency department visits, or hospitalizations [19].

Medical day care

Medical day care and prescribed pediatric extended care centers are other options for providing assistance for CMC. They allow the children to receive consistent medical care by trained medical professionals in a nonresidential setting. Care is often given for up to 12 hours a day, allowing parents to attend work. The centers also usually provide specialty services such as developmental therapies, occupational therapy, physical therapy, and speech therapy. In addition, staff can often provide parental training and education. Medical staff become very familiar with the CMC they care for, and their communication with the PCPs and specialists can provide significant insight and guidance in managing children's chronic conditions. These centers reduce the feeling of isolation that families and CMC often experience, and offer them opportunities to develop relationships with other families in similar circumstances.

Pediatric palliative care

Another form of patient and family support is early integration into pediatric palliative care. The American Academy of Pediatrics recommends that children with life-threatening conditions and their families be introduced to palliative care early, at the time of diagnosis if possible, to provide holistic care to the families. Pediatric palliative care programs often address psychological, social, and spiritual concerns from a family-centered perspective. The goals of pediatric palliative care focus on symptom relief, quality of life, communication, relationship building, and goal-directed decision making in an interdisciplinary collaboration [20]. The pediatric palliative care group can serve as a resource throughout the illness, and some have community-based practices that bridge hospital, home, and pediatric hospice programs [21].

Peer-to-peer support groups

When children are first diagnosed with significant medical issues, parents often face challenges processing the information and accommodating to new lifestyle changes. They are often overwhelmed and worried about the future. It is common for parents to be intimated and hesitant to ask questions, or feel a sense of powerlessness. An example of families adjusting to having a CMC is those who have infants in the neonatal intensive care unit (NICU). Parents with infants in the NICU have an increased risk of postpartum depression, posttraumatic stress disorder, and anxiety [22]. Following the birth of an infant, between 10% and 15% of mothers and between 2% and 5% of fathers reportedly experience depression. If their infants are admitted to the NICU, the incidence of depression increases to 38% and 11% for mothers and fathers, respectively [23].

Peer-to-peer support groups between families can be a great resource for families. It may include direct parent mentoring from a volunteer parent who had similar experiences, or it may be a community-based group available for general advice. The development of social media platforms has made it easier for families with CMC, especially for those with rarer diagnoses, to connect with each other. The goal of support groups is for families to share their experiences in a safe environment, obtain validation of their feelings, and to gain perspective [24]. These programs may also serve as a platform for parents to have questions answered, and to provide encouragement to each other [22].

Studies have shown that parents who receive peer support have increased sense of confidence, well-being, and self-esteem, often leading to them feeling more empowered to care for their children [24].

TRANSITIONS IN CARE

Hospital discharge

The initial discharge home from the hospital is one of the biggest transitions for families with CMC. The role of the hospital is to train the families and caregivers to understand the medical diagnoses of their children; the medical equipment, including how to use it appropriately; and the various medications the children are on and the reason they are prescribed, what specialist prescribed them, and how to appropriately administer them at the correct time.

When considering discharge to home, a psychosocial assessment of the family should be done and include the following:

- Educational level of family members
- Home environment, including who is living in the home and who will be the primary caregiver
- Economic strains
- Religious or cultural beliefs that may affect care of the child
- Parental history that may affect care of the child
- Social support systems for the family
- Depression screening of mother
- Transportation challenges
- Location of the family if the child is in a large referral center with a wide catchment area

This assessment better enables physicians and other medical providers to proceed with discharge education and training by providing them with a better understanding of the challenges the family faces. Having checklists or road maps helps ensure that all teaching goals are met, that the family has a visual of what needs to be achieved in order to be ready for a safe discharge, and that all physicians and providers are aware of what teaching has been provided to the family.

Case management systems should be used to assist families in the administrative aspects of transition to home, and should include:

- Insurance: ensure child is on a plan or the family applies for Medicaid
- PCP: find a PCP comfortable with complex patients, and assigned to insurance plan
- Appointments: assist families in making all follow-up appointments
- Transportation: set up transportation for the first follow-up appointment if necessary
- Medications: ensure they are prescribed and in the family's possession before discharge
- Durable medical equipment: ensure it is delivered to the family and that the caregiver is trained in its operation
- Nursing: initiate orders and staffing

Identification of pediatricians comfortable with CMC is vital, and they should be given updates on each child before discharge. Having the patient enrolled in a complex care medical home may be valuable, although is not always possible if there are barriers such as transportation when working within a large catchment area. A randomized controlled trial showed a nearly 50% reduction in hospitalizations for CMC if they were enrolled in a complex care medical home with case management resources [25].

Transitions in development

CMC experience life event transitions much like healthy children; however, these transitions can be much more stressful. Depending on social and economic situations, they may need to be enrolled in daycare. The PCP must be comfortable making recommendations for mainstream daycare versus a medical daycare or prescribed pediatric care center if the extra services they provide are needed. The PCP is responsible for writing the initial prescribed pediatric extended care order and for signing plans of care for the patients during their enrollments. The pediatrician's role is also crucial when children become school aged. The child should be assessed for enrollment in mainstream classrooms with or without an individualized educational plan, special educational classrooms, local exceptional centers, or hospital homebound (in-home education) services. Pediatricians need to be familiar with options in the geographic location they service.

It is also important to consider the CMC's transition in health status. Some CMC have improvements in their health, lose the need for medical equipment, are weaned off medications, and are discharged from specialists. Although this is exciting, many families feel anxious about leaving a complex care medical home and transitioning to a community pediatrician. These improvements in health should be celebrated and the medical home should have a transition policy in place for these children. There should be a good relationship with community pediatricians who will accept them as patients to ensure seamless handoffs to capable physicians.

In contrast, some CMC need the extra care and support that can be offered by long-term care facilities. The pediatrician's role in supporting families when making this decision for placement is critical and pediatricians need to be aware of places in the community to refer families who are considering such options. The health of some CMC declines and hospice care may be needed. These transitions are more seamless when palliative or hospice is already a part of the child's care team, thus involving them early is helpful.

Transition to adult care

Transitioning CMC to adult care is an extremely important but challenging task for the pediatricians who provide their care. Every year approximately 500,000 children with special health care needs become adults. Between 80% and 90% of children with cerebral palsy now survive to 30 years of age, infants born with cystic fibrosis are expected to live to at least 47 years of age, and the prevalence of congenital heart disease has the highest rate of growth in transition-aged patients [26,27].

A practice should establish a timeline for transition in order to provide consistent care to families. Discussions regarding when and where a patient will be transitioned should be initiated with families 2 to 3 years before the anticipated date of transition, and the age at which to transition should be consistent throughout the practice. A transition plan should consider the following:

- Hospitals: families need to choose the hospital they would want their child admitted to under a general medicine service, and they need to know the age at which a patient can no longer be admitted to the pediatrics floors, because this varies between hospitals.
- Physicians: families need to choose physicians who are affiliated with their chosen hospitals. When the child reaches adolescence, pediatricians should discuss with families the age at which they will need to transition to adult care. Pediatricians and pediatric subspecialists should recommend providers in advance of transition to enable families to research and meet with them if they choose. There should be a seamless handover of medical records.
- Personal: families should plan the future with their children, including living situations, education, and job training. They may also need to consider guardianship.

SUMMARY

Due to advances in medicine and improved outcomes in pediatrics, the population of CMC is rapidly growing. Obstacles to providing these children with optimal medical care are vast because of their high medical resource use and time-intensive needs. Because more CMC are being cared for at home, developing outpatient pediatric complex clinics specialized in providing comprehensive care is key. Identifying these children in a timely manner for early interventions, creating outpatient clinics structured to support their needs, and providing their families with appropriate resources are only a few of the ways that pediatricians can improve quality of care and outcomes in the outpatient setting for CMC.

CLINICS CARE POINTS

- Identify CMC as early as possible to implement early interventions, maximize patient and family services, and improve long-term outcomes.
- Help families find a medical home able to accommodate their children's needs, and consider a pediatric complex clinic to ensure comprehensive and efficient care with adequate patient and family support.
- Plan early and thoroughly for transitions in care, such as the transition home from the hospital, or the transition from pediatric to adult care, in order to improve patient safety and family comfort levels.

References

[1] Perrin JM. Health services research for children with disabilities. Milbank Q 2002;80(2):303–24.

[2] Karpook JW, Mark. Five keys to success: advancing care models for children with complex medical needs. 2016. Available at: https://www.chartis.com/resources/files/Advancing-Care-Models-for-Children-with-Complex-Medical-Needs-Final-indd-002.pdf cited 2020.

[3] Cohen E, et al. Children with medical complexity: an emerging population for clinical and research initiatives. Pediatrics 2011;127(3):529–38.

[4] Berry JG, et al. Ways to identify children with medical complexity and the importance of why. J Pediatr 2015;167(2):229–37.

[5] Pordes E, et al. Models of care delivery for children with medical complexity. Pediatrics 2018;141(Suppl 3):S212–23.

[6] Kuo DZ, Houtrow AJ, Council on Children with Disabilities. Recognition and management of medical complexity. Pediatrics 2016;138(6):e20163021.

[7] Cohen E, et al. Status complexicus? The emergence of pediatric complex care. Pediatrics 2018;141(Suppl 3):S202–11.

[8] Vestal C. Improving medicaid for 'medically complex'' kids. 2015. Available at: https://www.pewtrusts.org/en/research-and-analysis/blogs/stateline/2015/1/08/improving-medicaid-for-medically-complex-kids [Accessed November 08, 2020].

[9] de Banate MA, Maypole J, Sadof M. Care coordination for children with medical complexity. Curr Opin Pediatr 2019;31(4):575–82.

[10] Van Cleave J, et al. Medical homes for children with special health care needs: primary care or subspecialty service? Acad Pediatr 2016;16(4):366–72.

[11] Agrawal R, et al. Barriers to care for children and youth with special health care needs: perceptions of Illinois pediatricians. Clin Pediatr (Phila) 2012;51(1):39–45.

[12] Han X, Luo Q, Ku L. Medicaid expansion and grant funding increases helped improve community health center capacity. Health Aff (Millwood) 2017;36(1):49–56.

[13] Foster CC, Mangione-Smith R, Simon TD. Caring for children with medical complexity: perspectives of primary care providers. J Pediatr 2017;182:275–282 e4.

[14] Ming DY, et al. The intersection of complex care and hospital medicine: opportunities to advance health for chronically ill populations. Hosp Pediatr 2020;10(8):715–8.

[15] Avritscher EBC, et al. Post-trial sustainability and scalability of the benefits of a medical home for high-risk children with medical complexity. J Pediatr 2019;206:232–9.e3.

[16] Bogetz JF, et al. Challenges and potential solutions to educating learners about pediatric complex care. Acad Pediatr 2014;14(6):603–9.

[17] Murphy N, Christian B. Disability in children and young adults: the unintended consequences. Arch Pediatr Adolesc Med 2007;161(10):930–2.

[18] National Survey of Children with Special Health Care Needs. 2018. Available at: https://www.childhealthdata.org/old-(pre-july-2018)/learn/NS-CSHCN [Accessed 2020].

[19] Simpser E, Hudak ML, C.O.C.H.F. Section on Home Care. Financing of pediatric home health care. Pediatrics 2017;139(3):e20164202.

[20] Truog RD, Meyer EC, Burns JP. Toward interventions to improve end-of-life care in the pediatric intensive care unit. Crit Care Med 2006;34(11 Suppl):S373–9.

[21] Kaye EC, et al. Pediatric palliative care in the community. CA Cancer J Clin 2015;65(4):316–33.

[22] Bracht M, et al. Implementing family-integrated care in the NICU: a parent education and support program. Adv Neonatal Care 2013;13(2):115–26.

[23] Gonulal D, et al. Both parents of neonatal intensive care unit patients are at risk of depression. Turk J Pediatr 2014;56(2):171–6.

[24] Ainbinder JG, et al. A qualitative study of parent to parent support for parents of children with special needs. Consortium to evaluate parent to parent. J Pediatr Psychol 1998;23(2):99–109.

[25] Mosquera RA, et al. Effect of an enhanced medical home on serious illness and cost of care among high-risk children with chronic illness: a randomized clinical trial. JAMA 2014;312(24):2640–8.
[26] Goodman DM, et al. Adults with chronic health conditions originating in childhood: inpatient experience in children's hospitals. Pediatrics 2011;128(1):5–13.
[27] 2017 patient registry annual data report. Cystic Fibrosis Foundation; 2018.

Advances in Pediatrics 68 (2021) 103–119

ADVANCES IN PEDIATRICS

Postoperative Management of Pediatric Patients

Melinda Murphy, MD*, Patricia O'Brien, MD, PhD, Matthew Gates, MD

Department of Pediatrics, University of South Florida Morsani College of Medicine, 2 TGH Circle, 5th Floor, Tampa, FL 33606, USA

Keywords

• Pediatric surgical patients • Children with complex medical conditions
• Monitoring infants after anesthesia • Pain control • VTE/DVT prophylaxis

OBJECTIVES

1. Describe the role of pediatric hospital medicine in the management of post-surgical patients.
2. Discuss routine postoperative management in pediatric patients: specifically monitoring, prophylaxis, and pain control.
3. Describe approaches that can prevent common complications in pediatric post-surgical patients.

INTRODUCTION

Pediatric surgery and pediatric hospital medicine have undergone dramatic expansion and growth over the past 20 years [1]. The first 12 pediatric surgery training programs in the United States were formally recognized in 1966; as of 2020, there were 55 North American pediatric surgery fellowships [2]. The rapid expansion of the workforce has led to increased availability of pediatric surgical services outside of specialized children's hospitals [3]. In the mid-1990s, pediatric hospital medicine was formed and has developed into its own subspecialty [4]. With the expansion of these 2 specialties, more children are undergoing complex surgical procedures in community hospital settings rather than in specialized centers [5].

As pediatric hospital medicine and pediatric surgery have grown, opportunities for collaboration between surgeons and hospitalists have increased.

*Corresponding author. *E-mail address:* Mshiver@usf.edu

https://doi.org/10.1016/j.yapd.2021.05.010

Forming partnerships is beneficial for many reasons, including the increasing medical complexity of patients needing hospital admission, time constraints on surgeons, and incentives to improve the quality of medical care. Involving hospitalists in the care of postsurgical patients not only improves surgeons' efficiency but several studies have indicated that hospitalist comanagement improves patient outcomes and decreases lengths of stay [6]. Having a physician covering the hospital exclusively has been shown to improve both cost and patient outcomes [7]. Almost all pediatric surgical procedures are straightforward and uncomplicated, but, for some children, particularly those with medical complexity, pediatric hospitalists should be familiar with the inherent risks of post operative complications of anesthesia and surgery.

ROLE OF THE PEDIATRIC HOSPITALIST

In order to build a meaningful relationship between surgical services and the hospitalist service, it is important to establish respective roles before entering into the care of a postsurgical patient. The pediatric hospitalist may be consulted to address one specific aspect of the patient's care, such as asthma management. Alternatively, the patient may be admitted to the pediatric hospitalist's service while the surgeon takes on the role of consultant in managing only acute operative concerns. More typically, there is a sharing of roles with each service addressing particular aspects of the patient's care [8]. This model of comanagement delegates specific tasks to each service. Fig. 1 details the variety of care needs that must be assigned in order to prevent confusion and miscommunication later [7,8].

The more granular tasks that must be assigned are specific to the surgical service, the medical complexity of the patient, and the type of surgery being completed. It is important to acknowledge that each surgeon has specific preferences so that the teams can work collaboratively to ensure that the patients are receiving appropriate and efficient care. Understanding the types of

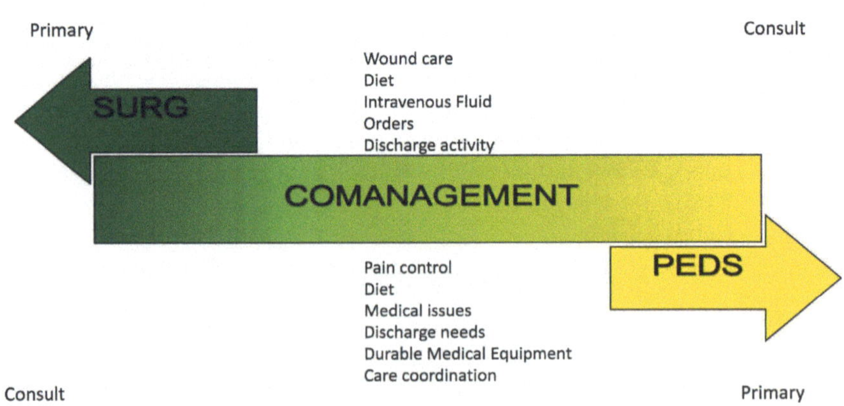

Fig. 1. Spectrum of care across services. PEDS, pediatrics; SURG, surgery.

operations the surgical team typically performs, the expected hospital course, and potential complications of the procedure is useful information for pediatric hospitalists. Pediatric hospitalists should engage the surgical service in conversation about these specific aspects of patient care before entering into a formal relationship with a surgical patient (Fig. 2) [7,8].

Disadvantages

Although there are many advantages of having pediatric hospitalists assist in caring for surgical patients, there are potential drawbacks. Adding an additional member to a patient's medical team increases the potential for miscommunication and confusion, and may prolong length of stay [9]. In adult patients, there was also an increase in postsurgical complications, specifically medication issues and infections [10]. Pediatric hospitalists should resist ordering nonurgent studies for patients admitted for surgical conditions. Avoiding unnecessary tests and imaging studies helps decrease potential complications and promotes a timely discharge.

COMMUNICATION

Communication is key to ensuring that the patients receive appropriate and complete care. The day-to-day care of postsurgical patients requires frequent and high-quality communication between all services in order to avoid unnecessary interventions, diagnostics, confusion between care givers, and extended lengths of stay [11]. Being admitted to the hospital is a stressful event regardless of the circumstances. Good communication helps decrease parental and child anxiety and distress. Table 1 lists typical events that can occur during a hospitalization that can lead to complications [11].

Family-centered rounds

Pediatric hospitalists have pioneered and embraced the practice of family-centered rounds (FCRs). Historically, daily hospital rounds involved the

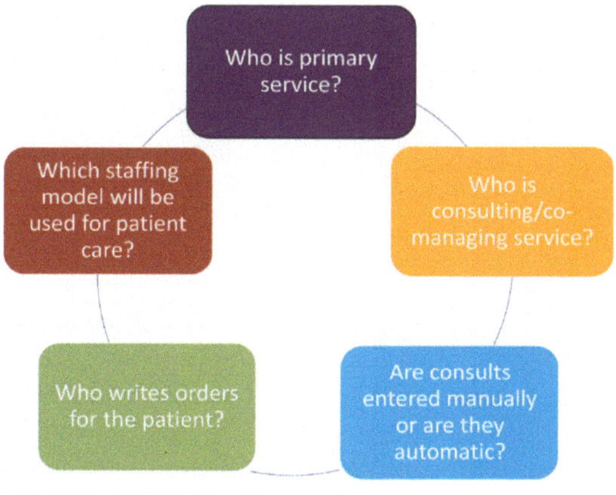

Fig. 2. Determining the roles of the various services caring for surgical patients.

Table 1
Clear communication decreases complications during hospitalization

Unnecessary or additional stressors	Unnecessary or harmful interventions
• Adult order sets used for pediatric patients • Pills ordered rather than liquids for pain medications • Poor communication or miscommunication to family	• Daily laboratory tests • Nonemergent tests or imaging studies that prolong length of stay • Medication errors

physician acting in an often-paternalistic manner when presenting the assessments and plans for the day with little to no opportunity for the patients and their guardians to interject or modify those plans. FCRs change that dynamic by including the patients and guardians as equal members of the medical team. Children as young as 2 years old can be engaged in discussing what is wrong and how the medical team and surgeons will help the child get better. Typically, FCR involves the physician team, nursing, and the patient's guardians discussing the patient's progress, concerns, and anticipated plan for the day. At the conclusion of the discussion, it is useful to confirm that the patient and guardians understand and agree with the medical plan and that all of their questions and concerns have been fully addressed [12]. When done well, FCRs can increase the family's involvement and understanding of what the issues are and help improve the communication between team members. It has also been shown to improve perceptions of patient safety. By using the technique of FCR with surgical patients, families feel reassured that the surgeon, the pediatrician, and the nurse all agree on the plan of care for the day [13].

Documentation

The primary means of communication among physicians is through documentation in the medical record. Regardless of how extensive pediatric hospitalists' involvement is in the care of surgical patients, they are the pediatricians in the hospital. Ensuring that a postsurgical patient receives care that is age and developmentally appropriate facilitates an improved patient experience and an event-free hospitalization. In addition to investigating pediatric-specific information, pediatric hospitalists should also review any existing orders written by the surgical team to ensure that they are appropriate for the patient's age and condition (Table 2).

Planning for discharge

The discharge planning for a surgical patient should begin before the procedure, especially for major orthopedic procedures where a prolonged recovery and assistive devices are expected to be needed. Physical therapy and case management can arrange for necessary medical equipment to be delivered before discharge. For children with complex medical needs who already receive therapies and home nursing, the orders for their home care may need to be updated with revised activity restrictions, pain medication regimens, and

Table 2
Recommended points to review in orders and components of the consult note

Review orders	Recommended components in consult note
Review all new medications to ensure type and dose are appropriate	Names of pediatrician (and specialists)
Diet: appropriate route and dose; particularly if receives feeds via enteral tube	Vaccination status (including tetanus if admitted with traumatic injury or burn)
Complete home medication reconciliation	Comorbidities
Order therapies and diet as appropriate	Development (eg, pills vs liquid medications, ability to engage and work with therapy)
Review nursing orders to notify MD, ensuring that vital sign ranges are age appropriate	Assess need for venous thromboembolism prophylaxis

changes to diet orders. Prescriptions for pain medications should be written and filled before discharge, particularly if prescribing narcotics. In addition, it must be clear which service will complete the discharge summary and communicate follow-up information to the child's pediatrician. The discharge summary should include all follow-up information, any pending laboratory or pathology results, complications that may occur, and the surgeon's contact information in case additional questions arise.

ROUTINE POSTSURGICAL MANAGEMENT CONSIDERATIONS

Respiratory

Acute respiratory issues account for most of the complications that can occur in young children during the immediate postoperative period [14]. These complications may be anesthesia related or may be caused by the type of surgery or procedure that was performed. Assessing for risk factors that can predict respiratory complications preoperatively and actively managing these risks in the perioperative and postoperative periods helps to mitigate and decrease the incidence of respiratory complications [15].

Anesthesia for young infants is particularly challenging. Because infants have a much higher risk of developing postanesthesia respiratory complications, they need extended observation postoperatively. Infants less than 12 months of age are more likely to experience laryngospasm, apnea, hypoxia, and cardiac arrest postanesthesia than older children, partly because they normally have increased vagal tone, which predisposes them to laryngospasm when the airway is manipulated. In addition, they tend to become hypoxic much faster than older children and adults; this can lead to catastrophic complications, including cardiac arrest, even in healthy infants [16]. Given the inherent risks of anesthesia, guidelines support intubation being completed by the most trained person available, ensuring that the young child is healthy before the procedure if it is an elective surgery, and having pediatric anesthesiologists immediately available in case of a complication.

In addition to laryngospasm, aspiration, postextubation croup, and hypoxic injury are well known potential complications of anesthesia [17]. The incidence of these events is inversely related to age, with premature infants being the most at risk. Anemia and low birth weight are additional independent risk factors for postanesthesia apneic events in neonates [18].

There is a range of guidelines and scoring systems that help anticipate anesthesia risks [19,20]. Although there are no universal protocols to guide which infants should have extended monitoring for respiratory complications, it is generally accepted that infants who are less than 45 weeks' corrected gestational age or those with underlying cardiac, pulmonary, or hematologic conditions should be monitored postoperatively for apnea or hypoxia for at least the first 12 to 24 hours following anesthesia [15]. Box 1 outlines known risk factors for respiratory complication related to anesthesia [15].

Children with sleep disordered breathing undergoing procedures of the upper airway also warrant particularly close monitoring postanesthesia. The nature of many ear, nose, and throat surgeries increases the risk for postoperative respiratory complications in addition to the risks associated with anesthesia. Children with chronic upper airway obstruction caused by adenoid or tonsil hypertrophy have a small but significant risk of postobstructive pulmonary edema [21]. This complication typically presents within 6 hours of relieving the chronically obstructive anatomy and presents with symptoms of respiratory distress and hypoxia. Treatment is generally supportive, with only rare instances of endotracheal intubation. Although infrequent, it is important that children at risk of this complication be monitored in a setting where they can be treated promptly and appropriately [15].

Postoperative pulmonary atelectasis can occur in the pediatric population just as it can in adults, but the incidence and severity are not well described. Although older, developmentally appropriate children can engage in incentive spirometry exercises and early ambulation to help prevent atelectasis, young

Box 1: Risk factors for respiratory complications following anesthesia

Prematurity (born at <37 weeks' gestation)
Low birth weight
Congenital heart disease
Asthma or chronic lung disease
Acute upper respiratory infection
Sleep disordered breathing or obstructive sleep apnea
Obesity (body mass index>95th percentile for age)
Tobacco use or exposure (includes vaping)
Anemia or transfusion dependent

children and those with developmental delays may not be able to cooperate with conventional methods. In these children, adequate (but not overly sedating) pain control is imperative to ensure that they can remain active and participate in recovery exercises as appropriate [22]. Many children's hospitals have child-life specialists who can be very helpful in engaging children in exercises such as blowing bubbles or pinwheels; however, these interventions have not been shown to improve recovery time or decrease frequency of pulmonary complications [23]. In children who cannot participate in such activities because of physical limitations or disease severity, respiratory therapy should be consulted on whether advanced airway clearance techniques or cough-assist devices should be used [24].

Venous thromboembolism prophylaxis

Venous thromboembolism (VTE) and deep vein thrombosis (DVT) are infrequent and preventable adverse events that can occur postoperatively. The precise frequency of VTE/DVT in children is not well known, but the rate of VTE/DVT in hospitalized children has increased over the past 20 years. Whether this phenomenon correlates with a true increase in incidence, an increase in the diagnosis of VTE/DVT, or a combination of factors is not clear [25]. Regardless, whenever a VTE/DVT event occurs it leads to increased morbidity and mortality [26], prolonged hospitalization, and increased costs [27]. VTE risks should be managed aggressively. Although there are no established pediatric-specific VTE risk factors, VTE/DVT is the second most common preventable adverse event in pediatric hospitals [28]. Table 3 outlines VTE risk factors [30].

There are numerous published guidelines to help clinicians recognize risk factors and manage them appropriately [29]. The authors have adapted VTE/DVT prophylaxis in postoperative pediatric patients based on several

Table 3
Risk factors for venous thromboembolism

Risk factors for VTE	
• Active cancer (or suspicion of cancer)	• Blood stream infection
• Obesity (body mass index >95th percentile for age)	• Major surgery (abdominal, pelvic, orthopedic surgery)
• History of nephrotic syndrome, antiphospholipid antibodies, or polycythemia	• Major trauma: more than 1 lower extremity long bone fracture, complex pelvic fractures, spinal cord injury
• Chemotherapy (especially asparaginase, bevacizumab, and high-dose dexamethasone)	• Central venous catheter (including nontunneled, tunneled, and percutaneously inserted peripheral catheters)
• Exogenous estrogen compounds (contraceptives) within past 2 mo	• History of congenital heart disease (nonbiological reconstruction)
• History of venous thrombosis or history of familial and/or acquired hypercoagulability	• History of inflammatory diseases (eg, inflammatory bowel disease, systemic lupus erythematosus)

guidelines using a risk-stratified approach [30]. Using the risk factors from Table 3, children are determined to be either low, moderate, or high risk for VTE/DVT. Prophylaxis, mechanical and/or chemical, is then ordered based on their risk level (Figs. 3 and 4).

Postoperative pain control

The plan for pain management should be discussed before undertaking a major surgical procedure. Factors to consider when making a pain plan include whether the child has had problems with pain control during prior procedures; whether the anticipated degree of pain associated with the planned procedure is mild, moderate, or severe; and whether regularly used pain medications are contraindicated [31]. Additional consideration should be given to the child's developmental level and underlying medical conditions. Children with seizure disorders may be more sensitive to additional sedating medications. Similarly, children with underlying nutritional or metabolic abnormalities and those with renal or bone disorders should receive lower doses of common over-the-counter pain relievers. This preoperative review serves the additional benefit of helping to set expectations for the family and decrease their anxiety before the surgery [32].

Nonpharmacologic interventions

Children are vulnerable because of their developmental stage resulting in a lack of understanding and anxiety when undergoing a procedure. Numerous studies reveal that clowns, animals, and play reduce anxiety, decrease opioid and pain medication use, and provide cost-saving effects on time in preoperative and postoperative areas and length of stay [33]. Child-life specialists can help patients of various developmental ages understand what is occurring in their bodies [34,35]. Addressing the psychological needs of patients and caregivers and providing strategies to cope with postoperative pain and frustration

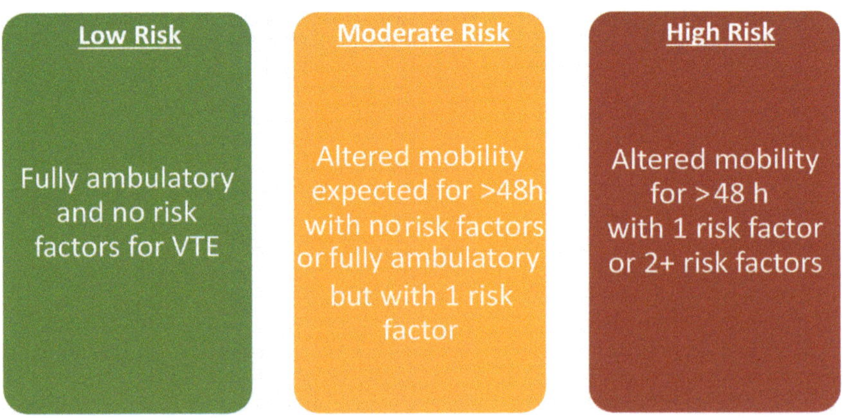

Fig. 3. Determine VTE risk level.

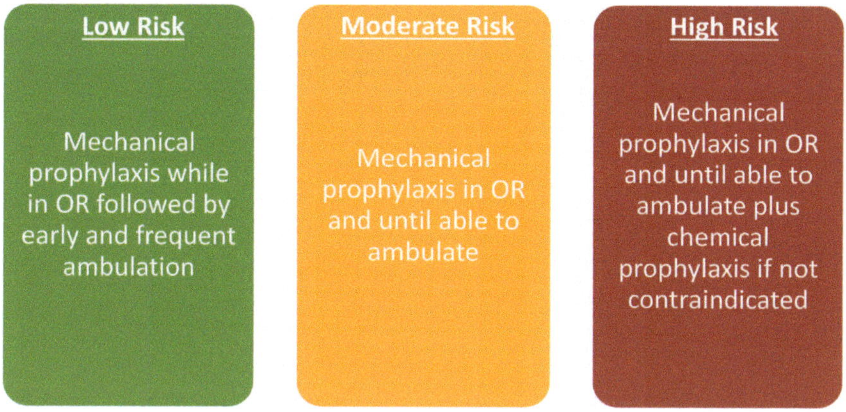

Fig. 4. VTE prophylaxis recommendations according to risk level Gradation of risk: low, medium and high and interventions recommended based on risk. Mechanical prophylaxis: serial compression devices (SCDs) and chemical prophylaxis usually enoxaparin. OR, operating room.

aids recovery while acknowledging the emotional component to the surgical intervention [36–38].

Pharmacologic management

A stepwise approach to pain management is ideal; the goals are to manage pain quickly and effectively with nonnarcotic agents and nonpharmacologic tools and to limit the use of opioids [39]. Mild postsurgical pain can typically be controlled with acetaminophen or nonsteroidal antiinflammatory drugs (NSAIDs) given on a regular schedule by mouth. Moderate postsurgical pain may require both acetaminophen and NSAIDs be given around the clock with opiate mediation available on an as-needed basis for breakthrough pain during the first 2 to 3 days after the procedure [40]. Severe postsurgical pain can be anticipated after major thoracic, abdominal, or orthopedic surgery and requires a multimodal approach. Patient-controlled analgesia (PCA) is sometimes an appropriate pain management tool in children who are developmentally and functionally able to recognize they are experiencing worsening pain and hit the button to administer a small bolus of intravenous opiate medication. Using NSAIDs and sometimes gabapentin on a scheduled basis helps decrease the dose and duration of opiate pain medications children require after a major surgery, thereby decreasing opioid-related toxicity and dose-related side effects [41–43].

Table 4 outlines regimens for mild, moderate, and severe postoperative pain management.

Nonsteroidal antiinflammatory drugs

As with all medications, pain medications each have potential side effects. NSAIDs have long been thought to increase the risk of postoperative bleeding

Table 4
Pain gradation: possible regimens for mild, moderate, and severe pain depending on patient tolerance for each medication

Pain agents	Mild	Moderate	Severe
Acetaminophen (PO/IV)	Scheduled	Scheduled	Scheduled
NSAIDs (PO/IV)	As needed	Scheduled	Scheduled
Valium	No	As needed	As needed/scheduled
Opioids: PO/IV	No	As needed/PO	PCA
Gabapentin	No	No	Scheduled

Gabapentin may be scheduled and ordered preoperatively and commenced in anticipation of possible nerve pain. Valium may be given intravenously or by mouth to treat muscle spasms [43].
Abbreviations: IV, intravenous; PO, by mouth.

and so were avoided. More recent reviews have not shown NSAIDs to increase bleeding following orthopedic procedures [44]; however, Diercks and colleagues [45] report that NSAIDs may increase the risk of bleeding following head and neck surgeries. Renal function must be considered when ordering NSAIDs. In addition, NSAIDs may have a negative impact on bone healing after trauma [46].

Opiates
Opioids are the most powerful drugs available to treat pain and are used to treat severe postsurgical pain. Although very effective at pain control, they are highly addictive and must be prescribed and used carefully. Opioids are available in numerous formulations and can be delivered orally, intravenously, or given regionally by the anesthesiologist. Prescribing and dosing narcotics is different in children versus adults because of children having a higher water content (increased volume of distribution), lower plasma protein levels, and faster hepatic metabolism [47]. The sedating effect of opioids is enhanced when used in combination with other medications, so extreme caution must be used when ordering both opiates and muscle relaxants, antianxiety medications, or antiepileptic medications. Hypoventilation and respiratory insufficiency are dose-related side effects of narcotics. Children receiving opiates should have continuous respiratory monitoring; capnography (end-tidal carbon dioxide monitoring) is a more reliable predictor of hypoventilation than pulse oximetry [48]. Any time an opiate is ordered, the reversal agent naloxone should be ordered and readily available at the bedside. Additional side effects from opiate use include pruritus, nausea, urinary retention, constipation, and intestinal ileus. Table 5 outlines these side effects and appropriate interventions.

Regional analgesia
Intrathecal, epidural, and peripheral nerve analgesia reduce the overall dose of narcotic medications received and allow transition to oral pain medication more quickly [49]. Regional anesthesia has also been shown to have fewer

Table 5
Side effects of opiate medications

Symptom	Monitoring/intervention
Nausea/vomiting	Ondansetron followed by promethazine; if severe, stop or switch to a different opiate medication and give low-dose benzodiazepine
Pruritis	Diphenhydramine or hydroxyzine; if severe, consider low-dose naloxone continuous IV
Constipation	Clean out before surgery to reduce stool load. Polyethylene glycol or docusate daily; encourage ambulation; if persists for >48 h, give sennoside medication and/or bisacodyl suppository and/or enema
Ileus	Bowel rest (nothing by mouth until resolves); nasogastric tube if vomiting; reduce narcotic dose; avoid giving bowel stimulants
Urinary retention	Monitor output; if no spontaneous void for more than 8 h, scan bladder and if >2 / 3 bladder volume perform straight catheterization to decompress
Respiratory depression	End-tidal CO_2 monitor and/or pulse oximetry. If symptoms develop, stop opiate, give supplemental O_2, and stimulate patient. For respiratory arrest, call code blue and begin cardiopulmonary resuscitation; give naloxone to reverse sedation

side effects and less stress response from surgical intervention [50]. Children with intrathecal or epidural analgesia are at risk for urinary retention, so a Foley catheter should remain in place until the epidural is discontinued.

Although intrathecal, epidural, and peripheral nerve analgesia are effective for pediatric patients, there remains the need for additional research into the management of postoperative pain in this population [51]. Postoperative pain monitoring and assessment in pediatric patients can be challenging because of developmental differences in age, parental concerns, behavioral challenges, the use of multiple standardized pain score tools and protocols, and communication challenges between nurses, patients, and parents [52–54]. In addition, concerns about the side effects of pain medications and the risks of addiction can result in poor postsurgical pain control and prolonged recovery time if the parents and medical team do not share similar goals for pain management [55].

COMPLICATIONS

Surgical complications in pediatric patients, including potential medications errors caused by miscommunication between medical teams, anesthesia-related respiratory events, VTE/DVT prevention, and complications related to medications, specifically narcotics, were discussed earlier. Fever and anemia are additional common complications that are frequently encountered.

Fever is a frequent event following major surgery but rarely indicates infection when it occurs within the first 2 days of the procedure [56]. Longer time intervals between the procedure and fever onset are more likely to indicate an infectious process. Evaluation should include a thorough review of the patient's medical history, home and current medications, operative report, and thorough physical examination. The differential of postoperative fever is broad and includes medication-related fevers, atelectasis and pneumonia, thrombophlebitis, and infection of the wound, blood, or urinary tract.

Postoperative anemia is influenced by the patient's preoperative health status, the type of surgery, and intraoperative blood loss and ongoing losses through drains that may be left in the surgical site. Estimated blood loss is often difficult to determine and may not be accurate. Patients with trauma and patients undergoing major orthopedic or large solid tumor surgeries tend to have more blood loss. Although there are no firm guidelines regarding when a patient requires a blood transfusion, factors to consider include whether there is any active bleeding, whether the patient is hemodynamically unstable, and whether the patient has any underlying conditions [57].

SPECIAL POPULATIONS

Scoliosis and spinal fusion

Pediatric patients undergoing spinal fusion for correction of scoliosis represent a significant segment of surgical patients who require inpatient postoperative treatment. Although surgical treatment of scoliosis is still considered to be a major procedure, advancements in surgical techniques and approaches have significantly decreased surgical risk over time [58]. Historically, patients undergoing spinal fusion have been managed postoperatively in the pediatric intensive care unit (ICU), primarily because of the high risk of complications and the prolonged duration of anesthesia required. However, recent studies suggest that many patients do not require ICU-level care following surgery and can be successfully managed on the pediatric inpatient ward service.

The primary factor to consider when evaluating the need for ICU care following spinal surgery is the cause of scoliosis: nonidiopathic (primarily

Box 2: Risk factors for intensive care unit admission in patients undergoing spinal fusion for scoliosis [57].

Black/African American race

Anterior or combined anterior/posterior approach

Preoperative ventilator dependence

Asthma or underlying structural pulmonary abnormality

Gross motor developmental delay

Underlying neuromuscular disorder

Total operating time greater than 270 minutes

neuromuscular) or idiopathic. Although idiopathic scoliosis is generally a diagnosis of exclusion, neuromuscular scoliosis is a broad category that includes patients whose scoliosis is caused by an underlying neurologic or neuromuscular condition, such as cerebral palsy or muscular dystrophy. In general, patients who are undergoing surgical treatment of idiopathic scoliosis can be managed on the general ward service, whereas patients with neuromuscular scoliosis (or other forms of nonidiopathic scoliosis) are at higher risk for complications and should be managed in the ICU [59,60].

Box 2 outlines additional risk factors that place patients at higher risk for complications and warrant consideration for intensive care monitoring during the postoperative period [57].

Common postoperative complications of spinal fusion

The most significant complication of scoliosis surgery is neurologic injury. Although most neurologic injury occurs intraoperatively, there remains a risk for delayed neurologic complications. This complication is very rare (estimated to be around 0.01%) [61,62] but should still be monitored for closely by both the pediatric and surgical teams. Dural tears are another complication of spinal fusion surgery and can be mitigated by bed rest in the immediate postoperative period [58].

Gastrointestinal issues, also common following spinal fusion surgery, occur in up to 77% of patients [59] and include a wide range of complications, including emesis and ileus. Other complications include significant intraoperative blood loss, VTE, and pulmonary complications [58,59].

Managing patients with scoliosis in the immediate postoperative period is best approached with a team effort consisting of the surgical team, anesthesia, pediatric hospitalists, nursing, therapy, pharmacy, and child life. Developing institutional practices that include standardized care pathways can decrease length of stay and improve outcomes in these patients [63]. Appropriate pain control and nutrition, an aggressive bowel regimen, and early ambulation all help promote an uncomplicated and brief hospitalization postoperatively [60].

SUMMARY

Caring for medically complex children in the hospital who have recently undergone surgical procedures is increasingly the responsibility of pediatric hospitalists. Building protocols and relationships with the surgical teams is essential to provide ideal care. The care of pediatric postoperative patients exists on a spectrum between primary, consultant, and shared comanagement with a clear definition of the role of each service. The pediatric hospitalist has expertise in quality improvement, patient safety, and family-centered care. Working collaboratively with the surgical team to manage pain and chronic medical conditions and prevent common postsurgical complications helps to ensure a safe hospitalization and an uneventful transition home.

CLINICS CARE POINTS

- Collaboration between pediatric surgical services and pediatric hospitalists enhances postoperative care of pediatric patients by ensuring pediatric-appropriate care and facilitating timely transition home.
- Assessing and actively managing risks for anesthesia-related respiratory complications, postsurgical complications, and VTE events improves morbidity, decreases length of stay, and improves quality of care during the hospitalization.
- Multimodal pain control using nonpharmacologic and opioid-sparing strategies decreases the risks of medication-related side effects and enhances postsurgical recovery.

DISCLOSURE

The authors have no conflicts of interest to disclose.

References

[1] Leape LL. A brief account of the founding of the American Pediatric Surgical association. J Pediatr Surg 1996;31(1):12–8.
[2] Pediatric Surgical Training Programs. In American Pediatric Surgical Association. 2020. Available at: https://apsapedsurg.org/continuing-education/early-career/fellowship-positions/pediatric-surgery-training-programs/. Accessed November 10, 2020.
[3] Zeller KA, Nakayama DK, Fraile K, et al. History of Pediatric Surgery. In: Waldhausen J, Powell D, Hirschl R, editors. Pediatric surgery NaT. East Dundee (IL): American Pediatric Surgical Association; 2020. Available at: https://www.pedsurglibrary.com/apsa/view/Pediatric-Surgery-NaT/829734/all/History_of_Pediatric_Surgery. Accessed November 10, 2020.
[4] Roberts KB, Fisher ER, Rauch DA. The history of pediatric hospital medicine in the United States, 1996-2019. J Hosp Med 2020;15(7):424–7.
[5] Ricketts TC, Adamson WT, Fraher EP, et al. Future supply of pediatric surgeons: analytical study of the current and projected supply of pediatric surgeons in the context of a rapidly changing process for specialty and subspecialty training. Ann Surg 2017;265(3):609–15.
[6] Simon TD, Eilert R, Dickinson LM, et al. Pediatric hospitalist comanagement of spinal fusion surgery patients. J Hosp Med 2007;2(1):23–30.
[7] Rappaport DI, Adelizzi-Delany J, Rogers KJ, et al. Outcomes and costs associated with hospitalist comanagement of medically complex children undergoing spinal fusion surgery. Hosp Pediatr 2013;3(3):233–41.
[8] Rappaport DI, Rosenberg RE, Shaughnessy EE, et al. Pediatric hospitalist comanagement of surgical patients: structural, quality, and financial considerations. J Hosp Med 2014;9(11): 737–42.
[9] Stevens JP, Hatfield LA, Nyweide DJ, et al. Association of variation in consultant use among hospitalist physicians with outcomes among medicare beneficiaries. JAMA Netw Open 2020;3(2):e1921750.
[10] Chen LM, Wilk AS, Thumma JR, et al. Use of medical consultants for hospitalized surgical patients: an observational cohort study. JAMA Intern Med 2014;174(9):1470–7.
[11] Rauch DA, COMMITTEE ON HOSPITAL CARE, SECTION ON HOSPITAL MEDICINE. Physician's role in coordinating care of hospitalized children. Pediatrics 2018;142(2): e20181503.
[12] Mittal V. Family-centered rounds. Pediatr Clin North Am 2014;61(4):663–70.

[13] Cox ED, Jacobsohn GC, Rajamanickam VP, et al. A family-centered rounds checklist, family engagement, and patient safety: a randomized trial. Pediatrics 2017;139(5):e20161688.
[14] Habre W, Disma N, Virag K, et al. Incidence of severe critical events in paediatric anaesthesia (APRICOT): a prospective multicentre observational study in 261 hospitals in Europe. Lancet Respir Med 2017;5(5):412–25 [published correction appears in Lancet Respir Med. 2017;5(5):e19] [published correction appears in Lancet Respir Med. 2017 Jun;5(6):e22].
[15] Egbuta C, Mason KP. Recognizing risks and optimizing perioperative care to reduce respiratory complications in the pediatric patient. J Clin Med 2020;9(6):1942.
[16] Bhananker SM, Ramamoorthy C, Geiduschek JM, et al. Anesthesia-related cardiac arrest in children: update from the Pediatric Perioperative Cardiac Arrest Registry. Anesth Analg 2007;105(2):344–50.
[17] Mir Ghassemi A, Neira V, Ufholz LA, et al. A systematic review and meta-analysis of acute severe complications of pediatric anesthesia. Paediatr Anaesth 2015;25(11):1093–102.
[18] Houck CS, Vinson AE. Anaesthetic considerations for surgery in newborns. Arch Dis Child Fetal Neonatal Ed 2017;102(4):F359–63.
[19] von Ungern-Sternberg BS, Boda K, Chambers NA, et al. Risk assessment for respiratory complications in paediatric anaesthesia: a prospective cohort study. Lancet 2010;376(9743):773–83.
[20] Mamie C, Habre W, Delhumeau C, et al. Incidence and risk factors of perioperative respiratory adverse events in children undergoing elective surgery. Paediatr Anaesth 2004;14(3):218–24.
[21] Fremont RD, Kallet RH, Matthay MA, et al. Postobstructive pulmonary edema: a case for hydrostatic mechanisms. Chest 2007;131(6):1742–6.
[22] Branson RD. The scientific basis for postoperative respiratory care. Respir Care 2013;58(11):1974–84.
[23] Morrow BM. Chest physiotherapy in the pediatric intensive care unit. J Pediatr Intensive Care 2015;4(4):174–81.
[24] Chiang J, Amin R. Respiratory care considerations for children with medical complexity. Children (Basel) 2017;4(5):41.
[25] Raffini L, Huang YS, Witmer C, et al. Dramatic increase in venous thromboembolism in children's hospitals in the United States from 2001 to 2007. Pediatrics 2009;124(4):1001–8.
[26] Faustino EV, Lawson KA, Northrup V, et al. Mortality-adjusted duration of mechanical ventilation in critically ill children with symptomatic central venous line-related deep venous thrombosis. Crit Care Med 2011;39(5):1151–6.
[27] Goudie A, Dynan L, Brady PW, et al. Costs of venous thromboembolism, catheter-associated urinary tract infection, and pressure ulcer. Pediatrics 2015;136(3):432–9.
[28] Lyren A, Brilli RJ, Zieker K, et al. Children's hospitals' solutions for patient safety collaborative impact on hospital-acquired harm. Pediatrics 2017;140(3):e20163494.
[29] Faustino EV, Raffini LJ. Prevention of hospital-acquired venous thromboembolism in children: a review of published guidelines. Front Pediatr 2017;5:9.
[30] Meier KA, Clark E, Tarango C, et al. Venous thromboembolism in hospitalized adolescents: an approach to risk assessment and prophylaxis. Hosp Pediatr 2015;5(1):44–51.
[31] Joshi GP, Kehlet H. Procedure-specific pain management: the road to improve postsurgical pain management? Anesthesiology 2013;118(4):780–2.
[32] Frizzell KH, Cavanaugh PK, Herman MJ. Pediatric Perioperative Pain Management. Orthop Clin North Am 2017;48(4):467–80.
[33] Kocherov S, Hen Y, Jaworowski S, et al. Medical clowns reduce pre-operative anxiety, post-operative pain and medical costs in children undergoing outpatient penile surgery: A randomised controlled trial. J Paediatr Child Health 2016;52(9):877–81.
[34] Inan G, Inal S. The impact of 3 different distraction techniques on the pain and anxiety levels of children during venipuncture: a clinical trial. Clin J Pain 2019;35(2):140–7.

[35] Kain ZN, Mayes LC, Caldwell-Andrews AA, et al. Preoperative anxiety, postoperative pain, and behavioral recovery in young children undergoing surgery. Pediatrics 2006;118(2): 651–8.
[36] Jennings JK, Doyle JS, Gilbert SR, et al. The use of chewing gum postoperatively in pediatric scoliosis patients facilitates an earlier return to normal bowel function. Spine Deform 2015;3(3):263–6.
[37] López-Jaimez G, Cuello-García CA. Use of chewing gum in children undergoing an appendectomy: A randomized clinical controlled trial. Int J Surg 2016;32:38–42.
[38] Petersen PC, Balakrishnan B, Vitola B, et al. Case report series of a novel application of neostigmine to successfully relieve refractory ileus status post-pediatric orthotopic liver transplantation. Pediatr Transplant 2019;23(7):e13564.
[39] Sheffer BW, Kelly DM, Rhodes LN, et al. Perioperative pain management in pediatric spine surgery. Orthop Clin North Am 2017;48(4):481–6.
[40] Michelet D, Andreu-Gallien J, Bensalah T, et al. A meta-analysis of the use of nonsteroidal antiinflammatory drugs for pediatric postoperative pain. Anesth Analg 2012;114(2): 393–406.
[41] Peng PW, Wijeysundera DN, Li CC. Use of gabapentin for perioperative pain control – a meta-analysis. Pain Res Manag 2007;12(2):85–92.
[42] Trzcinski S, Rosenberg RE, Vasquez Montes D, et al. Use of gabapentin in posterior spinal fusion is associated with decreased postoperative pain and opioid use in children and adolescents. Clin Spine Surg 2019;32(5):210–4.
[43] Ferland CE, Vega E, Ingelmo PM. Acute pain management in children: challenges and recent improvements. Curr Opin Anaesthesiol 2018;31(3):327–32.
[44] Cozowicz C, Bekeris J, Poeran J, et al. Multimodal pain management and postoperative outcomes in lumbar spine fusion surgery: a population-based cohort study. Spine (Phila Pa 1976) 2020;45(9):580–9.
[45] Diercks GR, Comins J, Bennett K, et al. Comparison of ibuprofen vs acetaminophen and severe bleeding risk after pediatric tonsillectomy: a noninferiority randomized clinical trial. JAMA Otolaryngol Head Neck Surg 2019;145(6):494–500.
[46] Lisowska B, Kosson D, Domaracka K. Positives and negatives of nonsteroidal anti-inflammatory drugs in bone healing: the effects of these drugs on bone repair. Drug Des Devel Ther 2018;12:1809–14.
[47] Nowicki PD, Vanderhave KL, Gibbons K, et al. Perioperative pain control in pediatric patients undergoing orthopaedic surgery. J Am Acad Orthop Surg 2012;20(12):755–65.
[48] Langhan ML, Li FY, Lichtor JL. The impact of capnography monitoring among children and adolescents in the postanesthesia care unit: a randomized controlled trial. Paediatr Anaesth 2017;27(4):385–93.
[49] Li Y, Hong RA, Robbins CB, et al. Intrathecal morphine and oral analgesics provide safe and effective pain control after posterior spinal fusion for adolescent idiopathic scoliosis. Spine (Phila Pa 1976) 2018;43(2):E98–104.
[50] Rubin K, Sullivan D, Sadhasivam S. Are peripheral and neuraxial blocks with ultrasound guidance more effective and safe in children? Paediatr Anaesth 2009;19(2):92–6.
[51] Chou R, Gordon DB, de Leon-Casasola OA, et al. Management of Postoperative Pain: A Clinical Practice Guideline From the American Pain Society, the American Society of Regional Anesthesia and Pain Medicine, and the American Society of Anesthesiologists' Committee on Regional Anesthesia, Executive Committee, and Administrative Council. J Pain 2016;17(2):131–57 [published correction appears in J Pain. 2016;17(4): 508-510. Dosage error in article text].
[52] Ceelie I, de Wildt SN, de Jong M, et al. Protocolized post-operative pain management in infants; do we stick to it? Eur J Pain 2012;16(5):760–6.
[53] Panjganj D, Bevan A. Children's nurses' post-operative pain assessment practices. Nurs Child Young People 2016;28(5):29–33.

[54] Quinn BL, Sheldon LK, Cooley ME. Pediatric pain assessment by drawn faces scales: a review. Pain Manag Nurs 2014;15(4):909–18.
[55] Merkel SI, Danaher JA, Williams J. Pain management in the post-operative pediatric urologic patient. Urol Nurs 2015;35(2):75–100.
[56] Corkum KS, Hunter CJ, Grabowski JE, et al. Early postoperative fever workup in children: utilization and utility. J Pediatr Surg 2018;53(7):1295–300.
[57] American Society of Anesthesiologists Task Force on Perioperative Blood Management. Practice guidelines for perioperative blood management: an updated report by the American Society of Anesthesiologists Task Force on Perioperative Blood Management*. Anesthesiology 2015;122(2):241–75.
[58] Lonner BS, Ren Y, Yaszay B, et al. Evolution of surgery for adolescent idiopathic scoliosis over 20 years: have outcomes improved? Spine (Phila Pa 1976) 2018;43(6):402–10.
[59] Abu-Kishk I, Kozer E, Hod-Feins R, et al. Pediatric scoliosis surgery–is postoperative intensive care unit admission really necessary? Paediatr Anaesth 2013;23(3):271–7.
[60] Malik AT, Yu E, Kim J, et al. Intensive Care Unit Admission Following Surgery for Pediatric Spinal Deformity: An Analysis of the ACS-NSQIP Pediatric Spinal Fusion Procedure Targeted Dataset. Glob Spine J 2020;10(2):177–82.
[61] Al-Mohrej OA, Aldakhil SS, Al-Rabiah MA, et al. Surgical treatment of adolescent idiopathic scoliosis: Complications. Ann Med Surg (Lond) 2020;52:19–23.
[62] Murphy RF, Mooney JF 3rd. Complications following spine fusion for adolescent idiopathic scoliosis. Curr Rev Musculoskelet Med 2016;9(4):462–9.
[63] Oetgen ME, Martin BD, Gordish-Dressman H, et al. Effectiveness and sustainability of a standardized care pathway developed with use of lean process mapping for the treatment of patients undergoing posterior spinal fusion for adolescent idiopathic scoliosis. J Bone Joint Surg Am 2018;100(21):1864–70.

Advances in Pediatrics 68 (2021) 121–142
ADVANCES IN PEDIATRICS

Inflammatory Bowel Disease in Children and Adolescents

Nathan S. Rubalcava, MD[a], Samir K. Gadepalli, MD, MS[a,b,*]

[a]Section of Pediatric Surgery, Department of Surgery, University of Michigan, Mott Children's Hospital, 1540 East Hospital Drive SPC 4217, Ann Arbor, MI 48109 – 4217, USA; [b]Susan B. Meister Child Health Evaluation and Research Center, Michigan Medicine, Ann Arbor, MI 48109, USA

Keywords

• Inflammatory Bowel disease • Crohn's disease • Ulcerative colitis • Early-onset IBD • Pediatric IBD

Key points

- Incidence of inflammatory bowel disease (IBD) is increasing in developed countries, and children are being diagnosed at earlier ages.
- The impact of IBD on children and their families is multifactorial: nutritional, psychosocial, developmental, and medical; therefore, a multidisciplinary approach to care is paramount to optimal care of children with IBD.
- Medical care for IBD in children should use a steroid-sparing approach with immunomodulators and biologic agents, individually tailored, and paying attention to psychosocial function, follow-up regarding fertility, and smooth transition from pediatric to adult care.
- In children with ulcerative colitis, long-term complications after surgical resection and reconstruction with J-pouch include pouchitis, incontinence, infertility, and unrecognized IBD-Unclassified or Crohn's disease requiring additional immunosuppressive therapy.
- Collaborative care IBD networks will allow new discoveries and enhanced care.

INTRODUCTION

Epidemiology

Inflammatory bowel disease (IBD) is a spectrum of conditions, including Crohn's disease (CD) and ulcerative colitis (UC), which can be characterized by chronic

*Corresponding author. Section of Pediatric Surgery, Department of Surgery, University of Michigan, Mott Children's Hospital, 1540 East Hospital Drive SPC 4217, Ann Arbor, MI 48109 – 4217. *E-mail address:* samirg@med.umich.edu

https://doi.org/10.1016/j.yapd.2021.05.005
0065-3101/21/

immune activation and inflammation of the gastrointestinal tract. Although IBD can be diagnosed at any age, 20% to 30% are diagnosed in childhood and young adulthood with an increased male predominance [1]. The true incidence and prevalence is approximately 2.1 to 15 per 100,000 for CD and 2.2 to 4.5 per 100,000 for UC [2]. Furthermore, the incidence in both CD and UC appears to be increasing in children of industrialized or Western nations [3,4]. Although data are lacking for undeveloped countries, the incidence of IBD is also increasing in newly industrialized countries of Asia, the Middle East, and South America [5,6].

Pathogenesis

The etiology of IBD in patients is believed to be multifactorial, with 3 main themes having emerged over the past 3 decades: individual genetics, environmental insults, and microbial influences [7]. Genetic predisposition can lead the immune system to mount a dysregulated response to the intestinal flora, following an environmental trigger inciting an accelerated mucosal barrier dysfunction [8,9]. Genes such as HLA-DRB1 and HLA-DQB have been identified as determinants that predispose patients to UC, whereas the IBD1 gene on 16q12 resulting in NOD2 mutation has been shown to be a contributor to the dysfunction in mucosal barrier integrity in CD. Yet, the rising incidence of IBD over the twentieth century in addition to the epidemiologic observations of higher prevalence in developed countries suggests contribution from environmental and dietary factors [10]. This has further led to intense investigation into the impact of the gut microbiome dysbiosis in IBD. Recent studies have shown patients with IBD have significant fluctuations and deviations from the healthy plane of microorganisms compared with healthy individuals without IBD, leading to a search for microbiomarkers that discriminate between CD and non-CD colitis [11,12].

Spectrum of disease

UC, CD, and IBD-Unclassified (IBD-U) are the most common forms of IBD. UC is characterized by continuous diffuse inflammation of the colon that will begin in the rectum and progress retrograde to the cecum and exhibit backwash ileitis or pancolitis [13]. CD can involve any portion of the gastrointestinal tract, although most commonly involves the terminal ileum, colon, and perianal region and can present as inflammatory, penetrating (fistulizing), or stricturing phenotype or any combination of the 3. A phenotype of CD that only involves the colon is more frequently seen in children than adults and can make it difficult to differentiate from UC at the time of diagnosis. The term IBD-U (previously known as indeterminate colitis) is reserved for those patients who have symptoms and findings of both CD from UC. Although these patients are often managed similar to UC, being able to identify problems associated with IBD-U is critical.

DIAGNOSIS

Presentation

The clinical presentation of IBD is often a constellation of heterogeneous symptoms. Children with UC frequently present with diarrhea (98%) and rectal bleeding (83%), whereas those with CD will present most frequently with weight loss/growth failure (55%–90%), abdominal pain, and diarrhea (67%–80%) [14,15]. An impact on growth and weight is a particular hallmark of pediatric IBD and can even precede the more common symptoms. Other symptoms are often related to severity of disease, such as anorexia, delayed puberty, weight loss, anxiety, and depression [16]. Perianal disease is reported in approximately 15% to 20% of children with CD with a cumulative probability of 26% at 5 years and 42% at 20 years [17]. There are several phenotypes, including anorectal/rectovaginal fistulae, perianal abscesses, fissures, skin tags, and strictures. Presence of 2 or more of these findings should raise the suspicion for underlying CD, especially in the setting of chronic weight loss [18]. Family history remains an important risk factor for IBD, with pediatric IBD more likely than adult-onset to have a positive family history of IBD [19].

Although IBD mainly affects the gastrointestinal tract, extraintestinal manifestations (EIM) can also occur [20]. In contrast to adults, children can present with EIM years before the onset of gastrointestinal symptoms, with as many as 28% of children having EIM at the time of diagnosis [21]. Manifestations can be musculoskeletal (arthritis, osteopenia), dermatologic (pyoderma granulosum, erythema nodosum), hepatobiliary (pancreatitis, primary sclerosing cholangitis), renal (uveitis, episcleritis, iritis), and hematologic (anemia, deep venous thromboembolism). Some EIMs parallel intestinal disease activity (episcleritis, erythema nodosum, arthritis), whereas others (primary sclerosing cholangitis, pyoderma granulosum) tend to be independent of intestinal inflammation [22].

Stratifying disease progression for purposes of clinical management, research, and effect of therapeutic interventions on outcomes have been improved by the development and validation of clinical scoring tools such as the Pediatric Crohn's Disease Activity Index (PCDAI) [23] (Table 1) and the Pediatric Ulcerative Colitis Activity Index (PUCAI) [24] (Table 2). The PCDAI is made up of subjective (patient symptoms) and objective (physical examination and laboratory investigation) components. Notably, PCDAI does not account for mucosal inflammation, which is a critical end-point in the management of CD. A PCDAI score less than 10 indicates inactive/mildly active disease, whereas a score $\geq$30 is considered moderately active disease. PUCAI, on the other hand, is exclusively subjective, with a score ranging from 0 to 85. Inactive disease is considered less than 10, moderate disease is $\geq$30, and severe disease is considered $\geq$65. The smallest change that should provoke a change in management, or the minimal important difference, is 20.

Very early onset IBD (VEO-IBD), defined as IBD diagnosed at younger than 6 years of age, is an atypical variant of IBD that is increasingly diagnosed in children [25]. Loss-of-function mutations in interleukin (IL)-10 and its receptor, and dysregulation in the nuclear factor kappa-light-chain-enhancer of activated B cells (NF-κB) pathway are just a couple of the near 60 monogenic mutations that have been associated with the development of VEO-IBD [25–27]. It should be emphasized that monogenic causes only make up 5% to 20% of VEO-IBD cases [28]. The clinical, endoscopic, and histologic

Table 1
Pediatric Crohn's Disease Activity Index (PCDAI)

History (recall, 1 wk)	
Abdominal pain:	
None	0
Mild	5
Moderate/Severe	10
Stools (per day):	
0–1 liquid, no blood	0
≤2 semi-formed with small blood/2–5 liquid, no blood	5
Gross bleeding, ≥6 liquid, or nocturnal diarrhea	10
Patient function:	
Well, no limitation of activities	0
Occasional difficulty in maintaining age-appropriate activities	5
Very poor, frequent limitation of activity	10
Laboratory	
Hematocrit (%):	
<10 y	
≥33	0
28–32	2.5
<28	5
11–19 y, female	
≥33	0
29–32	2.5
<29	5
11–14 y, male	
≥34	0
29–33	2.5
<29	5
15–19 y, male	
≥37	0
32–36	2.5
<32	5
ESR (mm/h):	
<20	0
20–50	2.5
>50	5
Albumin (g/dL):	
≥3.5	0
3.1–3.4	5
≤3.0	10
Examination	
Weight:	
Weight gain or voluntary weight stable/loss	0
Involuntary weight stable, weight loss 1%–9%	5
Weight loss ≥10%	10
Height (score "At diagnosis" OR "Follow-up"):	
At diagnosis:	
<1 channel decrease	0

(*continued on next page*)

Table 1
(*continued*)

Examination	
≥1, <2 channel decrease	5
>2 channel decrease	10
Follow-up:	
Height velocity ≥ −1 SD	0
Height velocity −2 SD < X < −1 SD	5
≤ −2 SD	10
Abdomen	
No tenderness, no mass	0
Tenderness, or mass without tenderness	5
Tenderness, involuntary guarding, definite mass	10
Perirectal disease	
None, asymptomatic tags	0
1–2 indolent fistulae, scant drainage, no tenderness	5
Active fistula, drainage, tenderness, or abscess	10
Extraintestinal manifestations:	
(Fever ≥38.5 for 3 d over past week, definite arthritis, uveitis, erythema nodosum, pyoderma gangrenosum)	
None	0
One	5
≥ Two	10
Total (0–100)	

Abbreviation: ESR, erythrocyte sedimentation rate; SD, standard deviation.

heterogeneity of VEO-IBD, especially in early childhood, make it difficult to differentiate it from CD or UC [3,29–31]. Approximately 30% of cases are classified as IBD-U. We recommend describing patients as CD-like or UC-like without completely committing the patient to one group or another to allow longer follow-up and better characterize the disease process. This may have implications in surgical management, specifically when deciding whether pouch construction is appropriate. Further, these patients frequently have complications and may have a change in their diagnosis from VEO-IBD [29]. Given that identification of these mutations may enable the possibility for a *curative* bone marrow transplant in the near future, children diagnosed with VEO-IBD should undergo genetic testing [28].

Laboratory investigations

Laboratory abnormalities in children with IBD are consistent with a chronic inflammatory state: anemia, hypoalbuminemia, and elevated inflammatory markers [32]. Anemia is from chronic rectal bleeding and hypoalbuminemia from ongoing protein losses secondary to the damaged colonic mucosa. Initial laboratory investigations are included in Box 1. Normal laboratory results do not rule out IBD, however, as up to 33% can have normal inflammatory markers [33]. Stool samples should be analyzed to rule out infectious etiologies for diarrhea, including *Clostridium difficile* and *Cytomegalovirus.*

Table 2
Pediatric ulcerative colitis activity index (PUCAI)

Abdominal pain:	
No pain	0
Pain can be ignored	5
Pain cannot be ignored	10
Rectal bleeding:	
None	0
Small amount only, <50% of stools	10
Small amount with most stools	20
Large amount (>50% of stool content)	30
Stool consistency of most stools:	
Formed	0
Partially formed	5
Completely unformed	10
Number of stools per 24 h:	
0–2	0
3–5	10
6–8	20
>8	30
Nocturnal stools (any episode causing wakening):	
No	0
Yes	10
Activity level	
No limitation	0
Occasional limitation of activity	5
Severe restricted activity	10
Total (0–85)	

Imaging

Imaging is essential for evaluating the extent of disease, severity, and potential complications, such as abscesses, fistulae, or strictures. Magnetic resonance enterography (MRE) with oral contrast is the current imaging modality of choice for diagnosis in children suspected of IBD. It provides high diagnostic accuracy compared with both endoscopy/histology or upper gastrointestinal contrast study (UGI) with small bowel follow-through and avoids the radiation exposure of computed tomography (CT). CT enterography (CTE) can demonstrate active CD inflammation similar to MRE with high sensitivity and specificity, although given the radiation exposure, should not be used for regular monitoring of disease. Ultrasound is a helpful adjunct but should be complemented with the more sensitive MRE. In patients with VEO-IBD, small bowel ultrasonography should be considered first-line, as MRE often requires anesthesia [34].

Endoscopic findings

When IBD is suspected in a child based on clinical presentation and laboratory investigation, prompt referral to a pediatric gastroenterologist is necessary for endoscopic evaluation [35]. The gold standard for diagnosis and classification

Box 1: Laboratory Investigations for Suspected Inflammatory Bowel Disease in Children

Serologic Evaluation

Complete blood cell count with differential

Inflammatory markers

- C-reactive protein (CRP)
- Erythrocyte sedimentation rate (ESR)

Complete metabolic/liver panel

- Alanine/Aspartate aminotransferase
- Alkaline phosphatase
- Bilirubin
- Albumin level

Fecal Evaluation

Gastrointestinal infectious panel

- Bacterial: *Escherichia coli, Clostridium difficile, Campylobacter, Salmonella, Shigella, Yersinia*
- Ova and parasites

Fecal calprotectin or lactoferrin

Fecal occult blood

of IBD is both esophagogastroduodenoscopy and colonoscopy with ileal and colonic biopsies. Endoscopically, the most important reliable feature in UC is continuous colonic mucosal inflammation that begins distally in the rectum without small bowel involvement (aside from backwash ileitis). Histologically, UC will demonstrate architectural distortion with basal lymphoplasmocytosis with no granulomas [15]. CD, on the other hand, has endoscopic features consistent with mucosal aphthous ulcers, cobble stoning, skip lesions, and linear or serpiginous ulceration. Histologically, noncaseating granulomas, transmural inflammation, and submucosal fibrosis are common in CD [35]. As with its clinical presentation, IBD-U can have endoscopic features consistent with either UC or CD, thus making a firm diagnosis of CD or UC uncertain despite a complete workup [36].

MANAGEMENT

Goals of management

The management of CD and UC is challenging and constantly evolving. In the era of biologics, the goal of management has transitioned from simply symptomatic improvement to inducing remission, healing the mucosa, augmenting growth, and ultimately modifying the natural history of IBD while minimizing treatment-related toxicity. The mainstay of therapy requires both medical and surgical management.

Medical management

Corticosteroids

Oral corticosteroids are effective at induction of remission in both CD and UC with an expected response rate of 60% to 80% after approximately 4 weeks. However, half of children will become steroid-dependent or ultimately require surgery [37]. In addition, steroids are not used for maintenance therapy because of the well-described list of significant side effects of long-term steroid use. Budesonide, a high-potency corticosteroid that is effective within the bowel lumen, but has extensive first-pass metabolism from the liver when absorbed, is used as a time-released formulation for induction of remission of mild to moderate CD and UC, although it is ineffective as maintenance therapy [38].

Aminosalicylates

Aminosalicylates (5-ASA) have been used for more than 40 years and provide an anti-inflammatory effect to the intestinal mucosa either orally via a time-released formulation or enema. The newer generation of 5-ASA (mesalamine, balsalazide disodium, and olsalazine sodium) are generally better tolerated than the older sulfasalazine and effective at both inducing remission and maintenance therapy in patients with mild to moderate UC [39]. A prospective observational study of 213 children with UC taking maintenance 5-ASA found that 40% remained in steroid-free remission at 1 year [40]. Although used frequently in CD, systematic reviews and consensus guidelines do not support their efficacy [41,42].

Immunomodulators

Thiopurines, such as Azathioprine (AZA) and 6-mercaptopurine (6-MP), and methotrexate are the main immunomodulators that have been used as maintenance therapy for more than 30 years. The landmark randomized clinical trial that established early introduction (within 8 weeks of initial diagnosis) of 6-MP to a regimen of corticosteroids found 6-MP reduced the need for corticosteroids and improved the maintenance of remission in children with CD [43]. Side effects of thiopurines, including myelotoxicity, hepatotoxicity, and allergic reaction, are dose-dependent and can impact the ability to maintain compliance with the treatment regimen. When taking AZA, the metabolite thiopurine S-methyltransferase (TPMT) should be monitored to optimize drug-dosing and minimize drug-related toxicity [44]. The primary safety concern of immunomodulators in children are opportunistic infections, teratogenic effects in pregnant patients, and malignancy [45].

Biologics

The era of biologics has revolutionized how we manage and understand CD and UC. Infliximab, an anti–tumor necrosis tumor factor (TNF) monoclonal antibody, is generally recommended for both induction and remission of CD. By neutralizing the TNF-alpha receptor, patients are able to achieve an 83% response rate and remission rate of 55% at 1 year [46,47].

Immunomodulators induce mucosal healing and are the only drugs with the ability to heal perianal fistulas in CD [48,49]. In a recent study by Adler and colleagues [48], young patients with CD treated with introduction of a steroid-sparing therapy, including immunomodulators and anti-TNF-α medications, was associated with a 59% lower risk of developing fistulizing complication than those not treated with steroid-sparing therapy. More importantly, anti-TNF agents allow for improved linear growth in children who suffer from growth failure [47]. When patients with CD develop antibodies to infliximab, adalimumab is a human monoclonal TNF-α antibody that is considered a second step of biologic therapy [50].

Vedolizumab (VEDO), an anti-integrin monoclonal antibody, is a newer biologic that has a slower response rate in CD compared with the other biologics, but is less effective in UC [51]. Ustekinumab (USTE), an IL-23 monoclonal antibody, is another recently available biologic that is used for refractory CD or progression while on medical therapy. In a recent study comparing outcomes in patients with CD taking VEDO versus USTE found that USTE was more likely to lead to steroid-free clinical remission, biochemical remission, and comparable safety outcomes [52].

Combination therapy

Recently, immunomodulators have been used in tandem with biologics to decrease antibody formation against anti-TNF. A recent retrospective study of 502 children by the Pediatric Inflammatory Bowel Disease Collaborative Research Group Registry, infliximab taken with an immunomodulator for at least 6 months increased the chance the patient would benefit from infliximab for 5 years [53]. Yet, with lack of high-quality studies in the pediatric population and concerns about health risks, particularly with the risk for lymphoproliferative disorders with prolonged thiopurine exposure, the North American Society for Pediatric Gastroenterology, Hepatology, and Nutrition has been unable to recommend combination therapy for all pediatric patients with IBD, but rather within the context of individualization and risk stratification [45].

Surgical management (Crohn's disease)

Historically, the inability to wean from steroids was a frequent indication for surgical intervention. With the introduction of biologics, this is less of an issue and, rather, children will undergo surgery after failure to control the disease, including growth failure, escalation in medical management, or development of antibodies to biologics. Complications such as strictures, obstruction, fistula disease (intestinal and perianal), bleeding, and sepsis are currently the primary indications for surgery in CD. In the only randomized controlled trial comparing medical versus surgical therapy for newly diagnosed nonstricturing ileocecal CD, Ponsioen and colleagues [54] enrolled 143 patients who failed at least 3 months of conventional therapy (corticosteroids and immunomodulators) and were randomized to either receive infliximab or a laparoscopic ileocecal resection. Half of the patients treated with infliximab eventually required surgery, while the remaining continued to require biologic therapy. Of the patients who underwent ileocecal resection, almost half no longer required medical therapy at 5 years. Ileocecal resection for limited (<40 cm limited segment) uncomplicated terminal ileitis should be considered a viable treatment option, which compares favorably to anti-TNF therapy.

Acute Crohn's colitis

Most operations for CD are not true emergencies. Absolute indications for emergent operation include perforation, peritonitis, exsanguinating hemorrhage, and complete obstruction. The goal of emergent surgery is to control ongoing sepsis and resect diseased bowel, if possible, while focusing on bowel preservation, given that surgery is not curative. For those with medically refractory segmental colitis, bowel preservation should remain the goal.

Stricturing disease

When medical management fails for single short strictures, bowel resection is recommended (Fig. 1). When longer strictures or multiple small bowel strictures are present, a stricturoplasty is ideal to preserve bowel length. A typical short-segment stricture (up to 10 cm) may be managed by opening the bowel longitudinally along the antimesenteric side and reapproximating transversely in 2 layers. A longer stricture up to 20 cm can be folded on itself with the stricture at the apex and then opened at the apex, using a linear stapler to staple and divide the tissue between the proximal and distal limbs, thus creating a common channel [29].

Fistulizing disease

Transmural inflammation can result in fistulizing disease between bowel, bowel to bladder, and bowel to abdominal wall. Given the efficacy of infliximab in healing fistulizing CD, patients should undergo a trial of infliximab before surgical management [48,55]. In addition, when an abscess is present, drainage of the collection along with antibiotic treatment is used as first-line therapy in addition to medical immunosuppression (Fig. 2). The goal of surgery for an enterocutaneous fistula should be resection of bowel and the skin to healthy tissue with primary anastomosis. Entero-enteral fistulas may be subclinical until a considerable amount of bowel is bypassed. With regard to fistulas, only the segment of bowel with active disease should be resected, with the bystander segment of bowel or bladder repaired primarily, thus preserving bowel length and minimizing morbidity.

Perianal disease

The treatment of perianal CD is difficult and requires local control of any active infection or abscesses in addition to medical optimization. Perianal abscesses that are superficial and 1 to 4 cm in size should be managed with incision and drainage with at least 1 counterincision to allow for drainage, breaking up of loculations, and irrigation. A silicon vessel loop is left in place between

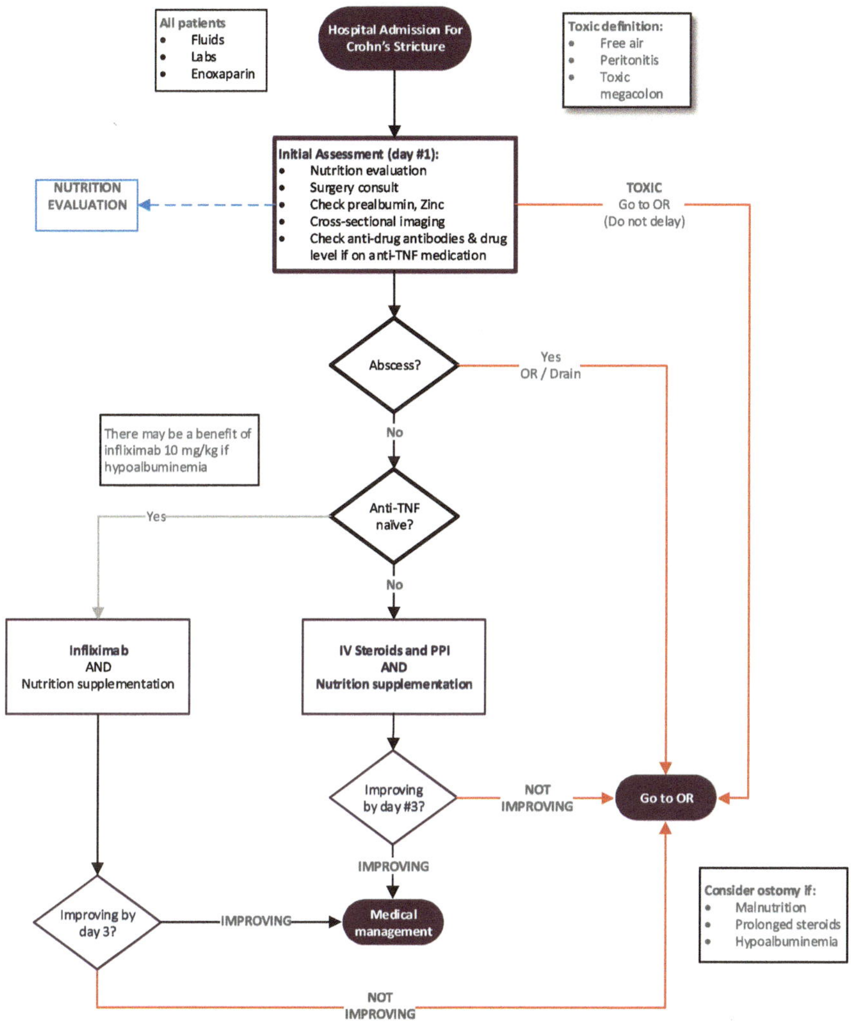

Fig. 1. Management of Crohn's stricture flowchart.

the incisions and secured to itself with silk ties [56]. Abscesses larger than 4 cm typically require more counterincisions and placement of a Penrose drain for thorough drainage. Although there is no consensus on the duration of seton placement, it can be left indefinitely depending on presence of ongoing symptoms and inflammation, as seen on MRI.

Similarly, fistulae that are identified, with or without a drainable abscess, should be managed with seton placement. Fistulotomy should be avoided due to the risk of nonhealing of the wound and incontinence. Compared with non-CD perianal fistulas, fistulotomy is an independent predictor of poorer quality of life [57].

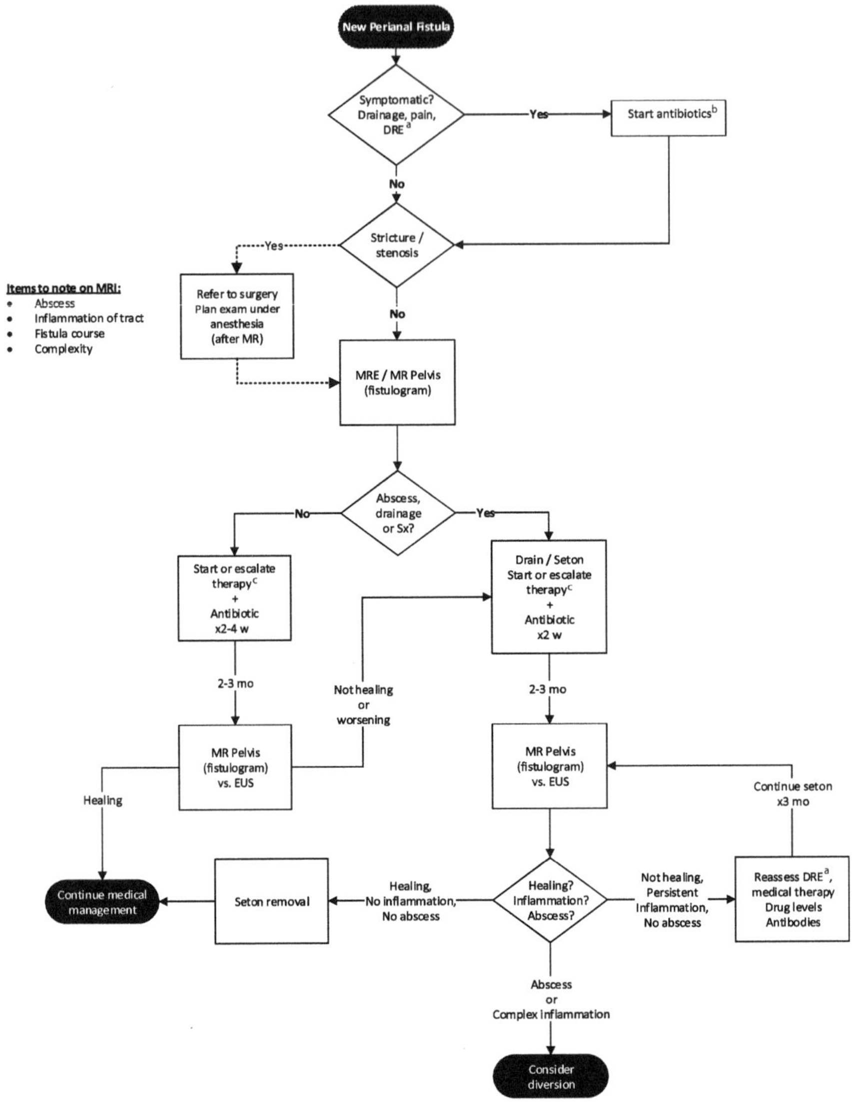

Fig. 2. Management of perianal fistula flowchart. Note, does not include rectovaginal fistulas. [a]Remember to perform *digital rectal exam* (DRE) to rule out stricture/stenosis. [b]Antibiotics: first choice Metronidazole, second choice Ciprofloxacin (if intolerant). [c]Escalation of therapy (if not already done): • Strongest evidence supports anti-TNF-α medication, • Consider high dose if hypoalbuminemic.

Surgical management (ulcerative colitis)

Acute setting

Similar to CD, most operations for UC are not true emergencies. Even in the setting of fulminant UC there is usually time to medically optimize patients for an operation (Fig. 3). Absolute indications for emergent operation include perforation, peritonitis, or exsanguinating hemorrhage. The goal of emergent surgery is to control ongoing sepsis or arrest hemorrhage and resect diseased bowel if possible without putting the patient at further risk. In UC, a subtotal colectomy is preferable to allow the option for restorative surgery in the future. Rarely, a total proctocolectomy may be necessary to control hemorrhage. In most emergent settings, a 3-stage approach is undertaken in which a colectomy and ileostomy is performed in the first stage; proctocolectomy with J-configuration ileoanal pouch anastomosis and ileostomy in the second stage; and takedown of ileostomy in the third stage. Many surgeons now use a double-stapled rather than a hand-sewn anastomosis, which may reduce operative time, especially by avoiding an often tedious submucosal dissection, while providing comparable outcomes to hand-sewn techniques [58,59].

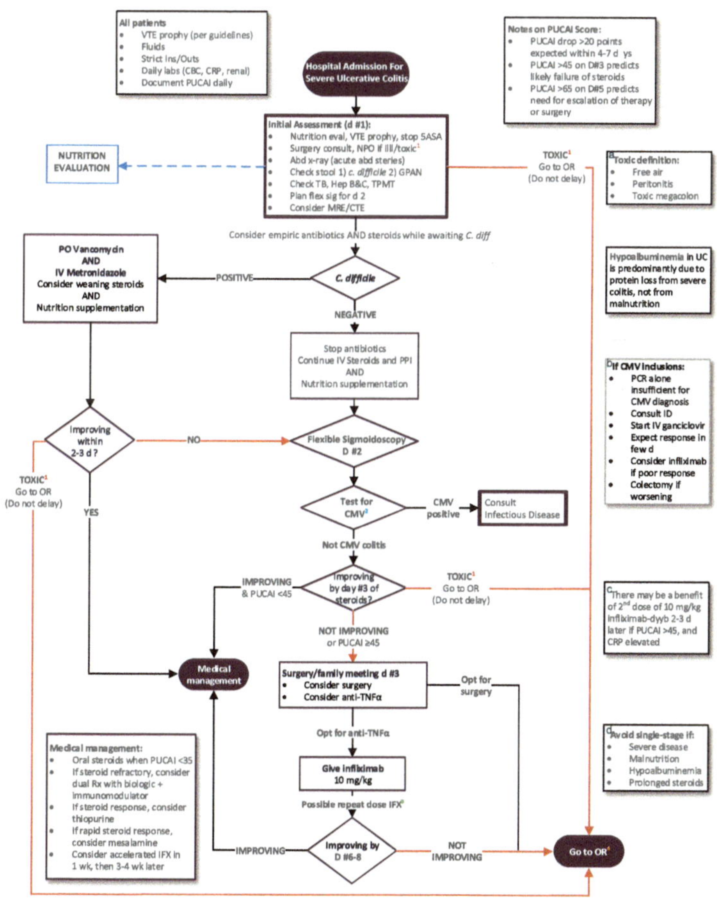

Fig. 3. Management of acute UC flowchart.

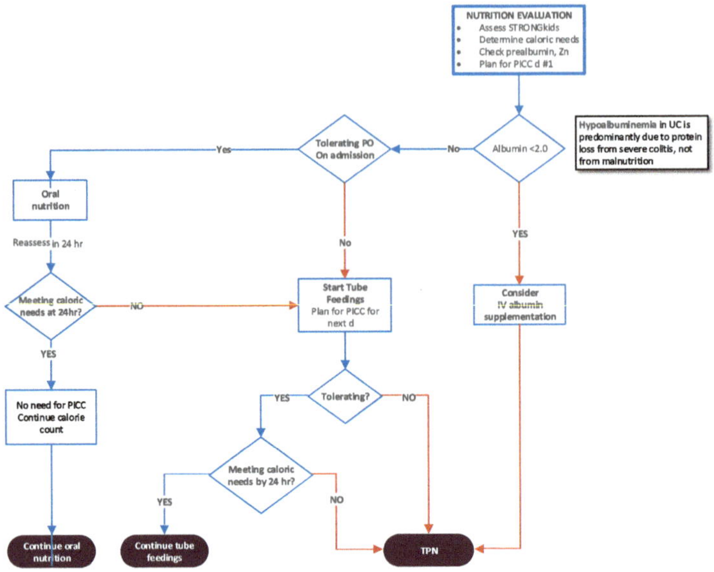

Fig. 3. (*continued*)

Elective setting

The 2-stage approach is the preferred method for patients with well-controlled disease and who are nutritionally stable. This approach includes a restorative proctocolectomy with ileoanal pouch anastomosis and diversion at the first stage and ileostomy closure as the second stage.

Relative contraindications to performing a 2-stage approach include severe proctitis (which may interfere with adequate dissection), high-dose steroids (which can impair healing of the anastomosis), and poor nutritional status. In the setting of these morbidities, a subtotal colectomy with diversion should be performed. Literature is beginning to emerge about the efficacy of a modified (or variant) 2-stage approach for these sicker patients over the traditional 2-stage approach [60,61]. In the modified or "reverse" 2-stage approach, an initial subtotal colectomy with ileostomy is performed followed by the ileoanal pouch anastomosis without an ileostomy. By performing the colectomy with ileostomy in the first stage, the patient can recover from the physiologic and nutritional impact of the disease before undergoing pouch creation [88].

Complications

Despite advances in surgical technique, there is a higher risk of postoperative infectious and anastomotic complications following bowel surgery for IBD compared with non-IBD conditions. Since biologics were first approved for pediatric IBD in 2006, hospitalizations in pediatric IBD have decreased, yet cumulative abdominal surgery rates have remained static or minimally increased [62,63]. Specifically for UC, it is difficult to determine if this reflects a more severe disease-process over time or evidence that biologic therapy does not significantly alter the natural history in children who become refractory to standard medical management. As such, children with UC who fail biologic therapy are presumably sicker with more severe disease at the time of colectomy. Whether preoperative biologic therapy contributes to postoperative complications remains unclear [64–66].

Pertaining to UC and pouch creation, risk of complications has been described as high as 76% [67]. Early complications occur anywhere from weeks to months following the initial colectomy and include leak, bleeding, wound infection, and small bowel obstruction. Strictures may occur that require dilation. Late complications pertain to function of the pouch, including pouchitis, incontinence, and impact on fertility. Pouchitis occurs in 25% to 70% of patients following pouch construction [68]. Most of those with pouchitis will experience looser and more frequent stools, mild to moderate incontinence, and intermittent bloody stools [69]. A course of metronidazole is often diagnostic and treats the acute pouchitis. Chronic pouchitis must be differentiated from CD of the pouch, which has become an increasingly common diagnosis in patients with pouch dysfunction. Given the challenging nature of distinguishing these diagnoses, pouch complications need to be evaluated with endoscopy with biopsies, and imaging studies to distinguish CD of the pouch from postoperative complications. The impact of surgical management on fertility has been increasingly discussed, yet data regarding IBD and infertility is lacking [70–72]. In a study by Ban and colleagues [73], women diagnosed with CD had lower rates of fertility following flares and surgery. Notably, women with UC were found to have a 21% decrease in fertility following surgery compared with women without IBD. Similarly, men with IBD have lower birth rates after diagnosis compared with before diagnosis. Sexual dysfunction may contribute to infertility, with erectile dysfunction as high as 26% following proctocolectomy [74]. Other variables may contribute to lower birth rates in patients with IBD, including issues related to nutrition, IBD therapies, and voluntary childlessness [75]. More research around IBD and reproductive health is needed and the impact on fertility should be discussed with patients and parents as part of preoperative counseling [72,76].

OUTCOMES

Nutrition and growth

Chronic blood loss, intestinal malabsorption (macronutrients and micronutrients such as iron, folate, Vitamin B/D), poor oral intake, increased energy requirements due to chronic inflammation, and corticosteroid use place patients with IBD at high risk for chronic malnutrition. This is particularly pronounced in pediatric IBD, because growth failure occurs in approximately 40% of CD and 10% of UC [77]. A dietician is a critical pillar in the multidisciplinary IBD team caring for pediatric IBD patients to help with assessing malnutrition and closely monitoring linear growth.

Psychosocial

As with any chronic disease, quality of life can be impacted significantly due to both the severity of disease activity and non–disease-specific psychological issues related to chronic disease [78]. Children with IBD have lower quality of life, higher rates of anxiety and depression, and reduced social and extracurricular activity compared with children with other chronic conditions [79]. Screening for quality of life in addition to anxiety and depression should be routinely performed. Medical providers can actively advocate for patients by engaging social work early in the disease process and helping to create individualized plans for reducing missed school and promoting school attendance (eg, unrestricted access to the restroom, extended time for completing assignments) [80].

Colon cancer

Over the decades, literature has demonstrated a clear link between the chronic inflammation inherent to IBD and the increased risk of colorectal cancer. A population-based study in 2001 reported that UC conferred a relative risk of colorectal cancer of 2.75 (95% confidence interval 1.91–3.97) when compared with a matched-population cohort of 2672 patients [81]. Although the risk of colorectal cancer in CD is less studied, an administrative claims database between 1998 and 2010 reported a 1.6-fold increase in colorectal cancer in patients with CD and colonic distribution, but not ileocecal disease [82]. The risk increases over time, and higher risk is associated with a younger age of diagnosis, presence of pancolitis, or with primary sclerosing cholangitis. Due to this increased risk, screening colonoscopy with biopsy should begin 7 to 10 years after the onset of symptoms and continue every 3 to 5 years, with increased frequency in patients at higher risk or with suspicious lesions.

FUTURE DIRECTIONS

Exclusive enteral nutrition

Exclusive enteral nutrition (EEN) is recommended as first-line therapy to induce remission of CD in children with active luminal disease, regardless of disease location. EEN allows for mucosal healing, which is essential for long-term remission [83,84]. EEN is included and recommended in contemporary consensus clinical guidelines from ESPGHAN, ESPEN, and NASPHGAN [85,86].

Collaborative care networks

Collaborative care networks, such as ImproveCareNow (ICN), are crucial to the future of pediatric IBD. These collaborations of patients, families, clinicians, and researchers allow for a concerted effort in improving the care of children with IBD. With input from the different stakeholders, best practices have been widely promoted, insights into discovery of new pediatric IBD genetic markers and the microbiome gained, and alternative medical treatments and approaches to care developed. However, ICN does not currently include postcolectomy data, thereby limiting its reach and applicability to patients post-UC surgery. Expanding to include surgical UC patients and outcomes would have a tremendous impact on this multidisciplinary care model, ultimately leading to improved care of all children with IBD.

Transition from childhood to adulthood

Dealing with chronic diseases such as IBD can be difficult for children, adolescents, and young adults. As they become more mature with increased autonomy, their health care needs change. A structured transition program is necessary to provide education, to support adherence to management therapies, and to ensure transition to adult care [87]. This can be facilitated by multidisciplinary IBD clinics with combined adult and pediatric providers that ultimately allow adolescents and young adults with IBD to easily and confidently navigate the transition from pediatric to adult health.

Fecal microbiota transplantation

Given the role bacterial loading and microbiota play in the pathogenesis in IBD, fecal microbiota transplantation (FMT) is an area of intense interest and innovation. A recent systematic review of 4 studies with 277 patients found that short-term use of FMT is an effective and safe treatment to induce remission in active UC. Yet, FMT needs to be further investigated before it can be considered as routine therapy.

SUMMARY

The incidence and prevalence of pediatric IBD are increasing throughout the world. Children with IBD, especially those with VEO-IBD, may present differently from adult-onset IBD. As the number of novel therapies increase, patients are increasingly able to have a tailored treatment plan that allows for improved remission with associated mucosal healing. With multidisciplinary IBD clinics, the focus of treatment plans should be on remission while promoting growth, adherence to the care plan, and limiting the toxicity of steroids and other medications. Equally as important as the medical management is the psychosocial function and ensuring smooth transition of pediatric to adult care. Through new discoveries and the concerted effort of collaborative care networks, we will continue to strive for a day when children with IBD enjoy sustained remission with minimal drug toxicity, optimal growth, and psychosocial development, and pursuit of their goals without IBD defining their lives.

CLINICS CARE POINTS

- Because VEO-IBD is difficult to different from CD or UC, patients should be described as CD-like or UC-like to allow longer follow-up and better characterization of the disease process.
- Combination therapy of immunomodulators and biologics increases the chances of biologic success at for 5 years. Caution should be used given the risk of lymphoproliferative disorders with prolonged thiopurine exposure.
- Early use of steroid-sparing therapy in young children with CD is associated with significant lower risk of developing fistulizing complication.

- Modified 2-stage operation for UC allows more acute patients the opportunity to recover from the physiologic and nutritional impact of their disease before undergoing pouch creation.

Disclosure

The authors have nothing to disclose.

References

[1] Kaplan GG. The global burden of IBD: from 2015 to 2025. Nat Rev Gastroenterol Hepatol 2015;12(12):720–7.
[2] Abramson O, Durant M, Mow W, et al. Incidence, prevalence, and time trends of pediatric inflammatory bowel disease in Northern California, 1996 to 2006. J Pediatr 2010;157(2):233–9.e1.
[3] Molodecky NA, Soon IS, Rabi DM, et al. Increasing incidence and prevalence of the inflammatory bowel diseases with time, based on systematic review. Gastroenterology 2012;142(1):46–54.e42.
[4] Ye Y, Manne S, Treem WR, et al. Prevalence of inflammatory bowel disease in pediatric and adult populations: recent estimates from large national databases in the United States, 2007-2016. Inflamm Bowel Dis 2020;26(4):619–25.
[5] Victoria CR, Sassaki LY, Nunes HRDC. Incidence and prevalence rates of inflammatory bowel diseases, in midwestern of São Paulo State, Brazil. Arq Gastroenterol 2009;46(1):20–5.
[6] Ng SC, Tang W, Ching JY, et al. Incidence and phenotype of inflammatory bowel disease based on results from the Asia-Pacific Crohn's and Colitis Epidemiology study. Gastroenterology 2013;145(1):158–65.e2.
[7] Khor B, Gardet A, Xavier RJ. Genetics and pathogenesis of inflammatory bowel disease. Nature 2011;474(7351):307–17.
[8] Xavier RJ, Podolsky DK. Unravelling the pathogenesis of inflammatory bowel disease. Nature 2007;448(7152):427–34.
[9] Hugot JP, Dumay A, Barreau F, et al. Crohn's disease: is the cold chain hypothesis still hot? J Crohns Colitis 2020;26(6):1–15.
[10] Ng SC, Shi HY, Hamidi N, et al. Worldwide incidence and prevalence of inflammatory bowel disease in the 21st century: a systematic review of population-based studies. Lancet 2017;390(10114):2769–78.
[11] Halfvarson J, Brislawn CJ, Lamendella R, et al. Dynamics of the human gut microbiome in inflammatory bowel disease. Nat Microbiol 2017;2(February):1–7.
[12] Pascal V, Pozuelo M, Borruel N, et al. A microbial signature for Crohn's disease. Gut 2017;66(5):813–22.
[13] Najarian RM, Ashworth LA, Wang HH. Microscopic/''' Backwash ''' ileitis and its association with colonic disease in new onset pediatric ulcerative colitis. J Pediatr Gastroenterol Nutr 2019;68(6):835–40.
[14] Benchimol EI, Bernstein CN, Bitton A, et al. Trends in epidemiology of pediatric inflammatory bowel disease in Canada: distributed network analysis of multiple population-based provincial health administrative databases. Am J Gastroenterol 2017;112(7):1120–34.
[15] Kugathasan S, Judd RH, Hoffmann RG, et al. Epidemiologic and clinical characteristics of children with newly diagnosed inflammatory bowel disease in Wisconsin: a statewide population-based study. J Pediatr 2003;143(4):525–31.
[16] Fuller MK. Pediatric inflammatory bowel disease. Surg Clin North Am 2019;99(6):1177–83.
[17] Adler J, Dong S, Eder SJ, et al. Perianal Crohn disease in a large multicenter pediatric collaborative. J Pediatr Gastroenterol Nutr 2017;64(5):e117–24.

[18] Singer AAM, Gadepalli SK, Eder SJ, et al. Fistulizing Crohn's disease presenting after surgery on a perianal lesion. Pediatrics 2016;137(3); https://doi.org/10.1542/peds.2015-2878.
[19] Childers RE, Eluri S, Vazquez C, et al. Family history of inflammatory bowel disease among patients with ulcerative colitis: a systematic review and meta-analysis. J Crohns Colitis 2014;8(11):1480–97.
[20] Rosen MJ, Dhawan A, Saeed SA. Inflammatory bowel disease in children and adolescents. JAMA Pediatr 2015;169(11):1053–60.
[21] Aloi M, Cucchiara S. Extradigestive manifestations of IBD in pediatrics. Eur Rev Med Pharmacol Sci 2009;13(Suppl. 1):23–32.
[22] Brown SR, Coviello LC. Extraintestinal manifestations associated with inflammatory bowel disease. Surg Clin North Am 2015;95(6):1245–59.
[23] Hyams J, Markowitz J, Otley A, et al. Evaluation of the pediatric Crohn disease activity index: a prospective multicenter experience. J Pediatr Gastroenterol Nutr 2005;41(4): 416–21.
[24] Turner D, Otley AR, Mack D, et al. Development, validation, and evaluation of a pediatric ulcerative colitis activity index: a prospective multicenter study. Gastroenterology 2007;133(2):423–32.
[25] Arai K. Very early-onset inflammatory bowel disease: a challenging field for pediatric gastroenterologists. Pediatr Gastroenterol Hepatol Nutr 2020;23(5):411.
[26] Kotlarz D, Beier R, Murugan D, et al. Loss of interleukin-10 signaling and infantile inflammatory bowel disease: implications for diagnosis and therapy. Gastroenterology 2012;143(2):347–55.
[27] Zaidi D, Wine E. Regulation of nuclear factor kappa-light-chain-enhancer of activated B cells (NF-κβ) in inflammatory bowel diseases. Front Pediatr 2018;6:1–9.
[28] Ouahed J, Spencer E, Kotlarz D, et al. Very early onset inflammatory bowel disease: a clinical approach with a focus on the role of genetics and underlying immune deficiencies. Inflamm Bowel Dis 2020;26(6):820–42.
[29] Kim A, Gadepalli S. Inflammatory bowel disease. In: Davenport M, Geiger J, editors. Operative pediatric surgery. 8th edition. Boca Raton: CRC Press; 2020. p. 440–51.
[30] Uhlig HH. Monogenic diseases associated with intestinal inflammation: implications for the understanding of inflammatory bowel disease. Gut 2013;62(12):1795–805.
[31] Kelsen JR, Russo P, Sullivan KE. Early-onset inflammatory bowel disease. Immunol Allergy Clin North Am 2019;39(1):63–79.
[32] Mack DR, Langton C, Markowitz J, et al. Laboratory values for children with newly diagnosed inflammatory bowel disease. Pediatrics 2007;119(6):1113–9.
[33] Alper A, Zhang L, Pashankar DS. Correlation of erythrocyte sedimentation rate and C-reactive protein with pediatric inflammatory bowel disease activity. J Pediatr Gastroenterol Nutr 2017;65(2):e25–7.
[34] Watson TA, Petit P, Augdal TA, et al. European Society of Paediatric Radiology abdominal imaging task force: statement on imaging in very early onset inflammatory bowel disease. Pediatr Radiol 2019;49(6):841–8.
[35] Levine A, Koletzko S, Turner D, et al. ESPGHAN revised porto criteria for the diagnosis of inflammatory bowel disease in children and adolescents. J Pediatr Gastroenterol Nutr 2014;58(6):795–806.
[36] Matsui T. [Natural history of inflammatory bowel disease]. Nihon Shokakibyo Gakkai Zasshi 2007;104(8):1172–11782.
[37] Tung J, Loftus EV, Freese DK, et al. A population-based study of the frequency of corticosteroid resistance and dependence in pediatric patients with Crohn's disease and ulcerative colitis. Inflamm Bowel Dis 2006;12(12):1093–100.
[38] Cohen SA, Aloi M, Arumugam R, et al. Enteric-coated budesonide for the induction and maintenance of remission of Crohn's disease in children. Curr Med Res Opin 2017;33(7):1261–8.

[39] Quiros JA, Heyman MB, Pohl JF, et al. Safety, efficacy, and pharmacokinetics of balsalazide in pediatric patients with mild-to-moderate active ulcerative colitis: results of a randomized, double-blind study. J Pediatr Gastroenterol Nutr 2009;49(5):571–9.
[40] Zeisler B, Lerer ÃT, Markowitz J, et al. Outcome following aminosalicylate therapy in children newly diagnosed as having ulcerative colitis. J Pediatr Gastroenterol Nutr 2013;56(1):12–8.
[41] Ruemmele FM, Veres G, Kolho KL, et al. Consensus guidelines of ECCO/ESPGHAN on the medical management of pediatric Crohn's disease. J Crohns Colitis 2014;8(10):1179–207.
[42] Lim WC, Wang Y, Macdonald JK, et al. Aminosalicylates for induction of remission or response in Crohn's disease. Cochrane Database Syst Rev 2016;(7); https://doi.org/10.1002/14651858.CD008870.pub2.
[43] Markowitz J, Grancher K, Kohn N, et al. A multicenter trial of 6-mercaptopurine and prednisone in children with newly diagnosed Crohn's disease. Gastroenterology 2000;119(4):895–902.
[44] Lee MN, Kang B, Choi SY, et al. Relationship between azathioprine dosage, 6-thioguanine nucleotide levels, and therapeutic response in pediatric patients with IBD treated with azathioprine. Inflamm Bowel Dis 2015;21(5):1054–62.
[45] Day AS, Gulati AS, Patel N, et al. The role of combination therapy in pediatric inflammatory bowel disease: a clinical report from the North American Society for Pediatric Gastroenterology, Hepatology and Nutrition. J Pediatr Gastroenterol Nutr 2018;66(2):361–8.
[46] Hanauer SB, Feagan BG, Lichtenstein GR, et al. Maintenance infliximab in Crohn's disease: the ACCENT I randomised trial. Lancet 2002;359:1541–9.
[47] Hyams J, Crandall W, Kugathasan S, et al. Induction and maintenance infliximab therapy for the treatment of moderate-to-severe Crohn's disease in children. Gastroenterology 2007;132(3):863–73.
[48] Adler J, Lin CC, Gadepalli SK, et al. Association between steroid-sparing therapy and the risk of perianal fistulizing complications among young patients with Crohn disease. JAMA Netw Open 2020;3(6):e207378.
[49] Lee MJ, Parker CE, Taylor SR, et al. Efficacy of medical therapies for fistulizing Crohn's disease: systematic review and meta-analysis. Clin Gastroenterol Hepatol 2018;16(12):1879–92.
[50] Corica D, Romano C. Biological therapy in pediatric inflammatory bowel disease a systematic review. J Clin Gastroenterol 2017;51(2):100–10.
[51] Ledder O, Assa A, Levine A, et al. Vedolizumab in paediatric inflammatory bowel disease: a retrospective multi-centre experience from the paediatric IBD porto group of ESPGHAN. J Crohns Colitis 2017;11(10):1230–7.
[52] Biemans VBC, van der Woude CJ, Dijkstra G, et al. Ustekinumab is associated with superior effectiveness outcomes compared to vedolizumab in Crohn's disease patients with prior failure to anti-TNF treatment. Aliment Pharmacol Ther 2020;52(1):123–34.
[53] Grossi V, Lerer T, Griffiths A, et al. Concomitant use of immunomodulators affects the durability of infliximab therapy in children with Crohn's disease. Clin Gastroenterol Hepatol 2015;13(10):1748–56.
[54] Ponsioen CY, de Groof EJ, Eshuis EJ, et al. Laparoscopic ileocaecal resection versus infliximab for terminal ileitis in Crohn's disease: a randomised controlled, open-label, multicentre trial. Lancet Gastroenterol Hepatol 2017;2(11):785–92.
[55] El-Matary W, Walters TD, Huynh HQ, et al. Higher postinduction infliximab serum trough levels are associated with healing of fistulizing perianal Crohn's disease in children. Inflamm Bowel Dis 2019;25(1):150–5.
[56] Tsoraides SS, Pearl RH, Stanfill AB, et al. Incision and loop drainage: a minimally invasive technique for subcutaneous abscess management in children. J Pediatr Surg 2010;45(3):606–9.

[57] Yassin NA, Askari A, Warusavitarne J, et al. Systematic review: the combined surgical and medical treatment of fistulising perianal Crohn's disease. Aliment Pharmacol Ther 2014;40(7):741–9.
[58] Slieker JC, Daams F, Mulder IM, et al. Systematic review of the technique of colorectal anastomosis. JAMA Surg 2013;148(2):190–201.
[59] Kennedy RD, Zarroug AE, Moir CR, et al. Ileal pouch anal anastomosis in pediatric familial adenomatous polyposis: a 24-year review of operative technique and patient outcomes. J Pediatr Surg 2014;49(9):1409–12.
[60] Traynor MD, Yonkus J, Moir CR, et al. Altering the traditional approach to restorative proctocolectomy after subtotal colectomy in pediatric patients. J Laparoendosc Adv Surg Tech A 2019;29(10):1207–11.
[61] Zittan E, Wong-Chong N, Ma GW, et al. Modified two-stage ileal pouch-anal anastomosis results in lower rate of anastomotic leak compared with traditional two-stage surgery for ulcerative colitis. J Crohns Colitis 2016;10(7):766–72.
[62] Park KT, Sin A, Wu M, et al. Utilization trends of anti-TNF agents and health outcomes in adults and children with inflammatory bowel diseases: a single-center experience. Inflamm Bowel Dis 2014;20(7):1242–9.
[63] Ihekweazu FD, Fofanova T, Palacios R, et al. Progression to colectomy in the era of biologics: a single center experience with pediatric ulcerative colitis. J Pediatr Surg 2020;55(9): 1815–23.
[64] Kunitake H, Hodin R, Shellito PC, et al. Perioperative treatment with infliximab in patients with Crohn's disease and ulcerative colitis is not associated with an increased rate of postoperative complications. J Gastrointest Surg 2008;12(10):1730–7.
[65] Narula N, Charleton D, Marshall JK. Meta-analysis: peri-operative anti-TNFα treatment and post-operative complications in patients with inflammatory bowel disease. Aliment Pharmacol Ther 2013;37(11):1057–64.
[66] Mitsuya JB, Gonzalez R, Thomas R, et al. The effect of biologics on postoperative complications in children with inflammatory bowel disease and bowel resection. J Pediatr Gastroenterol Nutr 2019;68(3):334–8.
[67] Koivusalo A, Pakarinen MP, Rintala RJ. Surgical complications in relation to functional outcomes after ileoanal anastomosis in pediatric patients with ulcerative colitis. J Pediatr Surg 2007;42(2):290–5.
[68] Pakarinen MP, Natunen J, Ashorn M, et al. Long-term outcomes of restorative proctocolectomy in children with ulcerative colitis. Pediatrics 2009;123(5):1377–82.
[69] Rintala RJ, Lindahl HG. Proctocolectomy and J-pouch ileo-anal anastomosis in children. J Pediatr Surg 2002;37(1):66–70.
[70] Faye AS, Oh A, Kumble LD, et al. Fertility impact of initial operation type for female ulcerative colitis patients. Inflamm Bowel Dis 2020;26(9):1368–76.
[71] Rajaratnam SG, Eglinton TW, Hider P, et al. Impact of ileal pouch-anal anastomosis on female fertility: meta-analysis and systematic review. Int J Colorectal Dis 2011;26(11): 1365–74.
[72] Purewal S, Chapman S, Czuber-Dochan W, et al. Systematic review: the consequences of psychosocial effects of inflammatory bowel disease on patients' reproductive health. Aliment Pharmacol Ther 2018;48(11–12):1202–12.
[73] Ban L, Tata LJ, Humes DJ, et al. Decreased fertility rates in 9639 women diagnosed with inflammatory bowel disease: a United Kingdom population-based cohort study. Aliment Pharmacol Ther 2015;42(7):855–66.
[74] Allocca M, Gilardi D, Fiorino G, et al. Sexual and reproductive issues and inflammatory bowel disease: a neglected topic in men. Eur J Gastroenterol Hepatol 2018;30(3):316–22.
[75] Tavernier N, Fumery M, Peyrin-Biroulet L, et al. Systematic review: fertility in non-surgically treated inflammatory bowel disease. Aliment Pharmacol Ther 2013;38(8):847–53.

[76] Wierstra K, Sutton R, Bal J, et al. Innovative online educational portal improves disease-specific reproductive knowledge among patients with inflammatory bowel disease. Inflamm Bowel Dis 2018;24(12):2483–93.
[77] Heuschkel R, Salvestrini C, Beattie RM, et al. Guidelines for the management of growth failure in childhood inflammatory bowel disease. Inflamm Bowel Dis 2008;14(6):839–49.
[78] Assa A, Ish-Tov A, Rinawi F, et al. School attendance in children with functional abdominal pain and inflammatory bowel diseases. J Pediatr Gastroenterol Nutr 2015;61(5):553–7.
[79] Kunz JH, Greenley RN, Howard M. Maternal, paternal, and family health-related quality of life in the context of pediatric inflammatory bowel disease. Qual Life Res 2011;20(8): 1197–204.
[80] Carreon SA, Bugno LT, Wojtowicz AA, et al. School functioning in adolescents with inflammatory bowel diseases: an examination of disease and demographic correlates. Inflamm Bowel Dis 2018;24(9):1624–31.
[81] Bernstein CN, Blanchard JF, Kliewer E, et al. Cancer risk in patients with inflammatory bowel disease: a population-based study. Cancer 2001;91(4):854–62.
[82] Herrinton LJ, Liu L, Levin TR, et al. Incidence and mortality of colorectal adenocarcinoma in persons with inflammatory bowel disease from 1998 to 2010. Gastroenterology 2012;143(2):382–9.
[83] Grover Z, Burgess C, Muir R, et al. Early mucosal healing with exclusive enteral nutrition is associated with improved outcomes in newly diagnosed children with luminal Crohn's disease. J Crohns Colitis 2016;10(10):1159–64.
[84] Grover Z, Muir R, Lewindon P. Exclusive enteral nutrition induces early clinical, mucosal and transmural remission in paediatric Crohn's disease. J Gastroenterol 2014;49(4):638–45.
[85] Forbes A, Escher J, Hébuterne X, et al. ESPEN guideline: clinical nutrition in inflammatory bowel disease. Clin Nutr 2017;36(2):321–47.
[86] Critch J, Day AS, Otley A, et al. Use of enteral nutrition for the control of intestinal inflammation in pediatric Crohn disease. J Pediatr Gastroenterol Nutr 2012;54(2):298–305.
[87] Carroll MW, Kuenzig ME, Mack DR, et al. The impact of inflammatory bowel disease in Canada 2018: children and adolescents with IBD. J Can Assoc Gastroenterol 2019;2(Supplement_1):S49–67.
88 Rubalcava NS, Moreno NA, Adler J, et al. Does the timing of pouch creation in 2-stage operations for pediatric patients with ulcerative colitis matter? Journal of Pediatric Surgery 2021;56:1203–7; https://doi.org/10.1016/j.jpedsurg.2021.02.023.

Advances in Pediatrics 68 (2021) 143–170

ADVANCES IN PEDIATRICS

Updates in Juvenile Idiopathic Arthritis

Deborah McCurdy, MD[a], Miriam F. Parsa, MD, MPH[a,b,*]

[a]Division of Allergy/Immunology/Rheumatology, David Geffen School of Medicine, UCLA, Mattel Children's Hospital, 10833 Le Conte Avenue, MDCC 12-430, Los Angeles, CA 90095, USA; [b]Pediatric Rheumatology, Cottage Children's Medical Center, 400 West Pueblo Street, PO Box 689, Santa Barbara, CA 93110-0689, USA

Keywords

• Arthritis • Juvenile idiopathic arthritis (JIA) • Spondyloarthropathy • Biologics • JAK inhibitors • Bone health • Diet

Key points

- Autoimmune arthritis is a systemic disease that affects not only the joints but also other organs and growth and development.
- Juvenile Idiopathic Arthritis classification is evolving as we better understand the disease process through genetic studies.
- An increased understanding of cytokine dysregulation has led to biologic therapies that have advanced the field of rheumatology and improved JIA prognosis and outcomes.
- For patients with autoimmune disease, maintaining a healthy balance in nutrition with sufficient Vitamin D and calcium, exercise, and sleep should be a priority.

INTRODUCTION

Juvenile idiopathic arthritis (JIA) is a clinically heterogeneous group of arthritides that has been divided into categories in order to better understand pathogenesis and prognosis. By definition, the disease starts before 16 years of age and persists for longer than 6 weeks; however JIA has distinct disease categories that have different presentations and symptoms [1–3]. Advances in genetics and immune system pathways help clarify the differences in presentations and clinical courses and better define each category of JIA [4].

*Corresponding author. Pediatric Rheumatology, Cottage Children's Medical Center, 400 West Pueblo Street, PO Box 689, Santa Barbara, CA 93110-0689. *E-mail address:* mparsa@sbch.org

https://doi.org/10.1016/j.yapd.2021.05.014

Current understanding of disease pathogenesis has resulted in remarkable advances in the targeted therapies: the biologics and the JAK inhibitors (JAKinibs). These new medications have changed the disease course and outcome for children with JIA. Despite these advances, therapies are not effective in all patients and there still is no cure.

CLASSIFICATION

The International League Against Rheumatism (ILAR) defined categories of JIA to better stratify disease presentation, clinical course, and prognosis and to aid in designing clinical trials. The criteria for diagnosis for each category include clinical and laboratory findings that aid in optimizing therapy [1,5]. The final proposal changed the name from juvenile rheumatoid arthritis (RA) to JIA. The proposal included 7 disease categories based on the features present in the first 6 months of illness: systemic arthritis, rheumatoid factor (RF)-positive polyarthritis, RF-negative polyarthritis, oligoarthritis (divided into persistent oligoarthritis, in which arthritis remains confined to 4 or fewer joints throughout the whole disease course, and extended oligoarthritis, in which arthritis extends to more than >4 joints after the first 6 months of illness), PsA, enthesitis-related arthritis (ERA), and undifferentiated arthritis (Table 1).

The criteria will be modified as understanding of the disease process further clarifies the categories. In 2011, Ravelli and colleagues [6] published an article proposing a distinct category of antinuclear antibody (ANA)–positive patients should be included. This group of children have early onset of disease, strong female predominance, prevalence of asymmetric arthritis, and increased risk for uveitis and currently is divided between the oligoarticular and RF-negative polyarticular groups. More recently, Eng and colleagues [7] used unsupervised machine learning that uncovered data-driven joint patterns that predicted clinical phenotypes and disease trajectories. Seven joint patterns were identified and named pelvic girdle, fingers, wrists, toes, knees, ankles and indistinct and were felt to better categorize the JIA groups for research studies and to determine prognosis.

Emerging molecular data challenge the current ILAR categories. For example, there has been an assumption that childhood-onset arthritis is different from adult-onset arthritis; however, genetic studies have revealed more similarities than differences [8]. Genome-wide association studies (GWASs) evaluating systemic JIA (sJIA), discussed later, suggests an interplay of more innate immune system dysfunction and autoinflammation, rather than autoantibody formation seen in most JIA categories. The Pediatric Rheumatology International Trials Organization (PRINTO) international consensus has taken the first step toward more accurately defining categories. These 4 categories–sJIA, RF-positive JIA, enthesitis/spondylitis-related JIA, and early-onset ANA-positive JIA–have yet to be formally validated; however, they demonstrate the evolving nature of the classification process [9].

INCIDENCE AND PREVALENCE

JIA is one of the most common chronic diseases in the pediatric population worldwide and certainly the most common of the rheumatic diseases in children. In Europe, the incidence rates varied from 1.6 to 23 and prevalence from 3.8/100,000 to 400/100,000. In the United States, the incidence is estimated at more than 14 patients per 100,000 and the prevalence at 96 patients per 100,000 [10]. Oligoarticular onset is more common in European descent but less common in the African American and Asian populations [11,12]. Differences in disease categories among racial and ethnic groups also have been reported, such as African-American children, are more likely to have a polyarticular onset than in white children [12], and, among Japanese children, sJIA is more common than oligoarticular form [13].

GENETICS

The genetics of JIA is under intense study, with candidate genes found in association with each category. HLA still confers the highest risk, notably HLA-B27 antigen association with ERA and spondyloarthritis, although there are many non-HLA associations described. The first report of risk alleles in the development of sJIA was described by the International Childhood Arthritis Genetics (INCHARGE) consortium, who performed a GWAS using DNA from nearly 1000 sJIA patients from multiple continents. Presence of the major histocompatibility complex (MHC) class II locus as a risk allele implicates a role for adaptive immunity in sJIA pathogenesis. The strongest non-MHC association was found in an intergenic region of chromosome 1, which overlapped a large cluster of transcription factor-binding sites [14]. Further research by Ombrello and INCHARGE colleagues [15] described 24 genetic loci with significant associations with sJIA; a majority of these loci had not been previously associated with inflammatory arthritis, providing strong genetic evidence for a distinction between sJIA and other JIA categories.

JUVENILE IDIOPATHIC ARTHRITIS CATEGORIES

Arthritis is the cardinal feature of JIA and is defined as heat, swelling, pain on motion, and/or limitation of motion. One of the most informative clinical symptoms is the presence of morning stiffness and its duration. Many children with JIA are described as slow in the morning or may limp. Also, these children often experience gelling or stiffness after a period of inactivity. Based on the number and pattern of joint involvement, patients are placed in 1 of the ILAR categories.

Oligoarticular juvenile idiopathic arthritis

Oligo is derived from Greek and means *few*. Oligoarticular JIA affects 4 or fewer joints and is the most common category, affecting more than 50% of children. The peak incidence is between 1 year and 3 years of age and often affects toddlers. One of the initial parental concerns may be that their baby is not

Table 1
Juvenile idiopathic subtypes (International League Against Rheumatism, 2011) and clinical features and optimal treatments

Juvenile diopathic Arthritis Subtype	Joints Involved	Age at Onset (y)	Gender (Female:Male)	ANA Positive (%)	Other Organs Involved	Differential Diagnosis (Common)	Therapy	Prognosis
Oligo-JIA persistent	$\leq$4 Asymmetric (eg, knee and PIP)	2–4 yo	3–5:1	30–60	Uveitis, leg length discrepancy	Septic joint, bone tumor	NSAIDs Steroid injection	Joint instability Uveitis
Oligo-JIA extended	$\leq$4 for 6 mo but then >4 Asymmetric	2–4 yo	3–5:1	30–60	Uveitis, leg length discrepancy	Septic joint, bone tumor	NSAIDs Mtx Biologics–TNF-α	Joint instability Uveitis
Poly-JIA RF-negative	5 or more Aymmetric	2–4 yo	3:1	20	Uveitis, joint instability	Infectious, postinfectious Malignancy Metabolic arthropathy	NSAIDs Mtx Biologics–TNF-α	Joint instability Uveitis
Poly-JIA RF- positive	5 or more Symmetric	Teens	3:1	20	Rheumatoid nodules, vasculitis, multiple organs	Infectious, postinfectious Malignancy Metabolic arthropathy	NSAIDs Mtx Biologics–TNF-α	Joint instability Joint replacements
sJIA	Variable, usually polyarticular	Throughout childhood	1:1	<5	Multiple organs, MAS	Sepsis Leukemia Malignancy	Steroids NSAIDs Mtx Biologics-IL-1	Joint instability Organ damage
Psoriatic	Usually $\leq$4 Asymmetric dactylitis	3–11yo	1:1	20	Skin	Infectious, malignancy	NSAIDs Mtx	Joint instability Skin malignancy

	Involves axial spine						Biologics-TNF-α	
ERA	Usually ≤4 Lower extremities Affects the SI joint and LS spine	>6 yo	1:7	Negative	Uveitis, Posture and gait abnormalities	Infectious, postinfectious Malignancy	NSAIDs Mtx Biologics–TNF-α	Joint instability Uveitis
Undifferentiated	Peripheral and axial spine	Older children, adolescents	1:1	+/−	IBD, skin, vasculopathy, other organs	Infectious, Malignancy	Tx for IBD Mtx	GI Vasculitis

learning to walk or falls often. Girls are affected more than boys (3–5:1, female [F]/male [M] ratio).

Oligoarticular JIA is an asymmetric arthritis: for example, 1 knee (the most common joint involved), wrist, ankle, or elbow, and a smaller joint, such as 1 of the proximal interphalangeal (PIP) joints. The hips or shoulders are involved less commonly and usually there is no involvement of the neck or spine. In most children, the arthritis remains in 4 or fewer joints, but in 30% to 40% the arthritis may become extended after 6 months of disease and involve 5 or more joints. Extended oligoarticular JIA is more severe and similar to polyarticular JIA but continues with asymmetric joint involvement [16].

Complications

Chronicity. Chronic arthritis leads to chronic changes in the joint: flexion contractures, joint subluxation, and instability of the joint. A potential result is a limb length discrepancy with the affected limb growing faster because of increased blood flow to the affected joints. Untreated, the joint ultimately fuses, resulting in a shortened limb. Treatment is designed to prevent joint instability and limb length discrepancies.

Anterior uveitis. The ANA test is positive in 30% to 65% of children with oligoarticular JIA and is associated with anterior uveitis in 15% to 30%. Anterior uveitis is inflammation of the iris, anterior uveal tract, and adjacent ciliary body (Fig. 1). Often, there are no symptoms and, to prevent irreversible changes, ophthalmology visits are scheduled routinely. In 2019, the American College of Rheumatology (ACR) updated guidelines for uveitis screening, emphasizing the presence of a positive ANA when determining risk (Table 2). Because the onset of ocular inflammation typically is asymptomatic, high-risk children should be checked by a pediatric ophthalmologist or uveitis specialist every 3 months for 4 years. If there is no sign of uveitis for more than 4 years, the risk becomes moderate, and the ophthalmology appointments can be scheduled every 6 months for 3 years and then annually. Typically, local steroid eye drops are used to control the disease, but more than 50% of children with uveitis require methotrexate (MTX) and/or a biologic to control the inflammation and the therapy generally continues for more than 2 years [17]. Untreated anterior uveitis may lead to glaucoma, cataracts, and blindness [18]. Specifically, monoclonal tumor necrosis factor (TNF)-α inhibitors (adalimumab and infliximab) now are an important component in the treatment of uveitis. In severe uveitis, infliximab can produce rapid decrease in inflammation and is used to save vision. The fusion protein etanercept may be associated with the onset of uveitis and thus is not used in treatment of uveitis [17,18].

Temporomandibular joint arthritis. Although temporomandibular joint (TMJ) involvement can be associated with all JIA categories, it may be the sole joint involved. The TMJ joint is unique in that the condyle is separated from the joint space by only a thin layer of fibrocartilage of type I and type II collagen. This makes it more vulnerable to arthritis changes. Children with TMJ arthritis

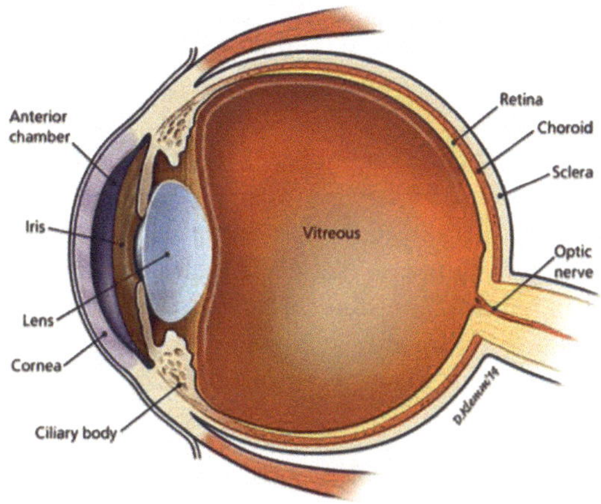

Fig. 1. Uveitis: the uvea located between the sclera and retina; the uvea consists of the iris, ciliary body, and choroid. (*Courtesy of* National Eye Institute; National Institutes of Health, *with permission.*)

often are asymptomatic; therefore, it has been suggested all children with JIA be screened for TMJ arthritis with magnetic resonance imaging [19]. Clinical symptoms include jaw pain, stiffness, clicking of the joint, and difficulty chewing. TMJ arthritis usually requires more aggressive therapies to prevent permanent destruction, including biologics [20]. Untreated, the problem worsens and may result in facial asymmetry and retrognathia with the need for operative correction or replacement.

Table 2
Ophthalmologic screening evaluation for juvenile idiopathic arthritis

Juvenile Idiopathic Arthritis Category	ANA–Positive and Onset Less at than 7 Years of Age and Duration Less than or Equal to 4 Years of Age	Antinuclear Antibody –Negative Onset at Greater than 7 Years of Age *OR* Duration Greater than 4 Years of Age
Oligoarticular	High risk	Low–moderate
Polyarticular, RF (−)	High risk	Low–moderate
PsA	High risk	Low–moderate
Undifferentiated arthritis	High risk	Low–moderate
Polyarticular, RF (+)	Low– moderate	Low–moderate
ERA	Low– moderate	Low–moderate
sJIA	Low–moderate	Low–moderate

High risk = every 3 mo screening.
Low–moderate risk = every 6 mo to 12 mo screening.
Data from Angeles-Han ST, Ringold S, Beukelman T, Lovell D, Cuello CA, Becker ML, et.al. 2019 American College of Rheumatology/Arthritis Foundation Guideline for the Screening, Monitoring, and Treatment of Juvenile Idiopathic Arthritis-Associated Uveitis. Arthritis Care Res (Hoboken). 2019 Jun;71(6):703-716. https://doi.org/10.1002/acr.23871. Epub 2019 Apr 25. PMID: 31021540; PMCID: PMC6777949.

Differential diagnosis
The differential includes infections and malignancy. A septic joint requires urgent treatment. If the onset of joint pain and swelling is sudden, unremitting, and associated with a fever, then the joint should be aspirated and cultured. In addition, radiographs should be obtained to evaluate the joint for effusions and chronic changes as well as to rule out a malignant tumor involving the bone. Musculoskeletal joint ultrasound increasingly is used in the diagnosis and management of JIA, because this dynamic imaging modality has been shown to be more sensitive than clinical examination and has other benefits over traditional imaging (eg, inexpensive, nonionizing, and assesses multiple joints at once and does not require sedation) [21,22].

Laboratory tests
The complete blood cell count (CBC) and acute phase reactants usually are normal. The test with the most prognostic significance is the ANA because it is associated with a greater risk for uveitis. The RF almost always is negative in oligoarthritis. Synovial fluid analysis shows 5000 white blood cells to 20,000 white blood cells with normal glucose and protein levels.

Treatment and prognosis
JIA is treated primarily with 5 categories of therapy: nonsteroidal anti-inflammatory drugs (NSAIDs), steroids (preferred locally), conventional synthetic disease-modifying antirheumatic drugs (DMARDs), targeted synthetic DMARDs, and biologic DMARDs (Table 3). Persistent oligoarticular JIA often responds to NSAIDs, but at times may require a joint injection with an intermediate-acting steroid preparation (triamcinolone) to quickly reduce the swelling and prevent damage. Joint injections may induce sustained remission in certain patients but, if this ideal response is not attained, may be repeated no more than twice per year. If nonresponsive to initial management, MTX is the second line of treatment. Because of the more aggressive and chronic nature of extended oligoarticular disease, biologic treatments may be needed to control the arthritis [23], discussed later.

Polyarticular juvenile idiopathic arthritis

Polyarticular JIA occurs in approximately 20% to 40% of patients with JIA, and these children have 5 or more joints affected by arthritis [24]. RF-negative polyarticular JIA is the most common (85%) and often presents in young girls (3:1, F/M) between 2 years and 4 years of age. The disease onset usually is insidious, with additional joints affected over time. The arthritis can be asymmetric but usually involves both sides of the body. The TMJ is affected in most patients. With the advent of biologics, spine complications are rarely seen. Unlike oligoarticular JIA, polyarticular JIA and sJIA are associated with marked inflammation and a catabolic state that results in growth failure (Fig. 2). RF-positive polyarticular JIA is most common in adolescent girls (10:1, F/M) of all ethnic backgrounds, with symmetric joint disease that involves the small

Table 3
Categories of juvenile idiopathic arthritis treatment, commonly used

Nonsteroidal Anti-inflammatory Drugs	Steroids	Conventional Synthetic Disease-Modifying Antirheumatic Drug	Biologic DMARD	Targeted Synthetic Disease-modifying Antirheumatic Drugs
Naproxen[a]	Triamcinolone hexacetonide[b] (for joint injection)	MTX[a]	Adalimumab	Tofacitinib
Ibuprofen		Leflunomide	Etanercept	Baricitinib
Celecoxib	Topical prednisolone (for uveitis)	Sulfasalazine	Rituximab	
Diclofenac	Oral prednisone (for severe flares)	Hydroxychloroquine	Golimumab	
Meloxicam			Tocilizumab	
			Abatacept	

[a] Commonly preferred first line in category.
[b] Triamcinolone hexacetonide is superior to triamcinolone acetonide in JIA outcomes but has not been readily available in the United States; therefore, triamcinolone acetonide has been used at higher doses.

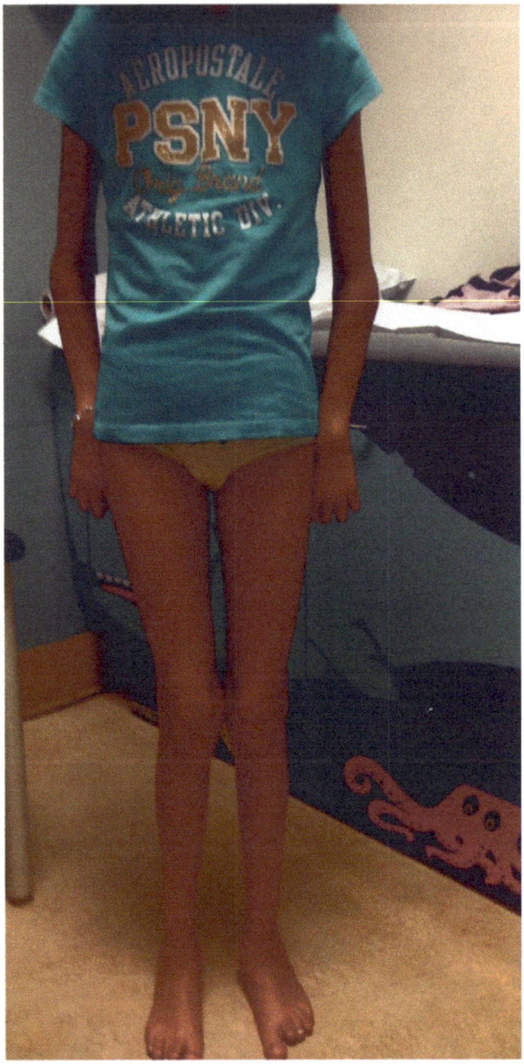

Fig. 2. RF-negative polyarticular JIA showing severe arthritis and cachexia when the inflammation is not well controlled.

and large joints, representing a spectrum of RA. The RF positivity is associated with more severe joint damage, as it is in RA [24].

Complications

Atlantoaxial subluxation. Especially those patients who have RF-positive polyarticular JIA or sJIA, it is important to assess for involvement of the cervical spine before surgery. The atlantoaxial or C1, C2 joints can be affected by arthritis resulting in damage to the integrity of the joint and subluxation. During intubation, a subluxed C1–C2 can cause spinal cord compression and possibly result in spinal cord damage. The diagnosis usually is made by plain films of the cervical spine in the neutral, flexed, and extended positions.

Extra-articular manifestations. Rheumatoid nodules are the most frequent extraarticular manifestation and occur most often in RF positive polyarticular JIA, with up to 30% of patients affected. The nodules portend a more severe disease course. As in RA, there are reports of vasculitis and Felty syndrome in RF-positive polyarticular JIA. Valvular heart disease and pulmonary parenchymal disease also have been seen and require more intensive therapies.

Differential diagnosis

The differential is broad, and a diagnosis is made after exclusion of infection, malignancy, and metabolic diseases. Infectious or postinfectious arthritis, as seen with viral infections or acute rheumatic fever, may have polyarticular joint involvement. In arthritis following a streptococcal infection, the arthritis usually is migratory. Malignancies, such as leukemia, may present with arthritis, but usually the laboratory tests are helpful in making the diagnosis. Metabolic and genetic disease may have associated arthropathies.

Laboratory tests

The CBC often shows anemia, usually the anemia of chronic disease, and may show a slightly increased white blood cell count. The erythrocyte sedimentation rate (ESR) and C-reactive protein (CRP) level often are increased. The ANA is positive in 50% and in younger children may be associated with anterior uveitis. Cyclic citrullinated peptide (CCP) antibody test is highly specific for polyarthritis seen in rheumatoid arthritis. Biomarkers promise to provide guidance in therapeutic decisions in the future. JIA activity is associated with activation of granulocytes and macrophages cells. The S100 proteins, calcium-binding proteins (such as calprotectin) that function as proinflammatory alarmins, are derived from phagocytes and are used as biomarkers; however, they currently are not commercially available [25].

Treatment and prognosis

Before 1999, children with polyarticular JIA usually had ongoing inflammation of their joints and required NSAIDs and MTX. Many had hours of morning stiffness and required intensive physical therapy to prevent contractures and atrophy. Since the advent of biologics, the prognosis has changed markedly. In 2018, an international group of experts outlined treatment goals for JIA, with the primary goal of assuring normal growth and development and avoidance of long-term systemic glucocorticoids [26]. One suggested measurement to monitor disease activity is through the use of the 10-point clinical Juvenile Arthritis Disease Activity Score, which measures active joint count, physician global disease activity score, and parent/patient global well-being score [27]. According to the updated 2019 ACR/Arthritis Foundation guidelines, patients first should be assessed for the presence of features that purport a poor prognosis, including cervical or hip arthritis, RF positivity, CCP positivity, and radiographic evidence of joint damage. Treatment is started early and stratified based on disease activity: mild, moderate/high. A DMARD is recommended for all polyarticular JIA patients at diagnosis, because monotherapy with NSAIDs rarely is successful. If there is an inadequate response to NSAIDs and MTX in 3 months, more aggressive treatment, usually with a TNF inhibitor, is indicated. Including a biologic DMARD and brief oral glucocorticoid course at disease onset is considered in the presence of severe polyarthritis or presence of poor prognostic factors [28].

There are many NSAIDs available, but usually naproxen is used first because of its safety profile and ease of use (twice per day dosing rather than 3–4 times per day). NSAIDs, MTX, and leflunomide (used when MTX not tolerated) may cause liver toxicity; therefore, liver function tests (LFTs) should be monitored. There are other available DMARDs, including sulfasalazine and hydroxychloroquine, but these are used less frequently in children. In 2020, the Food and Drug Administration (FDA) approved the use of tofacitinib, a JAKinib, in children age 2 years and older with polyarticular JIA. A more detailed discussion on JAKinibs and biologics are included later in chapter.

Systemic juvenile idiopathic arthritis

sJIA is included as a category of the ILAR classification of JIA and presents with high fevers, rash, lymphadenopathy, hepatosplenomegaly, and arthritis. As knowledge increased about the role of the innate immune system in inflammation and the autoinflammatory disease profile, sJIA appears to fit better into this category because it primarily is an innate, interleukin (IL-1) driven disease without associated autoantibodies [29,30]. The sJIA category includes the fewest number of children, making up 5% to 15% of all patients with JIA; however, it makes up the greatest mortality/morbidity of all JIA categories. The exact incidence is unknown; in Europe, the incidence is estimated at 0.3 per 100,000 to 0.8 per 100,000. There is no clear ethnic predilection. Boys and girls are affected equally and although sJIA can occur throughout childhood, the peak of onset is at 1 year to 5 years of age [31].

Fever is one of the most consistent presentations and, by definition, the fever must be greater than 39°C and return to less than 37°C between peaks for at least 3 days (called a quotidian fever). During the fever or at times of stress, the patients may have a salmon-colored rash that usually is nonpruritic and evanescent and may be difficult to see on dark skin tones. There may be a Koebner phenomenon that appears at the sites of trauma (Fig. 3). Criteria established by ILAR include arthritis and a quotidian fever of 2 weeks with 1 or more of the following: rash, lymphadenopathy, hepatosplenomegaly, and/or serositis. Arthritis may not be present at the time of the initial fever and may be delayed for up to 6 months and typically is polyarticular. The cardiac system may be involved in up to 30% of children and manifest as tachycardia, pericarditis, and pericardial effusions. Lymphadenopathy, hepatosplenomegaly, and hepatitis may be present. One curiosity is that approximately 50% of children with sJIA go into remission and it is not possible to predict this at onset. In contrast,

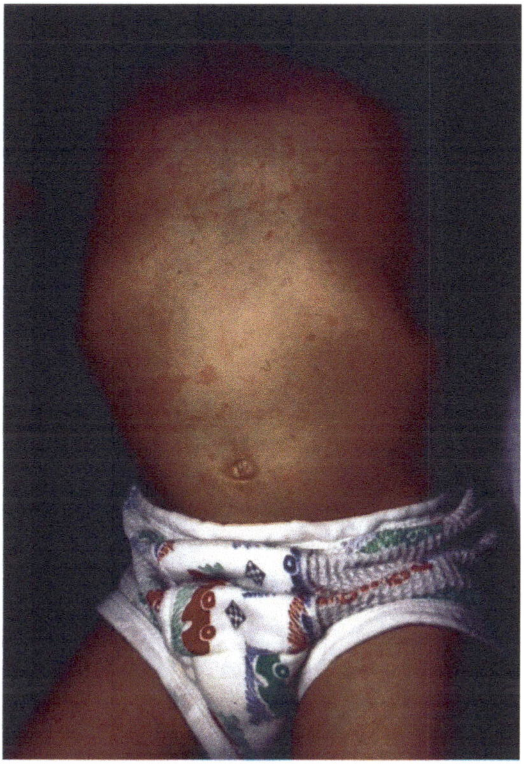

Fig. 3. The rash of sJIA with the Koebner phenomenon seen on the abdomen.

up to 8% develop macrophage activation syndrome (MAS), which previously was associated with mortality in more than 20% of children. Now, with earlier recognition and more aggressive therapy, mortality has decreased to 8% [32].

Macrophage activation syndrome

A frequent complication of sJIA is MAS that occurs as a full-blown picture in approximately 8% of children; however, a partial picture may be seen much more frequently. MAS may occur with infections, malignancies as well as systemic lupus erythematosus (SLE) and other autoimmune diseases; however, proportionately it is seen most commonly with sJIA and has been called a cytokine storm. There is accumulating evidence for a key role for free IL-18 as a driver to both sJIA and possibly MAS, and targeted treatment with a recombinant IL-18 binding protein currently is being studied [33]. In 2016, Ravelli and colleagues [34] published the European League Against Rheumatism/ACR/PRINTO classification criteria for MAS complicating sJIA (Box 1). The onset of MAS is sudden and severe and usually occurs early in the disease. The fever that was following a quotidian pattern becomes persistent and is associated with bruising and bleeding, mental status changes (including irritability,

Box 1: Criteria for macrophage activation syndrome in systemic juvenile idiopathic arthritis

Classification of MAS in sJIA (Ravelli and colleagues, 2016)

A febrile patient with known or suspected sJIA is classified as having MAS if the following criteria are met:

Ferritin greater than 684 ng/ml *and* any 2 of the following:

- Platelet count $\leq 181 \times 10^9$/L
- Aspartate aminotransferase greater than 48 U/L
- Triglycerides greater than 156 mg/dL
- Fibrinogen ≤ 360 mg/dL

seizures, and coma), lymphadenopathy, hepatosplenomegaly, and liver dysfunction. There is a precipitous decrease in at least 2 of 3 blood cell lines (leukocytes, erythrocytes, and platelets) and the ESR (secondary to hypofibrinogenemia). Tests that are helpful in the diagnosis of MAS include the CBC, comprehensive metabolic panel, ferritin, D-Dimer, fibrinogen, and triglycerides. In 2013, the ACR updated guidelines in response to the FDA approval of 2 important targeted therapies in sJIA. The guidelines include treatment recommendations of MAS complicating sJIA, such as intravenous (IV) methylprednisolone pulse therapy, cyclosporine A, and IL-1 inhibition [35]. Treatment should be started immediately, which requires early diagnosis.

Differential diagnosis

The differential of sJIA includes systemic infections and malignancies and a full work-up is indicated. At times, steroids are necessary to control the inflammation and a bone marrow test may be indicated to rule out malignancy before starting therapy.

Laboratory tests

There is marked increase in the levels of acute inflammatory markers in sJIA with high white counts with a shift to the left and high platelet counts, ESR, and CRP levels. The high platelet count helps in differentiating sJIA from leukemia. There usually is profound anemia that appears to be iron deficiency, but the bone marrow often shows adequate iron stores that are not being used secondary to inflammation. If a synovial aspiration is done, the cell count is 50,000/l L to 100,000/l L. Clinicians should be aware that these patients may develop MAS, especially early in the course of the disease. With persistent fevers and rash, a CBC, liver enzymes, ferritin, and D-dimer levels should be monitored to start treatment early if MAS is present.

Treatment and prognosis

Children with sJIA are the least likely to respond to the initial treatment with NSAIDs and MTX alone, although occasionally NSAIDs control children with mild sJIA. In 2013, the ACR updated guidelines in response to the results of 2 well-designed RCTs in 2012 that studied 2 important targeted therapies in sJIA: targeted anti–IL-1 monoclonal antibody (mAb) (canakinumab) and anti–IL-6 mAb (tocilizumab) [35–37]. Treatment guidelines categorize treatment recommendations based on the presence or absence of active systemic features, active joint count, and clinical assessment as well as if there is concern for MAS. Guidelines recommend early use of biologics to control systemic disease. For mild to moderate disease, NSAID monotherapy generally is not recommended for more than 1 week to 2 weeks as it is apparent whether systemic disease is controlled by this time. For moderate to severe disease, the current recommendation is to start IL-1 or IL-6 inhibitors early to control the systemic disease. Often, children with sJIA do not respond to TNF-a inhibitors. MTX often is used as a steroid-sparing agent, in particular in those children with significant arthritis. Glucocorticoids should not be used until the possibility of a malignancy has been excluded. The prognosis is guarded in many of these children. Although 80% respond favorably to treatment, 20% have ongoing disease and/or develop MAS despite treatment. Despite the recent advances in treatment, these children are still at increased risk for mortality (1% in North America), for permanent joint damage, and for increased morbidity related to cardiac involvement, CNS involvement, and MAS [32].

Juvenile psoriatic arthritis

The criteria for juvenile PsA (jPsA) as established by ILAR include psoriasis and 2 of the following: dactylitis (swelling of the entire digit), nail pitting or onycholysis, and/or psoriasis in a first-degree relative [38]. Psoriasis presents in 0.5% to 1% of children with arthritis. Children with jPsA have a presentation similar to oligoarticular JIA in the majority, but, unlike oligoarticular disease, jPsA can involve the shoulder, hip, spine, sacroiliac (SI) joint, and small joints. Treatment is similar to the treatment of JIA, with NSAIDs, MTX, and biologics, depending on the severity.

Enthesitis-related arthritis and juvenile ankylosing spondylitis

The ILAR criteria for ERA include arthritis or enthesitis and 2 or more of the following: onset of arthritis in boys more than 6 years old, SI joint or lumbosacral tenderness, presence of HLA-B27, family history of HLA-B27–associated diseases, and/or acute symptomatic anterior uveitis [39]. To make a diagnosis of juvenile ankylosing spondylitis (JAS), the axial skeleton must also be involved, most often the SI joint, and changes are noted on imaging. The exact incidence and prevalence are unknown, but ERA/JAS is much less common than JIA. ERA is more frequent in boys (1.4–7:1 M/F), but does occur in girls, usually with less severity. The onset is after 6 years of age, but the mean age of onset is 10 years to 13 years. The arthritis usually is oligoarticular, involving the lower extremities, including the hip. Tarsitis (inflammation of the tarsal joints) and enthesitis (inflammation at the attachment of ligaments and tendons) is seen in ERA. Involvement of the axial spine usually occurs later in the disease and is associated with HLA-B27 positivity. On forward flexion of the spine, there is decreased forward movement and flattening of the back. Other organ systems may be involved, most often uveitis, in 3% to 7% of children. Unlike the asymptomatic nature of anterior uveitis seen in oligoarticular JIA, HLA-B27 ocular disease is associated with acute onset of redness and pain. The treatment is similar to JIA, but often MTX is not as effective and TNF inhibitors are started earlier or in the place of MTX. The disease course is variable and remissions have been reported in up to 44% of patients. Damage to the hip and SI joints may occur, but often there is less axial involvement than is seen in adult-onset ankylosing spondylitis.

Undifferentiated

Other arthritis and arthropathies are included in this category, but the most common are the arthropathies associated with inflammatory bowel disease (IBD). This arthritis occurs in 7% to 21% of patients with IBD and may follow a polyarticular course but often also involves the SI joint and axial skeleton [40]. IBD-associated arthritis is considered to be peripheral SpA and coordination of medication management with pediatric gastroenterology is vital. Typically, arthritis symptoms improve when the IBD is controlled, but in a small percentage of children the arthritis persists and MTX is introduced. NSAIDs can be used judiciously in these cohort of patients.

BIOLOGIC THERAPIES

Cytokines are small proteins that bind to cellular receptors and affect cell signaling. They have a profound immunomodulatory role and, when dysregulated, can lead to a proinflammatory state and autoimmune disease. This increased understanding of cytokine immunoregulation has led to biologic therapies, including mAbs, inhibitors of cytokine binding, and enzyme inhibitors, each manufactured to block the binding of the cytokine to the receptor or to interfere with downstream activation induced by cytokine/receptor binding. This recent knowledge has resulted in a plethora of new therapies for autoimmune diseases with the potential for many powerful new immunomodulators that decrease inflammation and prevent the clinical manifestations of autoimmune disease.

Biologics usually are mAbs that when used for therapy have a name ending in "-mab". The antibody may be human with the name ending in "-umab" or a mixed human-murine chimeric antibody with the name ending in "-ximab". Fusion proteins, containing receptor domains or cell surface markers end in "-cept". The downstream JAK enzyme inhibitors end in "-nib" (Table 4).

Anti–tumor necrosis factor

One of the first cytokines known to be associated with inflammation was the TNF. TNF may remain on the cell surface or become soluble. TNF is produced by mainly by macrophages, but also by other cells of the immune system. TNF is a major proinflammatory mediator and may induce apoptosis. TNF-α has been identified as a cytokine with a major role in arthritis and vasculitis. As part of the proinflammatory function, TNF-α stimulates IL-1 secretion and induces cell proliferation and differentiation. mAbs to TNF-α have changed the course of arthritis. The efficacy of this group of medications is well studied in JIA. Infliximab (Remicade) works rapidly to decrease arthritis swelling and stiffness and is useful (although not approved by the FDA in children) for uveitis when other treatments fail. Etanercept (Enbrel), a fusion molecule is approved for children 2 years and older with JIA, adalimumab (Humira) a humanized mAb is approved for children 4 years and older with JIA, and golimumab (Simponi) is a humanized mAb IV infusion given every 8 weeks after induction, which was approved by the FDA in 2020 for poly JIA patients older than 2 years of age.

Anti–interleukin-1

The IL-1 proteins are another large cytokine family that activates signal transduction and inhibition leads to decreased pro-inflammatory transcription factors. The use of inhibitors to IL-1 has changed the disease course for those with sJIA, decreasing fevers, rashes, and joint pain. In many cases, the acute manifestations of MAS are controlled by IL-1 inhibitors and the morbidity and mortality are decreased. Anakinra (Kineret) is a recombinant version of the IL-1 receptor antagonist and competes with IL-1 for receptors on the cell surface. Rilonacept (Arcalyst) is a fusion protein that is made up of the ligand-binding domains of the extracellular portions of the IL-1 receptor linked to the Fc portion of human immunoglobulin G_1 (IgG_1). Rilonacept blocks IL-1α signaling by acting as a soluble decoy receptor that binds IL-1β and prevents its interaction with cell-surface receptors, whereas canakinumab (Ilaris) is a human mAb targeted at IL-1β.

Anti–interleukin-6

IL-6 is a proinflammatory cytokine that drives the production of other proinflammatory cytokines, such as TNF and IL-1. This combination of cytokines also induces the differentiation of type 17 helper T cell, which produces IL-17. IL-17 and TNF act together to promote activation of chondrocytes and fibroblast-like synoviocytes and production of metalloproteinases, which lead to joint destruction in RA. The beneficial effects of mAbs to IL-6, tocilizumab (Actemra), are well documented and currently are in use to treat polyarticular IJA and sJIA that is not responsive to initial treatments. Tocilizumab also may be useful in difficult to manage myositis.

Anti–interleukin-23 and anti–interleukin-17

IL-23 stimulates IL-17 and both are produced by helper T cells and are proinflammatory. IL-17 commonly is associated with the delayed-type hypersensitivity reaction and allergic responses but also with immune/autoimmune-related diseases. Recently, two mAbs, an anti–IL-17 antibody, secukinumab (Cosentyx) has been approved for the treatment of moderate to severe plaque psoriasis and PsA and the anti–IL-23 antibody ustekinumab (Stelara) has been used to effectively treat IBD and psoriasis by reducing IL-17.

Cellular immunomodulators

For a T cell to be activated, two signals must be presented by the antigen-presenting cell, the MHC combined with the antigen and the CD80 or

Table 4
Biologics used in pediatric rheumatic diseases

Target		Tumor Necrosis Factor Inhibitors			Interleukin-1 Inhibitors		Interleukin-6	Decreased T-cell Activation	B Cell	Type 17 Helper T Cells	JAK
Name Brand mame	Etaner -cept[1] Enbrel	Adalim -umab[2] Humira	Infli -ximab[3] Remicade	Anakinra Kineret	Rilona -cept[1] Arcalyst	Canakin -umab[2] Ilaris	Tociliz -umab[2] Actemra	Abata -cept[1] Orencia	Ritu -ximab[3] Rituxan	Ustekin -umab[2] Stelara	Tofaciti -nib Xeljanz
Dose	0.8 mg/ kg q wk SQ	15–30 kg 20 mg q 2 wk SQ >30 kg, 40 mg q 2 wk SQ	6–10 mg/kg q 2 wk × 2 then q mo IV	1 mg/ kg q wk SQ (higher doses may be required in MAS)	4.4 mg/kg SQ loading then 2.3 mg/kg SQ (max 160 mg)	4 mg/kg q 4 wk SQ	>2yo <30 kg 10–12 mg/ kg q 2–4 wk IV or SQ >30 kg 8 mg/kg q 2–4 wk IV or SQ	<75 kg 10 mg/ kg × 3 then q 4 wk IV or SQ	375 mg/ M_2 q 1 wk × 4 or 750 mg/M_2 q 2 wk × 2 IV	45 mg q 4 wk × 1 then q 12 wk SQ	5 mg po BID or 11 mg daily
Used to treat	JIA (oligo–ex poly), PsA, ERA, JAS	JIA (oligo–ex poly), PsA, ERA, JAS, uveitis	JIA (oligo–ex poly), PsA, ERA, JAS, uveitis, vasculitis (Takayasu)	JIA (systemic), periodic fevers	JIA (systemic), periodic fevers, gout	JIA (systemic), periodic fevers	JIA (poly, systemic)	JIA (oligo–ex poly), uveitis, arthritis of SLE, MCTD	SLE, ITP, Evan, CAPS, vasculitis (GPA, MPA), JIA (RF + poly)	PsA, Crohn	JIA (oligo–ex poly), ERA/JAS
Toxicity	Inj. site reaction, TB, fungal, MS, lymphoma, possibly uveitis	Inj. site reaction, TB, fungal MS, lymphoma	Inf. reaction, TB, fungal MS, lymphoma	Inj. site reaction, infection, high LFTs	Inj. site reaction, infection, high LFTs, lipids	Inj. site reaction, infection, high LFTs. neutropenia	Inf./hyper-sensitivity reactions, infection, TB, malignancy, MS, high lipids, GI perforation	Inj. site reaction	Inf. reaction, infections, progressive multifocal encephalo-pathy (JC polyoma virus)	Inj. site reaction, infection, TB, fungal, high LFTs	Infection, TB, fungal, high LFTs Avoid with liver disease

Used with other drugs	MTX 10–15 mg/M_2 q wk p or SQ	MTX 10–15 mg/M_2 q wk p or SQ	MTX 10–15 mg/M_2 q wk p or SQ	MTX cyclosporin 2.5–5 mg/kg/d	MTX 10–15 mg/M_2 q wk p or SQ	MTX 10–15 mg/M_2 q wk p or SQ	MTX 10–15 mg/M_2 q wk p or SQ	MTX 10–15 mg/M_2 q wk p or SQ	Other immune-suppressives	Other immune-suppressives	MTX 10–15 mg/M_2 q wk p or SQ

These are the most commonly used biologics as of this date; however, many more are being developed.

Names: 1-cept (fusion protein), 2-umab (humanized mAb), and 3-ximab (chimeric mAb).

The brand name is the name used in the United States. Anakinra: a recombinant form of IL-1Ra. Abatacept: $CTLA_4$ binds CD80/86 preventing the binding of CD28 to CD80/86. Dose: the usual doses, but each may be dosed differently or in higher doses with very active disease. Used to treat: the uses are expanding and each biologic may have additional uses. Oligoarticular (oligo). Extended polyarticular (ex poly). Toxicity: only the common ones are listed. Tuberculosis and hepatitis screens prior to start. See package inserts for full information. Injection (Inj). Infusion (Inf). Used with other drugs: the use of combined therapies increases the effectiveness in decreasing inflammation. With arthritis, MTX often is used in combined therapies; however, if not tolerated, leflunomide (Arava) may be used.

CD86 molecule (B7-1 and B7-2). Abatacept (Orencia) is a fusion protein made up of the Fc region of the immunoglobulin IgG1 fused to the extracellular domain of CTLA-4. Abatacept binds to the CD80 and CD86 molecule and prevents the second signal preventing T-cell activation. Abatacept is FDA approved for children greater than two years of age with JIA.

Anti-CD20

Rituximab (Rituxan) is a mAb against the protein CD20, which is found primarily on the surface of immune system B cells and in binding causes the B cell to undergo apoptosis. It has proved effective in non-Hodgkin lymphoma. In SLE, the B cells are the precursors to the plasma cells that produce antibodies. In antibody-mediated complications of SLE, JIA, JDM, and granulomatosis with polyarthritis, rituximab has been lifesaving.

Janus kinase inhibitors

Cytokines bind to their cell surface receptors that are bound on the cytoplasm to a kinase family, known as the Janus kinases (Jaks), and includes Tyk2, Jak1, Jak2, and Jak3. By blocking JAK, there is a decrease in multiple cytokines. Understanding of the JAK kinase pathway has allowed the creation of a unique therapeutic treatment of arthritis and other autoimmune diseases. These are not mAbs and are orally active. The JAKinibs include tofacitinib (Xeljanz) and has been tested in RA, IBD, and psoriasis as well as in renal transplantation rejection and dry eyes. In 2020, the FDA approved the use of tofacitinib in children age two years and older with polyarticular JIA. This is the first oral medication approved specifically for JIA in decades and has provided families with a much-anticipated noninjection option in MTX-refractory cases. Other JAKinibs inhibit primarily JAK1/JAK2 and include ruxolitinib (Jakafi) used for myelofibrosis and also for autoimmune diseases and baracitinib (Incyte) that has had promising clinical trials suggesting it may prove better than MTX for treatment of RA. Included in this review are the most commonly used biologics and JAKinibs used for the therapy for arthritis, but the future promises many new therapies, including biosimiliars, as well as therapies that target new pathways leading to arthritis.

DIET, ANTIBIOTICS, AND AUTOIMMUNITY

A major area of focus over the past decade is the role of the diet in the development of autoimmunity. Parents often get information from nonscientific reports, and children with arthritis are put on special diets that are restrictive, the most common being a dairy-free or gluten-free. Although there are clear implications of the gastrointestinal (GI) tract in the pathogenesis of certain types of arthritis, such as reactive arthritis, that follow certain bacterial infection and IBD-associated arthritis that is associated with inflammation in the small bowel and colon, there is no clear association with other JIA subtypes or other autoimmune diseases. In a meta-analysis of 204 articles that explored whether the introduction of allergic foods into the diet of infants was associated with allergies or autoimmunity, Ierodiakonou, and colleagues [41] reported that although the early introduction of eggs and peanuts resulted in reduced allergies to reduced egg and peanut allergies, the introduction of gluten was not associated with increased risk of celiac disease. None of these foods was associated with autoimmunity. Rare reports in the literature note that allergy to dairy products can cause abdominal pain and arthralgias that may mimic some aspects of JIA [42]. There are increasing numbers of reports that there is dysbiosis of the microbiome of children with arthritis, but there are no conclusive results to date.

The role diet plays on the GI tract microbiome is possible; however, the role of dairy and gluten specifically remains unknown [43–57]. There is parental perception, however, that a change in diet is beneficial. Little and colleagues [57] evaluated the prevalence of special diet adoption in JIA and parental perceptions of efficacy. In their study, approximately one-third of 261 patients had been tried on a special diet, including gluten-free, anti-inflammatory, and lactose-free, and approximately half of the parents reported improved pain or joint swelling [57]. Thus, the role of the diet in JIA remains an unanswered question, but, to date, elimination diets are not proven and may be harmful to a child's development.

In 2015, a study from the United Kingdom noted a link between antibiotic use and a 2-fold increase of JIA. The increased risk depended on the dose and was greatest for antibiotic exposures that occurred within 1 year of diagnosis. The investigators postulate that antibiotics cause an alteration of the intestinal microbiome, microorganisms found in the GI tract, with subsequent immune dysregulation [48].

Probiotics that are reported to provide the "good bacteria" to help to regulate the immune system often are tried in JIA. Several studies have reported that probiotic supplementation improved the disease activity and inflammatory status of patients with RA [58,59]. To date, the role of probiotics in the therapy for autoimmune disease is not clear and is not routinely suggested.

Currently, there is no cure for JIA; therefore, parents and patients frequently seek alternative therapies. Although these may have validity once studied, diets and alternative therapies should not preclude conventional treatments in severe or complicated disease. A healthy diet is important, however, and patients should be counseled on a healthy diet and exercise.

BONE HEALTH IN CHILDREN WITH JUVENILE IDIOPATHIC ARTHRITIS

Bone health in children with JIA is often compromised because of chronic inflammation, loss of muscle strength and the use of medications to control the disease, especially glucocorticoids. Inflammation profoundly affects the balance between osteoclasts and osteoblasts in bone remodeling and homeostasis. Osteoclasts, derived from hematopoietic stem cells, attach to the bone matrix and dissolve bone through phosphatases, lysosomal enzymes, and integrins. In the proinflammatory state seen with arthritis, there are high levels of

TNF-α, IL-β, and IL-6 that promote the production of osteoclasts and inhibit differentiation of osteoblast, increasing bone resorption and leading to osteopenia/osteoporosis [60–62].

Cholecalciferol (vitamin D_3) is essential for optimal bone health. Vitamin D_3 is produced by the dermis and epidermis when UV-B radiation converts 7-dehydrocholesterolin to cholecalciferol. Ergocalciferol (vitamin D_2) is made in mushrooms and yeast and is used in dietary supplements. Fish oils also are rich in vitamin D. Because 25-hydroxyvitamin D is stable for 3 weeks, this usually is the form tested for evaluation of vitamin D status. A deficiency in vitamin D results in a decline in the serum ionized calcium concentration, increased parathyroid hormone with increased production of osteoclasts, and lower blood phosphorus levels leading to osteoporosis. Vitamin D now is understood to have effects on more than calcium and bone homeostasis. Vitamin D can modulate both the innate and acquired immune systems [63–66]. A deficiency in vitamin D is associated with increased autoimmunity, and there are multiple studies suggesting that vitamin D deficiency is found in active SLE and arthritis and that a deficiency is associated with increased immune activation [67–69].

To optimize bone strength, weight bearing and muscle movement over the joint are necessary. In children with autoimmune disease, limitations in joint mobility and decreased energy secondary to the high catabolic state that occurs with inflammation may result in osteopenia [63]. In addition, corticosteroids may be a required part of treatment plan and can lead to osteopenia or osteoporosis. Trabecular bone that is the major constituent of the vertebral bodies is disproportionately affected compared with cortical bone [63]. Glucocorticoid therapy also is associated with an increased risk of avascular necrosis of bone, most often the femoral heads, leading to collapse and loss of the normal articular surface, resulting in pain and often the need for hip replacement.

Hypovitaminosis D in childhood is a public health problem in developed countries with contributing factors that include new lifestyle habits (many children staying indoors and exercising less during the COVID-19 pandemic) and the increased obesity in children and adolescents worldwide that lead to vitamin D deficiency [70]. A study in 2010 noted that the prevalence of vitamin D deficiency (levels below 15 ng/mL) was found in 9% and vitamin D insufficiency (levels below 30 ng/mL) was found in 15% of children and adolescents in the United States. Vitamin D deficiency was highest in non-Hispanic, African-descent adolescent girls (60%) and lowest in European-descent boys (1%) [71–73].

Current recommendations by Endocrine Society clinical practice guidelines are 400 IU daily in infants and children ages 0 to 1 year and 600 IU daily in children 1 year and older. The 25-hydroxyvitamin D blood level should be maintained consistently above 30 ng/mL. This may require doses up to 1000 IU in children and 2000 IU daily in adults [73,74]. Replacement doses suggested by an Australian and New Zealand consensus statement who are vitamin D deficient are suggested to be 1000 IU/d for infants less than 1 month old, 1000 to 5000 IU/d for infants 1 month to 12 months old, and greater than 5000 IU/d for children greater than 12 months old [75,76].

In children with JIA and severe osteopenia, bisphosphonate therapy, including alendronate, pamidronate, and clodronic acid, has been used, and studies suggest that there is an increase in the bone mineral density in the spine [77,78]. There are concerns about the use of bisphosphonates in children, however, including possible permanent effects on bone remodeling, impaired healing of fractures, possible damage to growth plates, and impaired linear growth. A notable adverse effect is osteonecrosis of the jaw.

SUMMARY

JIA is one of the most common of all chronic diseases in children. Unlike in adults, where there is essentially one presentation and clinical course, children with JIA, as it currently is defined, may present in six distinct categories. JIA nomenclature is evolving as more is learned about the genetics and respective pathophysiology of each category.

Oligoarticular JIA is the most common of all classes and is occurs most often in girls between 2 years and 4 years of age. The ANA is positive in approximately 60% of these patients and is associated with a greater risk of uveitis. Alongside the pediatric rheumatologist, the pediatric ophthalmologist plays a vital role in screening for occult uveitis. Teens with polyarticular JIA have a clinical course similar to adults with RA. sJIA now is understood to be an autoinflammatory disease with activation of the innate immune system. Children with sJIA rarely have autoantibodies; rather, they have high IL-1 and IL-18 levels that respond to IL-1 inhibition.

JIA categories of PsA, ERA, and JAS and other arthritis (eg, IBD-related spondyloarthropathies) share similar genetics and clinical course. In PsA, there usually is involvement of the skin or a family history of psoriasis. The course is most like oligoarticular JIA; however, axial arthritis may be present. ERA and JAS involves chronic inflammation of the entheses, peripheral joints, and axial skeleton: SI joints, hips, knees and ankles often are affected.

Research in JIA inflammation has opened the door to many new therapies, including anti-TNF and JAKinibs, while established therapies, including NSAIDs and MTX, continue to be used with frequency. The anti-TNF biologics are most helpful for all classes of JIA, except sJIA, where inhibition of IL-1 or IL-6 now is standard.

Regardless of the advances made in therapeutic targets, the importance of a healthy diet with sufficient calcium and vitamin D, exercise, and a good sleep cycle also should be prioritized for every child with chronic inflammation.

CLINICS CARE POINTS

- JIA is one of the more common chronic diseases in childhood, as common as type 1 diabetes mellitus. As such, pediatricians should be aware of the different presentations and diagnostic criteria and have an approach to initial therapy.
- As with all rheumatic diseases, diagnosis of JIA is one of exclusion: rule out infections, malignancy, and metabolic disease.
- The sooner JIA inflammation is under control, the less likely there will be joint damage. If a therapy is tried and there is insufficient response in 2 months, re-evaluate and reconsider other therapies.
- JIA is a systemic disease. Although JIA always affects the joints, it can affect other organs, especially the eye. In ANA-positive children under 7 years old, the patient should be sent to pediatric ophthalmology; this group is at high risk for asymptomatic uveitis.
- As the saying goes, "use it or lose it" children with arthritis should have a regular exercise program. Joint movement and weight-bearing activities are essential for maintaining range of motion and bone strength.
- As understanding of the genetics and immunology in JIA increases, new therapies are becoming standard of care and changing the prognosis of JIA.
- For pediatricians, a basic understanding of arthritis treatment, including biologics and JAKinibs, is essential in the assessment of medication side effects. It is imperative to order a QuantiFERON gold test or purified protein derivative test and a hepatitis panel with a hepatitis B surface antibody prior to starting therapy. Ideally, all immunizations should be up to date or the titer should be protective.
- For children with disease flares or limitations secondary to JIA, the public school system provides a 504 plan and, if necessary, an individualized education plan.

References

[1] Petty RE, Southwood TR, Manners P, et al. International League of Associations for Rheumatology classification of juvenile idiopathic arthritis: second revision, Edmonton, 2001. J Rheumatol 2004;31(2):390–2.
[2] Petty RE, Laxer RM. Wedderburn. Juvenile idiopathic arthritis. In: LR Petty RE, Laxer RM, Lindsley CB, et al, editors. Textbook of pediatric rheumatology. 7th edition. Philadelphia: Elsevier; 2016.
[3] Prakken B, Albani S, Martini A. Juvenile idiopathic arthritis. Lancet 2011;377(9783): 2138–49.
[4] Eng SW, Duong TT, Rosenberg AM, et al. REACCH OUTand BBOP Research Consortia The biologic basis of clinical heterogeneity in juvenile idiopathic arthritis. Arthritis Rheumatol 2014;66(12):3463.
[5] Merino R, de Inocencio J, Garcia-Consuegra J. Evaluation of revised international league of associations for rheumatology classification criteria for juvenile idiopathic arthritis in Spanish Children (Edmonton 2001). J Rheumatol 2005;32:559–61.
[6] Ravelli A1, Varnier GC, Oliveira S, et al. Antinuclear antibody-positive patients should be grouped as a separate category in the classification of juvenile idiopathic arthritis. Arthritis Rheum 2011;63(1):267–75.
[7] Eng SWM, Aeschlimann FA, van Veenendaal M, et al. Patterns of joint involvement in juvenile idiopathic arthritis and prediction of disease course: A prospective study with multilayer non-negative matrix factorization. PLoS Med 2019;16(2):e1002750.

[8] Nigrovic SR, Thompson S. Genetics and the classification of arthritis in adults and children. Arthritis Rheum 2018;70(1):7–17.
[9] Martini A, Ravelli A, Avcin T, et al. Pediatric Rheumatology International Trials Organization (PRINTO). Toward new classification criteria for juvenile idiopathic arthritis: first steps, pediatric rheumatology international trials organization international consensus. J Rheumatol 2019;46(2):190–7.
[10] Thierry S, Fautrel B, Lemelle I, et al. Prevalence and incidence of juvenile idiopathic arthritis: a systematic review. Joint Bone Spine 2014;81(2):112–7.
[11] Lawrence RC, Helmick CG, Arnett FC, et al. Estimates of the prevalence of arthritis and selected musculoskeletal disorders in the United States. Arthritis Rheum 1998;41(5):778.
[12] Schwartz MM, Simpson P, Kerr KL, et al. Juvenile rheumatoid arthritis in African Americans. Rheumatol 1997;24(9):1826.
[13] Fujikawa S, Okuni M. Clinical analysis of 570 cases with juvenile rheumatoid arthritis: results of a nationwide retrospective survey in Japan. Acta Paediatr Jpn 1997;39(2):245.
[14] Ombrello MJ, Remmers EF, Tachmazidou I, et al. HLA-DRB111 and variants of the MHC class II locus are strong risk factors for systemic juvenile idiopathic arthritis. Proc Natl Acad Sci U S A 2015;112:15970–5, 20.
[15] Ombrello MJ, Arthur VL, Remmers EF, et al. Genetic architecture distinguishes systemic juvenile idiopathic arthritis from other forms of juvenile idiopathic arthritis: clinical and therapeutic implications. Ann Rheum Dis 2017;76:906–13.
[16] Petty RE, Lindsley CB. Oligoarticular juvenile idiopathic arthritis. In: LR Petty RE, Laxer RM, Lindsley CB, et al, editors. Textbook of pediatric rheumatology. 7th edition. Philadelphia: Elsevier; 2016.
[17] Angeles-Han ST, Ringold S, Beukelman T, et al. 2019 American College of Rheumatology/ Arthritis Foundation Guideline for the Screening, Monitoring, and Treatment of Juvenile Idiopathic Arthritis-Associated Uveitis. Arthritis Care Res (Hoboken) 2019;71(6):703–16.
[18] Angeles-Han ST1, Pelajo CF, Vogler LB, et al, CARRA Registry Investigators. Risk markers of juvenile idiopathic arthritis-associated uveitis in the Childhood Arthritis and Rheumatology Research Alliance (CARRA) Registry. J Rheumatol 2013;40(12):2088–96.
[19] Weiss PF, Arabshahi B, Johnson A, et al. High prevalence of temporomandibular joint arthritis at disease onset in children with juvenile idiopathic arthritis, as detected by magnetic resonance imaging but not by ultrasound. Arthritis Rheum 2008;58(4):1189–96.
[20] Stoll ML, Kau CH, Waite PD, et al. Temporomandibular joint arthritis in juvenile idiopathic arthritis, now what? Pediatr Rheumatol Online J 2018;16(1):32.
[21] Magni-Manzoni S, Epis O, Ravelli A, et al. Comparison of clinical versus ultrasound-determined synovitis in juvenile idiopathic arthritis. Arthritis Rheum 2009;61(11): 1497–504.
[22] Janow GL, Panghaal V, Trinh A, et al. Detection of active disease in juvenile idiopathic arthritis: sensitivity and specificity of the physical examination vs ultrasound. J Rheumatol 2011;38(12):2671–4.
[23] Beukelman T, Patkar NM, Saag KG, et al. American College of Rheumatology Recommendations for the Treatment of Juvenile Idiopathic Arthritis: Initiation and Safety Monitoring of Therapeutic Agents for the Treatment of Arthritis and Systemic Features. Arthritis Care Res 2011;63(4):465–82.
[24] Rosenberg AM, Kiem GO. Polyarticular juvenile idiopathic arthritis. In: LR Petty RE, Laxer RM, Lindsley CB, et al, editors. Textbook of pediatric rheumatology. 7th edition. Philadelphia: Elsevier; 2016.
[25] Takeuchi T. Biomarkers as a treatment guide in rheumatoid arthritis. Clin Immunol 2018;186:59–62.
[26] Ravelli A, Consolaro A, Horneff G, et al. Treating juvenile idiopathic arthritis to target: recommendations of an international task force. Ann Rheum Dis 2018;77(6):819–28.
[27] Consolaro A, Giancane G, Schiappapietra B, et al. Clinical outcome measures in juvenile idiopathic arthritis. Pediatr Rheumatol 2016;14:23.

[28] Ringold S, Angeles-Han ST, Beukelman T, et al. 2019 American College of Rheumatology/ Arthritis Foundation Guideline for the Treatment of Juvenile Idiopathic Arthritis: Therapeutic Approaches for Non-Systemic Polyarthritis, Sacroiliitis, and Enthesitis. Arthritis Care Res (Hoboken) 2019;71(6):717–34.

[29] Pascual V, Allantaz F, Arce E, et al. Role of interleukin-1 (IL-1) in the pathogenesis of systemic onset juvenile idiopathic arthritis and clinical response to IL-1 blockade. J Exp Med 2005;201:1479–86.

[30] Ogilvie EM, Khan A, Hubank M, et al. Specific gene expression profiles in systemic juvenile idiopathic arthritis. Arthritis Rheum 2007;56:1954–65.

[31] DeBenedetti F, Schnieder R. Systemic juvenile idiopathic arthritis. In: LR Petty RE, Laxer RM, Lindsley CB, Wedderburn LR, editors. Textbook of pediatric rheumatology. 7th edition. Philadelphia: Elsevier.

[32] Davies R, Southwood T, Kearsley-Fleet L, et al. Mortality rates are increased in patients with systemic juvenile idiopathic arthritis. Arch Dis Child 2017;102:206–7.

[33] Yasin S, Schulert GS. Systemic juvenile idiopathic arthritis and macrophage activation syndrome: update on pathogenesis and treatment. Curr Opin Rheumatol 2018;30(5):514–20.

[34] Ravelli A, Minoia F, Daví S, et al. 2016 Classification Criteria for Macrophage Activation Syndrome Complicating Systemic Juvenile Idiopathic Arthritis: a European League Against Rheumatism/American College of Rheumatology/Paediatric Rheumatology International Trials Organisation Collaborat. Arthritis Rheumatol (Hoboken, Nj) 2016;68(3):566–76.

[35] Ringold S, Weiss PF, Beukelman T, et al. 2013 update of the 2011 American College of Rheumatology recommendations for the treatment of juvenile idiopathic arthritis: recommendations for the medical therapy of children with systemic juvenile idiopathic arthritis and tuberculosis screening among children receiving biologic medications. Arthritis Care Res (Hoboken) 2013;65(10):1551–63.

[36] Ruperto N, Brunner HI, Quartier P, et al, PRINTO; PRCSG. Two randomized trials of canakinumab in systemic juvenile idiopathic arthritis. N Engl J Med 2012;367(25):2385–95.

[37] De Benedetti F, Brunner HI, Ruperto N, et al, PRINTO; PRCSG. Randomized trial of tocilizumab in systemic juvenile idiopathic arthritis. N Engl J Med 2015;372(9):887.

[38] Nigrovic PA, Sundel RP. Psoriatic arthritis.. In: LR Petty RE, Laxer RM, Lindsley CB, et al, editors. Textbook of pediatric rheumatology. 7th edition. Philadelphia: Elsevier; 2016.

[39] Tse SML, Petty RE. Enthesitis related arthritis.. In: LR Petty RE, Laxer RM, Lindsley CB, et al, editors. Textbook of pediatric rheumatology. 7th edition. Philadelphia: Elsevier; 2016.

[40] Lindsley CB, Laxer RM. Arthropathies of Inflammatory Bowel Disease. In: LR Petty RE, Laxer RM, Lindsley CB, et al, editors. Textbook of pediatric rheumatology. 7th edition. Philadelphia: Elsevier; 2016.

[41] Ierodiakonou D, Garcia-Larsen V, Logan A, et al. Timing of allergenic food introduction to the infant diet and risk of allergic or autoimmune disease: a systematic review and meta-analysis. JAMA 2016;316(11):1181–92.

[42] Muñoz-Urribarri AB, Delgado Godos AG, Castillo Durand R, et al. Juvenile â€œidiopathicâ€ arthritis (JIA) as a manifestation of food allergy. Case study. Rev Gastroenterol Peru 2020;40(2):177–81, English.

[43] van Dijkhuizen EHP, Del Chierico F, Malattia C, et al. Microbiome analytics of the gut microbiota in patients with juvenile idiopathic arthritis: a longitudinal observational cohort study. Arthritis Rheumatol 2019;71:1000–10.

[44] Arvonen M, Vänni P, Sarangi AN, et al. Microbial orchestra in juvenile idiopathic arthritis: Sounds of disarray? Immunol Rev 2020;294(1):9–26.

[45] Klareskog L, Padyukov L, Lorentzen J, et al. Mechanisms of disease: genetic susceptibility and environmental triggers in the development of rheumatoid arthritis. Nat Clin Pract Rheumatol 2006;2(8):425–33.

[46] Catrina AI, Deane KD, Scher JU. Gene, environment, microbiome and mucosal immune tolerance in rheumatoid arthritis. Rheumatology (Oxford) 2014;55(3):391–402.

[47] McClure R, Massari P. TLR-dependent human mucosal epithelial cell responses to microbial pathogens. Front Immunol 2014; https://doi.org/10.3389/fimmu.2014.00386.
[48] Leifera CA, McConkey C, Li S, et al. Linking genetic variation in human Toll-like receptor 5 genes to the gut microbiome's potential to cause inflammation. Immunol Lett 2014;162(2):3–9.
[49] Horton DB, Scott FI, Haynes K, et al. Antibiotic exposure and juvenile idiopathic arthritis: a case-control study. Pediatrics 2015;136:e333.
[50] Sparks JA, Costenbader KH. Genetics, environment, and gene-environment interactions in the development of systemic rheumatic diseases. Rheum Dis Clin Northam 2014;40(4):637–57.
[51] McLean MH, Dieguez D Jr, Miller LM, et al. Does the microbiota play a role in the pathogenesis of autoimmune diseases? Gut 2015;64(2):332–41.
[52] Scher JU, Abramson SB. The microbiome and rheumatoid arthritis. Nat Rev Rheumatol 2011;7:569–78.
[53] Mu Q, Zhang H, Luo XM. SLE: another autoimmune disorder influenced by microbes and diet? Front Immunol 2015; https://doi.org/10.3389/fimmu.2015.00608.
[54] Taneja V. Arthritis susceptibility and the gut microbiome. FEBS Lett 2014;588(22):4244–9.
[55] Proal AD, Albert PJ, Marchall TG. The human microbiome and autoimmunity. Curr Opin Rheumatol 2013;25(2):234–40.
[56] Tejesvi MV, Arvonen M, Kangas SM, et al. Faecal microbiome in new-onset juvenile idiopathic arthritis. Eur J Clin Microbiol Infect Dis 2015;35(3):363–70.
[57] Little EM, Grevich S, Huber JL, et al. Parental perception of dietary intervention in juvenile idiopathic arthritis. J Altern Complement Med 2019;25(6):643–7.
[58] Vaghef-Mehrabany E, Alipour B, Homayouni-Rad A, et al. Probiotic supplementation improves inflammatory status in patients with rheumatoid arthritis. Nutrition 2014;30(4):430–5.
[59] Mandel DR, Eichas K, Holmes J. Bacillus coagulans: a viable adjunct therapy for relieving symptoms of rheumatoid arthritis according to a randomized, controlled trial. BMC Complement Altern Med 2010;10:1.
[60] Teitlebaum SL. Osteoclasts: what do they do and how do they do it? Am J Pathol 2007;170(2):427–35.
[61] Clements TL, Rosen CJ. The insulin like growth factor system and bone. Insulin-like growth factors. Austin (TX): Landes Bioscience; 2003.
[62] Kogianni G, Noble BS. The biology of osteocytes. Curr Osteoporos Rep 2007;5(2):81–6.
[63] Cimaz R, Ward L. The impact of rheumatic disease and their treatment on bone strength and development in childhood. In: Textbook of pediatric rheumatology. Philadelphia: Elsevier; 2016.
[64] Aranow C. Vitamin D and the immune system. J Investig Med 2011;59(6):881–6.
[65] Dusso AS, Brown AJ, Slatopolsky E. Vitamin D. Am J Physiol Ren Physiol 2005;289(1):F8–28.
[66] Ritterhouse LL, Crowe SR, Niewold TB, et al. Vitamin D deficiency is associated with an increased autoimmune response in healthy individuals and in patients with systemic lupus erythematosus. Ann Rheum Dis 2011;70:1560–74.
[67] Robinson AB, Tangpricha V, Yow E, et al. APPLE Investigators. Vitamin D deficiency is common and associated with increased C-reactive protein in children and young adults with lupus: an Atherosclerosis Prevention in Pediatric Lupus Erythematosus substudy. Lupus Sci Med 2014;1(1):e000011.
[68] Lee YH, Bae SC, Choi SJ, et al. Associations between vitamin D receptor a meta-analysis. Mol Biol Rep 2011;38:3643–51.
[69] Finch SL, Rosenberg AM, Vatanparast H. Vitamin D and juvenile idiopathic arthritis. Pediatr Rheumatol Online J 2018;16(1):34.
[70] Antonucci R, Locci C, Clemente MG, et al. Vitamin D deficiency in childhood: old lessons and current challenges. J Pediatr Endocrinol Metab 2018;31(3):247–60.

[71] Melamed ML, Kumar J. Low levels of 25-hydroxyvitamin D in the pediatric populations: prevalence and clinical outcomes. Ped Health 2010;4(1):89–97.
[72] Holick MF. Sunlight and vitamin D for bone health and prevention of autoimmune diseases, cancers, and cardiovascular disease. Am J Clin Nutr 2004;80(6 Suppl):1678S–88S.
[73] Holick MF, Binkley NC, Bischoff-Ferrari HA, et al. Evaluation, treatment, and prevention of vitamin D deficiency: an Endocrine Society clinical practice guideline. J Clin Endocrinol Metab 2011;96(7):1911–30.
[74] Bouillon R. Comparative analysis of nutritional guidelines for vitamin D. Nat Rev Endocrinol 2017;13(8):466–79.
[75] Misra M, Pacaud D, Petryk A, et al. Vitamin D deficiency in children and its management: review of current knowledge and recommendations. Pediatrics 2008;122(2):398–417.
[76] Chang SW, Lee HC. Vitamin D and health - The missing vitamin in humans. Pediatr Neonatol 2019;60(3):237–44.
[77] Munns C, Zacharin MR, Rodda CP, et al. Prevention and treatment of infant and childhood vitamin D deficiency in Australia and New Zealand: a consensus statement. Med J Aust 2006;185(5):268–72.
[78] Iqbal SM, Qamar I, Zhi C, et al. Role of bisphosphonate therapy in patients with osteopenia: a systemic review. Cureus 2019;11(2):e4146.

Advances in Pediatrics 68 (2021) 171–194
ADVANCES IN PEDIATRICS

Vitamin D Update in the Pediatric Population

Lindsey A. Warner, MD, MS[a,c], Rachel L. Sewell, MD[a,c], Nina S. Ma, MD[b,c,*]

[a]Children's Hospital Colorado, University of Colorado School of Medicine, 13123 East 16th Avenue, B158, Aurora, CO 80045, USA; [b]Bone and Mineral Metabolism Program, Section of Endocrinology, Children's Hospital Colorado, University of Colorado School of Medicine, 13123 East 16th Avenue, B265, Aurora, CO 80045, USA; [c]Department of Pediatrics, University of Colorado School of Medicine, Aurora, CO, USA

Keywords

• Vitamin D • Ergocalciferol • Cholecalciferol • Bone • Fracture • Infants • Children • Supplementation

Key points

- Risk factors for vitamin D deficiency include preterm and exclusively breastfed infants, darker skin, decreased sun exposure and sunscreen use, obesity, malabsorption disorders, and medications that increase vitamin D catabolism.
- Serum 25-hydroxyvitamin D is the analyte of choice and the best indicator of vitamin D status.
- There is not a standard definition of optimal vitamin D status in infants and children.
- Current evidence supports vitamin D supplementation for the prevention of rickets and vitamin D deficiency in preterm and exclusively breastfed infants.
- The association between vitamin D and bone health is most evident in children with the lowest vitamin D levels; there are mixed results regarding the ability of higher vitamin D targets to prevent fractures or increase bone mass.

INTRODUCTION

Cutaneous synthesis of vitamin D is responsible for 80% to 100% of circulating vitamin D concentrations [1,2]. 7-Dehydrocholesterol undergoes photochemical conversion to vitamin D_3 (cholecalciferol) in the basal layer of the

*Corresponding author. University of Colorado School of Medicine, 13123 East 16th Avenue, B265, Aurora, CO 80045. *E-mail address:* nina.ma@childrenscolorado.org

https://doi.org/10.1016/j.yapd.2021.05.008

epidermis with ultraviolet B exposure. The geographic latitude, seasonal tilt of the earth, and an individual's melanin pigment determine how much vitamin D is generated in the skin. Vitamin D is naturally found in fatty fish, cod liver oil, and egg yolks, and there are various vitamin D_2 (ergocalciferol) and D_3–fortified foods and supplements [3]. Vitamin D from the skin and dietary sources are converted by 25-hydroxylase in the liver to 25-hydroxyvitamin D [25(OH)-D], the major storage form of vitamin D in circulation. In the kidney, 25(OH)-D is converted by 1α-hydroxylase to 1,25-dihydroxyvitamin D [1,25(OH)$_2$-D], the active form of vitamin D. The expression and activity of 1α-hydroxylase is upregulated by hypophosphatemia and parathyroid hormone (PTH), a key regulator of calcium homeostasis. 1,25(OH)$_2$-D (calcitriol) increases serum calcium concentrations through several mechanisms. Calcitriol binds vitamin D receptors in the small intestine and facilitates active absorption of calcium [4] and phosphorus [5], promotes calcium reabsorption in the renal distal convoluted tubule, and activates osteoclasts that break down bone matrix, releasing calcium and phosphorus into the bloodstream. The subsequent increase in ionized calcium concentrations causes negative feedback to decrease PTH level and the activation step of vitamin D to calcitriol.

It is well documented that severe vitamin D deficiency, such as a serum 25(OH)-D concentration less than 12 ng/mL, can cause rickets in children and osteomalacia in adults [6]. Vitamin D deficiency rickets remains a global challenge, with moderate to high prevalence reported in regions including Africa, East and South Asia, Europe, and the Middle East [7]. An increasing prevalence of nutritional rickets has also been reported in high-income nations, partially driven by changes in the ethnic composition of pediatric populations and increasing numbers of immigrant and refugee children from the Middle East, Africa, and South Asia [8]. The estimated annual incidence of rickets per 100,000 young children has been reported to be 9 to 12 in Canada [9], 7.5 in the United Kingdom [10], and 24 in the United States [8,11]. In general, incidence rates of rickets are highest among breastfed children with intermediate to darker skin pigmentation and residing at northern latitudes [8,9].

Youth with obesity and lifestyle factors such as spending more time indoors, wearing sun-protective lotion and clothing, and consuming less vitamin D from foods or supplements are at greater risk of vitamin D deficiency [12]. Between 1988 to 1994 and 2001 to 2006, there was a 15% to 16% decline in mean serum 25(OH)-D concentrations among US adolescents, and the prevalence estimates of serum 25(OH)-D less than 30 nmol/L (<12 ng/mL) increased from 3% to 8% for ages 12 to 15 years and from 5% to 11% for ages 16 to 19 years [13]. It is encouraging that a more recent report concluded that the percentage of the US population at risk of vitamin D deficiency (<30 nmol/L or <12 ng/mL) remained stable from 2003 to 2014 [14].

The early recognition of vitamin D deficiency in pediatric populations is important to prevent rickets and to optimize bone mass accrual. It is well accepted that severe vitamin D deficiency negatively affects pediatric bone health. However, vitamin D has not consistently correlated with clinical outcomes such as fracture and bone mineral density (BMD). More research is required to determine the optimal vitamin D status in infants and children, and the standardization of vitamin D assays is needed as well. This article reviews the recent pediatric literature on vitamin D and skeletal health outcomes.

DEFINITION OF HYPOVITAMINOSIS D

The optimal 25(OH)-D concentration is debated. The Institute of Medicine (IOM) and the Endocrine Society published different guidelines for the evaluation and treatment of vitamin D deficiency in 2011. The IOM focused on skeletal health outcomes and recommended greater than or equal to 20 ng/mL as sufficient for the general population [15]. The Endocrine Society issued recommendations that included the general healthy population as well as cohorts with chronic conditions and suggested that 25(OH)-D concentrations between 21 and 29 ng/mL represented insufficiency and greater than or equal to 30 ng/mL was vitamin D sufficient [16]. Both groups agreed that 25(OH)-D concentrations less than 20 ng/mL constitute vitamin D deficiency.

The higher vitamin D targets issued by the Endocrine Society were based on adult studies. The evidence in children and adolescents is insufficient to determine that a 25(OH)-D concentration greater than 30 ng/mL is consistently associated with greater health benefits, particularly at a population level. Therefore, certain groups, such as the American Academy of Pediatrics (AAP) and the Pediatric Endocrine Society, did not increase their recommended daily intake of vitamin D and use a target 25(OH)-D concentration of greater than or equal to 20 ng/mL [17,18]. More research is needed to determine an optimal serum 25(OH)-D threshold for children and adolescents. Meanwhile, certain professional groups and pediatric bone experts may support the use of higher vitamin D targets in at-risk youth in clinical practice until more data become available [12].

PEDIATRIC AT-RISK GROUPS

Several pediatric groups are at increased risk of clinically significant hypovitaminosis D. Exclusively breastfed infants are at risk for declining concentrations of vitamin D if they are not supplemented with vitamin D [17,18]. Youth with decreased sun exposure because of limited outdoor physical activity, chronic illness, and sunscreen or coverage through clothing are more reliant on dietary intake of vitamin D because of decreased cutaneous synthesis of vitamin D [1]. Similarly, individuals with darker skin have increased melanin pigment, which mitigates the skin's ability to use sunlight to produce vitamin D [19]. Increased adiposity in obese individuals sequesters vitamin D and dysregulates its release into the circulation [20,21]. The Endocrine Society suggested that patients with obesity may require 2 to 3 times greater intake of vitamin D compared with their age group [16]. Patients with gastrointestinal disorders may have decreased absorption of macronutrients and micronutrients, including vitamin D, a fat-soluble vitamin, and individuals with severe liver disease may have decreased capacity to 25-hydroxylate vitamin D. Patients consistently receiving certain medications are also at increased risk for vitamin D deficiency. Several types of medications, including antiepileptics (eg, phenytoin, carbamazepine, phenobarbital), glucocorticoids, antibiotics, antiretrovirals, antihypertensives, and antineoplastic drugs act as pregnane X receptor (PXR) ligands [16,22]. Activation of PXR leads to increased catabolism of 25(OH)-D and calcitriol [22]. At-risk groups benefit from surveillance monitoring of their vitamin D status and supplementation to prevent vitamin D deficiency.

VITAMIN D ASSAYS

Serum 25(OH)-D is the analyte of choice and the best indicator of vitamin D status because of its stability and longer half-life of 25 days [23]. In contrast, calcitriol's half-life is 4 to 6 hours and it circulates in significantly lower concentrations, making it more challenging to measure [23]. Also, secondary hyperparathyroidism can increase calcitriol concentrations in patients with hypovitaminosis D via increased renal 1α-hydroxylation. The tight regulation of 1,25$(OH)_2$-D production makes it a less accurate measure of overall vitamin D status.

Available methods to measure 25(OH)-D include various immunoassays, high-performance liquid chromatography, and liquid chromatography–tandem mass spectrometry (LC-MS/MS) [23]. The different assays that are used to evaluate 25(OH)-D have contributed to challenges when defining vitamin D status and developing evidence-based guidelines for clinical practice. In 2010, the Office of Dietary Supplements of the National Institutes of Health organized the Vitamin D Standardization Program (VDSP) to standardize laboratory measurement of 25(OH)-D, and VDSP-recommended assay performance limits were established as a coefficient of variation (CV) less than or equal to 10% [ie, 25(OH)-D measurement variability] and bias less than or equal to 5% in relation to reference values [ie, trueness of a 25(OH)-D measurement] [24]. A comparison study of 15 different laboratories showed that only 50% of immunoassays achieved a CV less than or equal to 10% and 38% reached a bias less than or equal to 5%, whereas almost all LC-MS/MS results met VDSP criteria [25]. Different approaches have been used to improve the analytical performance of immunoassays for 25(OH)-D, but problems with sensitivity and specificity remain [26]. Presently, the desired method to accurately assess vitamin D status is LC-MS/MS [23,25–27]. However, immunoassays are commonly used clinically because of time and throughput concerns. There has been significant effort during the last 10 years to improve standardization of 25(OH)-D assays to reduce bias and facilitate comparability of measurements between laboratories, although more work is needed [28,29].

Related to 25(OH)-D assay standardization, there are specific clinical conditions when certain immunoassays may not perform properly. For instance, a significant proportion of total vitamin D can include C3 epimers in infants [30]. The clinical significance of C3 epimers is not well understood, but epimeric interference caused by cross reactivity can overestimate and lead to inaccurate laboratory assessments of vitamin D status [31]. Therefore,

25(OH)-D measurements in infants should be performed using a platform that differentiates between 25(OH)-D and vitamin D epimers [27]. Certain immunoassays may also underperform during physiologic states that alter vitamin D–binding protein concentrations, emphasizing the importance of testing immunoassays against a VDSP-standardized method to ensure comparable results [28].

VITAMIN D AND CLINICAL OUTCOMES

Fractures

Recent studies examining the relationship between vitamin D status and fracture were reviewed (Table 1). Although some studies support a role for higher vitamin D concentrations or supplementation to prevent fractures, other studies did not find an association. The 11 studies reviewed were identified using PubMed advanced search for human-based studies, with subjects from birth to age 18 years old, from 2010 to October 2020, and using key terms ("Vitamin D" OR "Cholecalciferol" OR "Ergocalciferol" [Title]) AND ("Fracture" [Title/Abstract]). Studies were included if subjects were healthy children, the total number of subjects exceeded 30, and outcome measures included fracture or fracture severity, and serum 25(OH)-D.

Several studies observed a positive relationship between vitamin D deficiency and fracture or fracture severity. Liu and colleagues [32] conducted one of the largest case-control studies (695 cases and 224 controls) and found the average serum 25(OH)-D level was significantly lower in children with upper limb fractures (24.5 ng/mL) compared with healthy controls (28.1 ng/mL). Karpiński and colleagues [33] also reported significantly lower median concentrations of vitamin D in their fracture group (12 ng/mL) compared with the control group (16 ng/mL). Hosseinzadeh and colleagues [34] did not report a statistically significant difference in mean 25(OH)-D levels between patients requiring surgical management of low-energy forearm fractures and the nonsurgical management group. However, a higher percentage of patients were vitamin D deficient in the surgical group (50%) compared with the nonsurgical group (17%), and vitamin D deficiency [25(OH)-D <20 ng/mL] was associated with a 3.8-fold greater risk of surgical management. A prospective case-control study in an urban population with diverse racial backgrounds showed that lower 25(OH)-D levels were associated with increased fracture risk after multivariate regression analysis [35]. Sixty-five percent of the fracture group had vitamin D deficiency or insufficiency, and, after controlling for confounders, there was a nearly 3-fold increase in fracture risk with vitamin D insufficiency [25(OH)-D 20–30 ng/mL] [35]. Accordingly, the investigators suggested targeting a 25(OH)-D concentration greater than or equal to 30 ng/mL because the increased fracture risk with vitamin D levels less than 30 ng/mL implied real health consequences. Minkowitz and colleagues [36] also noted a skeletal disadvantage in youth when their vitamin D levels were low. Although a relationship between 25(OH)-D and fracture occurrence was not identified, mean vitamin D concentrations decreased with increasing fracture severity

Table 1
Vitamin D status and fractures

Reference	Fracture group	Control group	Prevalence of vitamin D deficiency (<20 ng/mL); insufficiency (21–29 ng/mL)	Results
Schilling et al, [37] 2011	N = 118 infants (age<2 y) admitted to hospital with fracture (Philadelphia, PA)	None	FG: 8% (deficiency); 31% (insufficiency)	Suboptimal vitamin D status was not more common in children with fracture or multiple vs single fracture
Perez-Rossello et al, [38] 2012	N = 40 infants (age 8–24 mo) presenting to primary care for a well-child check (Boston, MA)	None	FG: 100% (deficiency)	Rachitic changes and definite demineralization were uncommon; zero fractures
Ceroni et al, [39] 2012	N = 100 youth (age 10–16 y) admitted to the hospital with first limb fracture (Geneva, Switzerland)	N = 50 healthy youth presented to the hospital as patients' visitors or volunteers	FG: 12% (deficiency); 36% (insufficiency) CG: 6% (deficiency); 34% (insufficiency)	No influence of low vitamin D status on limb fracture or lumbar spine and heel BMC/BMD
Contreras et al, [41] 2014	N = 100 children (age 1–18 y) presenting to a pediatric emergency department with fracture (Winston-Salem, NC)	N = 100 children evaluated for various problems that did not result in fracture	FG: 20% (deficiency); 43% (insufficiency) CG: 22% (deficiency); 42% (insufficiency)	No relationship between vitamin D deficiency and fracture risk
Minkowitz et al, [36] 2017	N = 369 children (age 2–18 y) presenting with fracture (Morristown, NJ)	N = 662 healthy children presenting to pediatrician or siblings of patients with fractures	FG: 20% (deficiency); 27% (insufficiency) CG: 18% (deficiency); 50% (insufficiency)	No association between 25(OH)-D and fracture; however, children with lower vitamin D levels had higher risk of more severe fractures
Anderson et al, [42] 2017	N = 206 children (age<6 y) recruited from a fracture clinic (Toronto, Ontario, Canada)	N = 342 matched controls from the TARGet Kids! primary-care research network	FG: 5% (deficiency) CG: 4% (deficiency)	No association between serum 25(OH)-D and fracture risk; however, vitamin D supplementation decreased odds of fracture

Thompson et al, [35] 2017	N = 60 children (age 2–14 y) presenting with fracture requiring sedation or anesthesia (Chicago, IL)	N = 60 children undergoing nonfracture orthopedic procedures	FG: 10% (deficiency); 55% (insufficiency) CG: 13% (deficiency); 32% (insufficiency)	Lower 25(OH)-D level associated with increased fracture risk; nearly 3-fold increased fracture risk with vitamin D insufficiency (20–30 ng/mL)
Karpiński et al, [33] 2017	N = 100 children (age 3–18 y) hospitalized because of fracture (Poland)	N = 127 children hospitalized for other reasons without fracture	FG: 97% CG: 93%	Patients with fracture had significantly lower median 25(OH)-D levels (12 ng/mL) compared with controls (16 ng/mL)
Ramirez et al, [40] 2019	N = 107 Hispanic children (age 1–18 y) (Puerto Rico)	N = 94 children with bone/joint pain without fracture	FG: 11% (deficiency); 35% (insufficiency) CG: 6% (deficiency); 48% (insufficiency)	No relationship between serum 25(OH)D and fracture risk
Hosseinzadeh et al, [34] 2020	N = 100 children (age 3–17 y) with low-energy forearm fractures prospectively enrolled from a single hospital and categorized as requiring surgery or nonsurgical management (Miami, FL)	None	FG: 21% (deficiency); 49% (insufficiency)	50% of the surgical management group were vitamin D deficient compared with 17% of the nonsurgical management group; 3.8-fold increased risk of surgical management with vitamin D deficiency
Liu et al, [32] 2020	N = 695 children (age 1–15 y) admitted for upper limb fracture (Shenyang, China)	N = 224 healthy children presenting for regular health check	FG: 40% (deficiency); 34% (insufficiency) CG: 35% (deficiency); 27% (insufficiency)	Patients with fractures had significantly lower serum 25(OH)-D levels

Abbreviations: CG, control group; FG, fracture group.

using the Abbreviated Injury Scale. Also, patients with vitamin D levels between 20 and 30 ng/mL were at more than 2-fold greater risk of presenting with a higher severity fracture, and, when vitamin D levels were between 12 and 30 ng/mL, patients were at more than 6-fold risk of presenting with more severe fractures compared with youth with vitamin D levels greater than or equal to 40 ng/mL. The investigators suggested a minimal target 25(OH)-D level of at least 40 ng/mL because their study found an increased risk for more severe fractures even at vitamin D levels of 30 to 40 ng/mL [36].

In contrast with the 5 studies outlined earlier, 6 studies did not find a strong correlation between vitamin D status and fracture. In an observational study of children younger than age 2 years and admitted with fracture to an urban pediatric hospital, vitamin D insufficiency was common [8% and 31% had 25(OH)-D levels <20 and 21–29 ng/mL, respectively] [37]. However, suboptimal vitamin D status was not more prevalent in children with fracture compared with a previously reported sample of healthy children. Moreover, the incidence of vitamin D insufficiency was similar whether children presented with a single fracture or multiple fractures. From a prospective sample of healthy infants and toddlers (aged 8–24 months) with vitamin D deficiency [25(OH)-D ≤20 ng/mL], Perez-Rossello and colleagues [38] examined bilateral wrist and knee radiographs for the presence of rachitic changes and demineralization. A fracture questionnaire and follow-up telephone interview were also conducted 2 to 3 years after the initial clinical encounter. In these children, rachitic changes and definite demineralization were uncommon, and there were zero fractures [38].

Ceroni and colleagues [39] evaluated the relationship between vitamin D status and first appendicular fracture in older children and adolescents (aged 10–16 years). There were no significant differences in the baseline serum 25(OH)-D levels between adolescents with upper and lower limb fractures and healthy controls, although the fracture groups showed mean 25(OH)-D levels of 32.1 ng/mL and 30.5 ng/mL for upper and lower limb fractures, respectively, which are in the vitamin D sufficiency range. Also, a correlation was not detected between serum 25(OH)-D and lumbar spine BMD (ascertained by dual energy x-ray absorptiometry [DXA]) and a low but significant inverse relationship was found between 25(OH)-D and spine bone mineral content (BMC) and calcaneal BMD z scores. The investigators note that their study failed to show an influence of low vitamin D status on spine and heel BMC and/or BMD, suggesting that other variables, such as pubertal status, race, or genetics, are confounding the relationship of vitamin D and bone mass accrual in adolescent youth [39]. When vitamin D levels and fracture risk were examined exclusively among Hispanic children (mean age, 8.6 years), a direct relationship between low vitamin D level and the incidence of low-energy fracture was also not established [40]. Similar to this study, Ramirez and colleagues [40] reported mean 25(OH)-D levels in both fracture and control groups in the sufficient range (33 ng/mL and 32 ng/mL, respectively). Also, the reported prevalence of vitamin D deficiency and insufficiency among

Hispanic youth living in Puerto Rico was similar to that of white youth living in Switzerland, an unexpected finding because Puerto Rico is located closer to the equatorial line and other studies have reported lower 25(OH)-D concentrations in Hispanic children [39,40].

Contreras and colleagues [41] examined the relationship between vitamin D deficiency and fracture risk in a prospective case-control study involving a diverse patient population and fracture types resulting from minor accidental injuries. Median 25(OH)-D levels were not statistically different between fracture and control groups (26.7 ng/mL vs 25.45 ng/mL), and vitamin D sufficiency was not a significant predictor of fracture after adjusting for male sex and season of enrollment. In secondary analyses, reported milk intake and multivitamin use were higher in youth with sufficient vitamin D levels greater than or equal to 30 ng/mL.

Similarly, in a large study of young children (age<6 years) with fracture (N = 206) and matched controls (N = 343), a significant association between 25(OH)-D and fracture risk was not identified, although the prevalence of vitamin D deficiency (<20 ng/mL) was low at 5% and 4% in fracture and control groups, respectively [42]. In contrast, children reported to regularly take a vitamin D supplement were shown to have a 58% reduction in the odds of fracture, a counterintuitive finding because serum 25(OH)-D and multivitamin use did not associate with fracture risk in this study. The investigators speculated that the practice of vitamin D supplementation may associate with certain healthy lifestyle characteristics or protective parenting that were not measured or accounted for in their analysis, and that there are differences between vitamin D supplements and multivitamins with regard to vitamin D dose and frequency of intake [42].

The reviewed studies also had secondary analyses and additional findings. For instance, of the 2 studies that evaluated fracture severity, only 1 found that overweight/obesity increased the likelihood of vitamin D deficiency and fracture requiring surgical management [34,36]. Minkowitz and colleagues [36] did not report an association between body mass index and vitamin D status. Studies that evaluated seasonal variation generally found that serum 25(OH)-D levels were highest in summer and autumn, and lowest in winter and spring. This finding was most evident in the study by Liu and colleagues [32], which reported 65.1% to 67.3% prevalence of vitamin D deficiency in winter and 14.7% to 24% prevalence in autumn. Most, but not all, studies that accounted for skin pigmentation found lower serum 25(OH)-D levels in children with darker skin [34–36,41]. Interestingly, when the 2 countries located at higher latitudes are considered, they yielded different results. A low prevalence of vitamin D deficiency and no association between serum 25(OH)-D and fracture were reported in Canada [42], whereas, in Poland [33], the median 25(OH)-D levels were low and patients with fracture had significantly lower median 25(OH)-D levels compared with controls. These data suggest that severe vitamin D deficiency associates with fracture risk and support the importance of public health measures for vitamin D supplementation that are well established in Canada [43] and underway in Poland [44]. In addition, Karpiński and colleagues [33] examined the impact of vitamin D receptor polymorphisms on serum vitamin D levels in children with low-energy fractures. Higher vitamin D levels were associated with the recessive aa genotype of ApaI and the dominant TT genotype of TaqI polymorphism.

Taken together, the recent pediatric vitamin D literature reports heterogenous results regarding the ability of vitamin D status in children to predict fracture risk. Five of the 11 studies reviewed here reported lower serum 25(OH)-D levels in children with fracture or more severe fracture. With minimal risk and modest evidence of benefit, it may be sensible to target 25(OH)-D levels greater than 30 ng/mL. Additional research is necessary to arrive at a standard definition of optimal vitamin D status in youth.

Bone imaging

Recent studies examining the relationship between vitamin D and bone health assessed by imaging modalities such as DXA, peripheral quantitative computed tomography (pQCT), and radiographs were reviewed (Table 2). Studies were identified using PubMed advanced search for human-based studies, in subjects from birth to age 18 years, 2010 to October 2020, and using key terms ("Vitamin D" OR "Cholecalciferol" OR "Ergocalciferol" [Title]) AND ("Bone" OR "Fracture" [Title/Abstract]). For the scope of this update article, vitamin D treatment trials were included if subjects were healthy children, total number of subjects exceeded 30, and primary outcome measures included bone imaging (radiographs, DXA, pQCT). Studies of premature infants located in the neonatal intensive care unit were also included because they constitute a significant proportion of pediatric practice and have increased risk of metabolic bone disease.

The importance of vitamin D during early infancy is well accepted. Preterm infants are at risk for vitamin D deficiency [45,46], and studies have shown a correlation between 25(OH)-D levels and gestational age at delivery [47–49]. However, the optimal 25(OH)-D target for premature infants is not well defined and various professional organizations recommend different doses of vitamin D [50].

Preterm infants fed an isocaloric, protein-enriched, and mineral-enriched postdischarge formula (PDF) showed increased gains in BMC during the first 6 months postterm compared with infants fed a standard term formula (TF) or human milk (HM) [51]. Van de Lagemaat and colleagues [52] showed that higher vitamin D intake and increases in 25(OH)-D levels associated with increased bone accretion in PDF-fed infants, suggesting that increased bone accretion in preterm infants is related to improved vitamin D status. PDF-fed preterm infants had significantly higher intake of dietary calcium and phosphorus as well, so vitamin D may play a partial or adjunctive role in the presence of adequate calcium and phosphorus availability to improve bone accretion in preterm infants between term and 6 months' corrected age (CA). The vitamin

Table 2
Vitamin D treatment trials with bone imaging outcomes

Reference	Study type and N	Participant characteristics	Intervention	Duration	Bone imaging	Effect of intervention
Ward et al, [58] 2010	Double-blind RCT N = 73 I: 37 C: 36	Postmenarchal girls aged 12–14 y recruited from an inner-city, multiethnic, all-girls school (Manchester, United Kingdom)	Four doses of 150,000 IU D_2 orally every 3 mo	1 y	DXA pQCT	25(OH)-D level was higher in the intervention group (56 nmol/L) vs controls (15.8 nmol/L); no effect of supplementation was shown on bone mass, geometry, or strength
Soliman et al, [61] 2011	Vitamin D treatment trial N = 40	Adolescents aged 11–17 y randomly selected from primary-care clinic and found to have 25(OH)-D <10 ng/mL; 65% (26 out of 40) had radiographic rickets (Doha, Qatar)	Intramuscular injection of cholecalciferol (10,000 IU/kg, max 600,000 IU)	1 y	Radiograph of wrist or knee	Mean 25(OH)-D level increased from 9.3 ng/mL to 27.7 ng/mL after treatment, although most had 25(OH)-D <20 ng/mL after 6 mo; 92% (24out of 26) had complete healing of radiographic rickets within 6–12 mo
Abrams et al, [54] 2012	Vitamin D intervention trial N = 38 Hispanic: 19 White: 19	Term infants of healthy mothers recruited from 2 hospitals (Houston, TX)	400 IU D_3 oral daily	3 mo	DXA	400 IU/d was sufficient to increase 25(OH)-D level to >30 ng/mL in white and Hispanic infants at 3 mo; however, there was no significant relationship between changes in 25(OH)-D and BMC

(continued on next page)

Table 2
(*continued*)

Reference	Study type and N	Participant characteristics	Intervention	Duration	Bone imaging	Effect of intervention
Al-Shaar et al, [60] 2013	Double-blind RCT N = 338 Low dose:113 High dose:114 Placebo: 111	Healthy girls and boys aged 10–17 y recruited from 4 schools (Beirut, Lebanon)	Placebo, 1400, or 14,000 IU D_3 oral weekly	1 y	DXA-derived hip structural analysis	Vitamin D supplementation improved bone mass and several structural bone parameters in adolescent girls, but not boys; a vitamin D dose effect was not detected
van de Lagemaat et al, [52] 2013	RCT N = 139 HM: 46 TF: 41 PDF: 52	Infants born at ≤32 wk and/or with birth weight ≤1500 g (Amsterdam, Netherlands)	PDF (median 445 IU/d), TF (median 380 IU/d), or HM + 200 IU vitamin D/d	From term age (40 wk) to 6 mo CA	DXA	PDF-fed infants had higher 25(OH)-D concentrations than TF-fed and HM-fed infants at 6 mo CA (103 vs 92.8 vs 95.6 nmol/L, respectively); greater vitamin D intake and serum 25(OH)-D level in PDF-fed infants associated with increased bone accretion during the first 6 mo after term

Gallo et al, [55] 2013 Gallo et al, [56] 2016	Double-blind RCT N = 132 400 IU: 39 800 IU: 39 1200 IU: 38 1600 IU: 16 Observational 3-y follow-up study N = 87 400 IU: 25 800 IU: 25 1200 IU: 26 1600 IU: 11	Healthy, term, breastfed infants aged 1 mo (Montreal, Quebec, Canada)	400 IU, 800 IU, 1200 IU, or 1600 IU D_3 oral daily	11 mo	DXA	25(OH)-D ≥50 nmol/L was achieved with all dosages in 97% of infants at 3 mo and was sustained in 98% at 12 mo; the 1600-IU/d dosage was discontinued at 3 mo because of 25(OH)-D ≥100 ng/mL. Spine, femur, and whole-body BMC did not differ by vitamin D dosage up to age 1 y, and >400 IU/d did not provide additional bone health benefit at age 3 y
Natarajan et al, [53] 2014	Double-blind RCT N = 96 400 IU: 48 800 IU: 48	Infants born at 28–34 wk receiving at least 100 mL/kg/d of enteral feeds by age 2 wk (New Delhi, India)	400 or 800 IU D_3 oral daily	Until 3 mo CA	DXA	Lower percentage of vitamin D deficiency among infants treated with 800 IU/d at 40 wk (38% vs 67%) and at 3 mo (12.5% vs 35%); serum 25(OH)-D level was higher in the 800-IU group at 40 wk (22.6 vs 15.7 ng/mL) and at 3 mo. BMC and BMD were not significantly different between groups at 3 mo CA. One infant in the 800-IU group had 25(OH)-D of 141 ng/mL at 3 mo CA

(*continued on next page*)

Table 2
(*continued*)

Reference	Study type and N	Participant characteristics	Intervention	Duration	Bone imaging	Effect of intervention
Hanson et al, [47] 2015	RCT N = 32 400 IU: 16 800 IU: 16	Infants born at <32 wk (Omaha, NE)	400 or 800 IU D_3 oral daily	8 wk	DXA	Mean 25(OH)-D level increased in both groups after 8 wk (54.1 vs 65.7 ng/mL for 400 and 800 IU/d, respectively). Free vitamin D correlated with 25(OH)-D; increasing free vitamin D level at birth associated with improved total-body BMC at term CA
Anderson-Berry et al, [50] 2017	Double-blind RCT N = 32 400 IU: 16 800 IU: 16	Infants born at 24–32 wk (Omaha, NE)	400 or 800 IU D_3 oral daily	8 wk	DXA	Median 25(OH)-D level increased in both groups and more significantly in the 800-IU group at 4 wk (105.3 vs 84.6 nmol/L). No difference in BMD seen between groups at term CA, but infants in the 400-IU group were more likely to have BMC <10%

Karlsland Åkeson et al, [62] 2018	Double-blind RCT N = 206 Fair skin: 108 Dark skin: 98	Healthy children aged 5–7 y from well-baby clinics and schools in November and December (Umea [northern] and Malmo [southern], Sweden)	80 (placebo), 400, or 1000 IU milk-based D_3 oral daily	3 mo in winter	DXA	BMC and BMD were higher in dark-skinned children despite lower 25(OH)-D levels. Changes in BMC and BMD did not differ between intervention and placebo groups in fair-skinned children, but femoral neck BMC increased more among dark-skinned children in the 400-IU and 1000-IU groups compared with placebo
Rosendahl et al, [57] 2018	RCT N = 975 I: 486 C: 489	Healthy, term infants, age 2 wk to 24 mo (Helsinki, Finland)	400 or 1200 IU D_3 oral daily	24 mo	Bone strength (CA)	At 24 mo, mean 25(OH)-D level was higher in 1200-IU/d group (47.16 vs 34.7 ng/mL), but no differences observed between groups in bone strength measures

Abbreviations: C, control; CA, corrected age; HM, human milk; I, intervention; max, maximum; PDF, isocaloric, protein-enriched, and mineral-enriched formula; RCT, randomized controlled trial; TF, term formula.

D intake for PDF-fed infants was 445 IU/d, which is consistent with current supplementation guidelines. None of the infants at 6 months' CA had vitamin D deficiency or insufficiency.

In another study of preterm infants that randomized patients born at less than 32 weeks to receive 400 IU/d or 800 IU/d of vitamin D_3 (in addition to a parenteral multivitamin while on parenteral nutrition and enteral vitamin D from human milk fortifier or preterm formula), median 25(OH)-D levels increased in both groups to 84.6 nmol/L (33.8 ng/mL) and 105.3 nmol/L (41.1 ng/mL) at 4 weeks and 114.1 nmol/L (45.6 ng/mL) and 138.78 nmol/L (55.5 ng/mL) at 8 weeks in the 400-IU and 800-IU groups, respectively [50]. A total-body DXA scan was performed at term CA and a difference was not observed in BMD between groups. However, a higher proportion of infants in the 400-IU/d group had BMC measures less than 10%, suggesting that the higher vitamin D supplementation dose of 800 IU/d may have a positive impact on bone health in high-risk preterm infants that are hospitalized in the neonatal intensive care unit (NICU). Hanson and colleagues [47] further evaluated the relationship between vitamin D and BMC in preterm infants at the time of discharge from the NICU. Mean 25(OH)-D levels at birth (17.3 ng/mL) increased after 8 weeks of vitamin D_3 supplementation to 54.1 ng/mL and 65.7 ng/mL in the 400-IU/d and 800-IU/d groups, respectively. Free vitamin D, which represents the fraction of vitamin D that is not bound to vitamin D–binding protein or albumin and estimates the biologically active component of vitamin D, was highly correlated with 25(OH)-D concentrations and improved BMC at term CA [47]. More research is needed to determine whether higher vitamin D supplementation in preterm infants yields greater or sustained skeletal benefits with longer-term follow-up.

Similar to the studies discussed earlier, Natarajan and colleagues [53] showed higher serum 25(OH)-D levels in preterm infants treated with 800 IU/d compared with 400 IU/d, and a lower percentage of vitamin D deficiency [25(OH)-D <20 ng/mL] among infants treated with 800 IU/d at 40 weeks' postmenstrual age and at 3 months' CA. However, in contrast with the studies discussed earlier, BMC and BMD were not significantly different between groups at 3 months' CA. In addition, 1 infant in the 800-IU group had a 25(OH)-D level of 141 ng/mL at 3 months' CA, although without hypercalcemia, hypercalciuria, or nephrocalcinosis. Vitamin D toxicity is a rare event, but awareness that this dosage may occasionally result in vitamin D excess is important and a careful assessment of vitamin D status is sensible in neonates receiving higher doses of vitamin D. Larger controlled trials that examine the optimal vitamin D status and supplementation for preterm infants are needed, and this remains an area of ongoing research.

In healthy, term infants, the 4 studies reviewed in this update article did not find a significant correlation between vitamin D supplementation and improved bone-related outcomes. Abrams and colleagues [54] evaluated the effect of 400 IU/d of D_3 supplementation on total-body BMC and BMD in breastfed Hispanic and white infants. Vitamin D deficiency was common at birth (60%), and serum 25(OH)-D levels were lower in Hispanic infants (17 ng/mL) compared with white infants (23 ng/mL). After 3 months of vitamin D supplementation, mean 25(OH)-D levels increased to greater than 30 ng/mL regardless of ethnicity and the starting value of 25(OH)-D. These data suggested that 400 IU/d may be adequate to increase 25(OH)-D levels in healthy infants living in a southern US climate during the first few months of life. However, improvements in 25(OH)-D level do not correlate with changes in BMC.

Gallo and colleagues [55] examined the effects of higher oral vitamin D supplementation (400, 800, 1200, or 1600 IU/d) on vitamin D status in breastfed infants at a northern latitude of residence (Montreal, Quebec, Canada). All dosages achieved 25(OH)-D levels greater than or equal to 50 nmol/L ($\geq$20 ng/mL) in 97% of infants at 3 months, and this was sustained in 98% at 12 months. Only the 1600-IU/d group increased 25(OH)-D levels to greater than or equal to 75 nmol/L ($\geq$30 ng/mL) in 97.5% of infants at 3 months, which was the study's primary end point, but, because 93% of infants had hypervitaminosis D [25(OH)-D level $\geq$250 nmol/L or $\geq$100 ng/mL] by 3 months, the 1600-IU/d group was discontinued. Although a dose-response relationship was observed in 25(OH)-D levels, BMC did not differ by vitamin D dosage up to age 1 year and greater than 400 IU/d did not provide additional bone health benefit at age 3 years [56].

Recently, Rosendahl and colleagues [57] published a large, 2-year study of 975 northern European infants randomized to 400 IU/d or 1200 IU/d of vitamin D_3. Mean 25(OH)-D concentrations were 33.13 ng/mL and 46.07 ng/mL at 12 months and 34.7 ng/mL and 47.16 ng/mL at 24 months in the 400-IU/d and 1200-IU/d groups, respectively. A higher percentage of children at age 24 months had 25(OH)-D levels greater than 30 ng/mL in the 1200-IU/d group (95.4%) compared with the 400-IU/d group (70.5%), although none of the participants developed severe hypercalcemia or a 25(OH)-D levels greater than 100.16 ng/mL. A primary outcome measure for this study was bone strength ascertained by pQCT at age 24 months, and a significant difference in bone strength measures was not observed between groups.

There are generally mixed results among vitamin D treatment trials with bone imaging outcomes in older children and adolescents. Ward and colleagues [58] examined the effect of intermittent, high-dose vitamin D_2 over 1 year on musculoskeletal health in a multiethnic group of postmenarchal women. The intervention group (150,000 IU every 3 months for 4 doses) achieved higher 25(OH)-D levels compared with controls (56 nmol/L vs 15.7 nmol/L); however, no significant effect of vitamin D supplementation was observed on DXA and pQCT measures of bone mass, geometry, and strength. Assessments of muscle function were also performed and although no effect was seen on maximum muscle force or power, a 5% increase in movement efficiency was detected in the intervention group, suggesting that vitamin D supplementation may indirectly improve musculoskeletal health in adolescents with vitamin D deficiency. The lack of effect of vitamin D supplementation on bone outcomes in postmenarchal women may partially be caused by the timing of the intervention relative to completion of skeletal growth and peak rate of bone accrual, because other studies have shown a positive impact of vitamin D on musculoskeletal parameters in girls at premenarchal stages [59]. Al-Shaar and colleagues [60] performed post hoc analyses of the El-Hajj Fuleihan and colleagues [59] vitamin D treatment trial to further examine the effect of vitamin D supplementation on bone geometry. Although vitamin D supplementation improved bone mass and hip geometry in the overall group of adolescent girls, significant correlations were not detected in subgroup analyses by pubertal status or in boys. The baseline 25(OH)-D level was less than 20 ng/mL in most participants for both girls and boys (83.2% and 80.1%, respectively), and a notable proportion had severe deficiency with 25(OH)-D levels less than 10 ng/mL (33.5% of girls and 13.5% of boys), but higher 25(OH)-D levels at study entry in boys compared with girls, among other reasons, may partially explain the sex-specific effect of vitamin D supplementation in this study.

In a prospective study of 40 adolescents with severe vitamin D deficiency [25(OH)-D level <10 ng/mL) and 65% (26 out of 40) of the cohort with radiographic rickets, 1 megadose of vitamin D (10,000 IU/kg, maximum dose 600,000 IU) was shown to improve clinical symptoms of vitamin D deficiency (85% [34 out of 40]), increase mean 25(OH)-D levels from 9.3 ng/mL to 27.7 ng/mL at 3 months, and improve radiographic rickets within 6 to 12 months (92% [24 out of 26]) [61]. After 6 months, most subjects were reported to have 25(OH)-D levels less than 20 ng/mL, suggesting that, after successful treatment of vitamin D deficiency, maintenance vitamin D supplementation is necessary to prevent recurrent deficiency states.

In contrast with the studies discussed earlier, Karlsland Åkeson and colleagues [62] investigated the effects of daily vitamin D at more conservative dosages on BMC and BMD in younger children (aged 5–7 years). Fair-skinned and dark-skinned children received placebo, 10 μg (400 IU), or 25 μg (1000 IU) for 3 winter months. Despite lower 25(OH)-D levels, BMC and BMD were higher in dark-skinned children, suggesting perhaps a more powerful effect of race/ethnicity on bone mass compared with vitamin D. Femoral neck BMC increased more in the intervention groups compared with placebo among dark-skinned children, and in those who improved their vitamin D status the most, suggesting an effect of vitamin D on bone in those with the lowest levels of vitamin D. To that end, BMC and BMD did not differ between intervention and placebo groups in fair-skinned children with a baseline mean 25(OH)-D level of 63 nmol/L (25.2 ng/mL).

In summary, our review of newly published research during the past 10 years continues to support vitamin D supplementation for a bone health benefit in youth with the lowest vitamin D levels, consistent with the systematic review and meta-analysis article published by Winzenberg and colleagues [63] in 2011, and the more recent review by Laing and Lewis [64] in 2018. Overall, the evidence is mixed and less conclusive to universally recommend vitamin D supplementation in healthy children with adequate vitamin D levels. The heterogeneous results reported in pediatric vitamin D trials may be explained by differences in patient characteristics, including age, race/ethnicity, pubertal status, and baseline vitamin D status, as well as differences in the vitamin D supplementation regimens and outcome measures that are studied. More research is needed in larger pediatric populations to validate higher vitamin D targets in healthy children and adolescents. The tolerable upper intake of vitamin D in infants may also deserve further study because of rare reports of hypervitaminosis D.

CURRENT SUPPLEMENTATION GUIDELINES

Infants

The vitamin D content in human breast milk is low, particularly in vitamin D–deficient mothers and during winter months [18,65]. Thus, in exclusively or primarily breastfed infants, vitamin D supplementation is recommended to prevent rickets and vitamin D deficiency. In 2008, the AAP published revised guidelines for vitamin D intake and recommended a minimum of 400 IU of vitamin D daily for infants and children beginning soon after birth [18]. This vitamin D dosage has been shown to maintain serum 25(OH)-D levels greater than 50 nmol/L (20 ng/mL) in breastfed infants [66] and is congruent with the IOM specification of adequate intake for children aged 0 to 12 months [15]. Supplementation should continue until the infant transitions to 1 L/d of vitamin D–fortified formula or milk [18].

Hollis and colleagues [67] recently showed in a randomized, double-blind, comparative effectiveness trial that maternal vitamin D supplementation with 6400 IU/d of D_3 for 6 months supplied breast milk with sufficient vitamin D to satisfy the nursing infant's requirement, and suggested that maternal vitamin D supplementation with 6400 IU/d of D_3 offered an alternative strategy to direct infant supplementation of 400 IU/d of D_3. More studies to validate the safety and effectiveness of high-dose vitamin D supplementation in lactating women are awaited before high-dose vitamin D can be universally recommended to breastfeeding women [18].

Children and adolescents

The recommended daily intake of vitamin D in children and adolescents varies considerably, depending on how the optimal serum 25(OH)-D level is defined and the presence of risk factors [15,16]. In general, 600 to 1000 IU/d of vitamin D is enough to provide skeletal health benefits and prevent vitamin D deficiency, although higher doses may be required in youth with obesity or malabsorption, in those taking medications that accelerate vitamin D catabolism, and to acutely treat vitamin D deficiency states. There are various strategies to treat and prevent vitamin D deficiency, and choosing a specific approach may be informed by cost and patient adherence [12].

EXTRASKELETAL EFFECTS OF VITAMIN D

The study of vitamin D and extraskeletal effects is a growing area of significant interest, although it is beyond the scope of this review article. In brief, the landmark Vitamin D and Omega-3 Trial (VITAL) [68] recruited almost 26,000 adults, aged 50 years and older, who were randomized to receive 2000 IU/d of vitamin D with and without omega-3 supplementation. After 5 years, vitamin D did not significantly reduce cancer, heart attack, or stroke incidence, although there was a suggestion of lower cancer mortality in patients who later developed cancer. It is yet to be determined whether similar findings would be observed in a pediatric population and there is no study of this magnitude that has been undertaken to date.

SUMMARY

Vitamin D is crucial for mineral homeostasis and skeletal health. Adequate intake of vitamin D is necessary to prevent vitamin D deficiency, which is commonly seen in healthy and vulnerable pediatric populations. At present, there is no standard definition of optimal vitamin D status in infants and children, although many important pediatric studies have been published during the past decade that examine the relationship between vitamin D and pediatric bone health. It is our review and synthesis of the current evidence that supports the importance of vitamin D supplementation in breastfed and premature infants and in treating vitamin D levels in older youth that are clearly in the deficiency range. More research is needed in large, pediatric populations to validate higher vitamin D targets and supplementation, and the implementation of standardized vitamin D assays may help to define the optimal 25(OH)-D level in children. In addition, there is significant interest in the nonskeletal benefits of vitamin D. Better understanding of the importance of vitamin D in other systems may further influence the definition of vitamin D sufficiency in the future.

Acknowledgments

Dr N.S. Ma was supported by the Ed and Jeannette Kerr Family Endowed Chair in Endocrinology at Children's Hospital Colorado.

Disclosure

L.A. Warner and R.L. Sewell have no commercial or financial conflicts of interest to report. N.S. Ma is a site investigator for industry-funded clinical trials, including Ascendis Pharma, Ultragenyx Pharmaceutical Inc., and Amgen Inc. She had a 1-time consulting agreement with Ascendis Pharma from 15 August 2019 to 30 September 2019 and received a 1-time honorarium from the Muscular Dystrophy Association as an invited speak (2 November 2019). N.S. Ma receives peer-reviewer royalties from UpToDate. She serves on the Scientific Advisory Board for Sophie's Neighborhood, a 501(c)(3) organization for research and treatment development for multicentric carpotarsal osteolysis (MCTO). Sophie's Neighborhood supports some of N.S. Ma's work related to MCTO.

References

[1] O'Neill CM, Kazantzidis A, Ryan MJ, et al. Seasonal changes in Vitamin D-effective UVB availability in Europe and Associations with population serum 25-hydroxyvitamin D. Nutrients 2016;8(9):533.
[2] Kimlin MG. Geographic location and vitamin D synthesis. Mol Aspects Med 2008;29(6): 453–61.
[3] Holick MF. Vitamin D deficiency. N Engl J Med 2007;357(3):266–81.
[4] Christakos S, Dhawan P, Porta A, et al. Vitamin D and intestinal calcium absorption. Mol Cell Endocrinol 2011;347(1–2):25–9.
[5] Harrison HE, Harrison HC. Intestinal transport of phosphate: action of vitamin D, calcium, and potassium. Am J Physiol 1961;201(6):1007–12.
[6] Bouillon R, Marcocci C, Carmeliet G, et al. Skeletal and extraskeletal actions of vitamin D: current evidence and outstanding questions. Endocr Rev 2019;40(4):1109–51.
[7] Thacher TD, Fischer PR, Strand MA, et al. Nutritional rickets around the world: causes and future directions. Ann Trop Paediatr 2006;26(1):1–16.
[8] Thacher TD, Pludowski P, Shaw NJ, et al. Nutritional rickets in immigrant and refugee children. Public Health Rev 2016;37(1):1–10.
[9] Ward LM, Gaboury I, Ladhani M, et al. Vitamin D–deficiency rickets among children in Canada. CMAJ 2007;177(2):161–6.
[10] Callaghan AL, Moy R, Booth IW, et al. Incidence of symptomatic vitamin D deficiency. Arch Dis Child 2006;91(7):606–7.
[11] Thacher TD, Fischer PR, Tebben PJ, et al. Increasing incidence of nutritional rickets: a population-based study in Olmsted County, Minnesota. Paper presented at: Mayo Clinic Proceedings 2013;88(2):176–83.
[12] Ma N, Gordon C. The truth about vitamin D and adolescent skeletal health. Adolesc Med State Art Rev 2012;23(3):457.
[13] Ganji V, Zhang X, Tangpricha V. Serum 25-hydroxyvitamin D concentrations and prevalence estimates of hypovitaminosis D in the US population based on assay-adjusted data. J Nutr 2012;142(3):498–507.
[14] Herrick KA, Storandt RJ, Afful J, et al. Vitamin D status in the United States, 2011–2014. Am J Clin Nutr 2019;110(1):150–7.
[15] Institute of Medicine Committee to Review Dietary Reference Intakes for Vitamin D, Calcium. The National Academies Collection: reports funded by National Institutes of Health. In: Ross AC, Taylor CL, Yaktine AL, et al, editors. Dietary reference intakes for calcium and vitamin D. Washington, DC: National Academies Press (US); 2011 Copyright © 2011, National Academy of Sciences.
[16] Holick MF, Binkley NC, Bischoff-Ferrari HA, et al. Evaluation, treatment, and prevention of vitamin D deficiency: an Endocrine Society clinical practice guideline. J Clin Endocrinol Metab 2011;96(7):1911–30.
[17] Misra M, Pacaud D, Petryk A, et al. Vitamin D deficiency in children and its management: review of current knowledge and recommendations. Pediatrics 2008;122(2):398–417.
[18] Wagner CL, Greer FR. Prevention of rickets and vitamin D deficiency in infants, children, and adolescents. Pediatrics 2008;122(5):1142–52.
[19] Clemens T, Henderson S, Adams J, et al. Increased skin pigment reduces the capacity of skin to synthesise vitamin D3. Lancet 1982;319(8263):74–6.
[20] Walsh JS, Bowles S, Evans AL. Vitamin D in obesity. Curr Opin Endocrinol Diabetes Obes 2017;24(6):389–94.
[21] Wortsman J, Matsuoka LY, Chen TC, et al. Decreased bioavailability of vitamin D in obesity. Am J Clin Nutr 2000;72(3):690–3.
[22] Gröber U, Kisters K. Influence of drugs on vitamin D and calcium metabolism. Dermatoendocrinol 2012;4(2):158–66.
[23] Altieri B, Cavalier E, Bhattoa HP, et al. Vitamin D testing: advantages and limits of the current assays. Eur J Clin Nutr 2020;74:231–47.

[24] Sempos CT, Vesper HW, Phinney KW, et al. Vitamin D status as an international issue: national surveys and the problem of standardization. Scand J Clin Lab Invest 2012;72(sup243):32–40.
[25] Wise SA, Phinney KW, Tai SS, et al. Baseline assessment of 25-hydroxyvitamin D assay performance: a vitamin D standardization program (VDSP) interlaboratory comparison study. J AOAC Int 2017;100(5):1244–52.
[26] Fraser WD, Tang JC, Dutton JJ, et al. Vitamin D measurement, the debates continue, new analytes have emerged, developments have variable outcomes. Calcif Tissue Int 2020;106(1):3–13.
[27] Gallo S, Comeau K, Agellon S, et al. Methodological issues in assessing plasma 25-hydroxyvitamin D concentration in newborn infants. Bone 2014;61:186–90.
[28] Giustina A, Adler R, Binkley N, et al. Consensus statement from 2nd International Conference on Controversies in Vitamin D. Rev Endocr Metab Disord 2020;21(1):89–116.
[29] Rabenberg M, Scheidt-Nave C, Busch MA, et al. Implications of standardization of serum 25-hydroxyvitamin D data for the evaluation of vitamin D status in Germany, including a temporal analysis. BMC Public Health 2018;18(1):845.
[30] Singh RJ, Taylor RL, Reddy GS, et al. C-3 epimers can account for a significant proportion of total circulating 25-hydroxyvitamin D in infants, complicating accurate measurement and interpretation of vitamin D status. J Clin Endocrinol Metab 2006;91(8):3055–61.
[31] Al-Zohily B, Al-Menhali A, Gariballa S, et al. Epimers of Vitamin D: a review. Int J Mol Sci 2020;21(2):470.
[32] Liu T, Wang E, Li Q, et al. High prevalence of vitamin D insufficiency in Chinese children with upper limb fractures. Genes Dis 2020;7(3):408–13.
[33] Karpiński M, Galicka A, Milewski R, et al. Association between Vitamin D receptor polymorphism and serum Vitamin D levels in children with low-energy fractures. J Am Coll Nutr 2017;36(1):64–71.
[34] Hosseinzadeh P, Mohseni M, Minaie A, et al. Vitamin D status in children with forearm fractures: incidence and risk factors. J Am Acad Orthop Surg Glob Res Rev 2020;4(8):e20.00150-5.
[35] Thompson RM, Dean DM, Goldberg S, et al. Vitamin D insufficiency and fracture risk in urban children. J Pediatr Orthop 2017;37(6):368–73.
[36] Minkowitz B, Cerame B, Poletick E, et al. Low Vitamin D levels are associated with need for surgical correction of pediatric fractures. J Pediatr Orthop 2017;37(1):23–9.
[37] Schilling S, Wood JN, Levine MA, et al. Vitamin D status in abused and nonabused children younger than 2 years old with fractures. Pediatrics 2011;127(5):835–41.
[38] Perez-Rossello JM, Feldman HA, Kleinman PK, et al. Rachitic changes, demineralization, and fracture risk in healthy infants and toddlers with vitamin D deficiency. Radiology 2012;262(1):234–41.
[39] Ceroni D, Anderson De La Llana R, Martin X, et al. Prevalence of vitamin D insufficiency in Swiss teenagers with appendicular fractures: a prospective study of 100 cases. J Child Orthop 2012;6(6):497–503.
[40] Ramirez N, Ortiz-Fullana JL, Arciniegas N, et al. Vitamin D levels and fracture risk among Hispanic children. Eur J Orthop Surg Traumatol 2019;29(3):531–6.
[41] Contreras JJ, Hiestand B, O'Neill JC, et al. Vitamin D deficiency in children with fractures. Pediatr Emerg Care 2014;30(11):777–81.
[42] Anderson LN, Heong SW, Chen Y, et al. Vitamin D and fracture risk in early childhood: a case-control study. Am J Epidemiol 2017;185(12):1255–62.
[43] Calvo MS, Whiting SJ. Survey of current vitamin D food fortification practices in the United States and Canada. J Steroid Biochem Mol Biol 2013;136:211–3.
[44] Rusińska A, Płudowski P, Walczak M, et al. Vitamin D Supplementation guidelines for general population and groups at risk of Vitamin D deficiency in Poland-Recommendations of the Polish Society of Pediatric Endocrinology and Diabetes and the expert panel with

participation of national specialist consultants and representatives of scientific societies-2018 update. Front Endocrinol (Lausanne) 2018;9:246.
[45] Hanson C, Armas L, Lyden E, et al. Vitamin D status and associations in newborn formula-fed infants during initial hospitalization. J Am Diet Assoc 2011;111(12):1836–43.
[46] Dawodu A, Nath R. High prevalence of moderately severe vitamin D deficiency in preterm infants. Pediatr Int 2011;53(2):207–10.
[47] Hanson C, Lyden E, Nelson A, et al. Response of vitamin D binding protein and free vitamin D concentrations to vitamin D supplementation in hospitalized premature infants. J Pediatr Endocrinol Metab 2015;28(9–10):1107–14.
[48] Monangi N, Slaughter JL, Dawodu A, et al. Vitamin D status of early preterm infants and the effects of vitamin D intake during hospital stay. Arch Dis Child Fetal Neonatal Ed 2014;99(2):F166–8.
[49] Burris HH, Van Marter LJ, McElrath TF, et al. Vitamin D status among preterm and full-term infants at birth. Pediatr Res 2014;75(1):75–80.
[50] Anderson-Berry A, Thoene M, Wagner J, et al. Randomized trial of two doses of vitamin D3 in preterm infants <32 weeks: dose impact on achieving desired serum 25(OH)D3 in a NICU population. PLoS One 2017;12(10):e0185950.
[51] van de Lagemaat M, Rotteveel J, van Weissenbruch MM, et al. Increased gain in bone mineral content of preterm infants fed an isocaloric, protein-, and mineral-enriched postdischarge formula. Eur J Nutr 2013;52(7):1781–5.
[52] van de Lagemaat M, Rotteveel J, Schaafsma A, et al. Higher vitamin D intake in preterm infants fed an isocaloric, protein- and mineral-enriched postdischarge formula is associated with increased bone accretion. J Nutr 2013;143(9):1439–44.
[53] Natarajan CK, Sankar MJ, Agarwal R, et al. Trial of daily vitamin D supplementation in preterm infants. Pediatrics 2014;133(3):e628–34.
[54] Abrams SA, Hawthorne KM, Rogers SP, et al. Effects of ethnicity and vitamin D supplementation on vitamin D status and changes in bone mineral content in infants. BMC Pediatr 2012;12:6.
[55] Gallo S, Comeau K, Vanstone C, et al. Effect of different dosages of oral vitamin D supplementation on vitamin D status in healthy, breastfed infants: a randomized trial. JAMA 2013;309(17):1785–92.
[56] Gallo S, Hazell T, Vanstone CA, et al. Vitamin D supplementation in breastfed infants from Montréal, Canada: 25-hydroxyvitamin D and bone health effects from a follow-up study at 3 years of age. Osteoporos Int 2016;27(8):2459–66.
[57] Rosendahl J, Valkama S, Holmlund-Suila E, et al. Effect of higher vs standard dosage of vitamin D3 supplementation on bone strength and infection in healthy infants: a randomized clinical trial. JAMA Pediatr 2018;172(7):646–54.
[58] Ward KA, Das G, Roberts SA, et al. A randomized, controlled trial of vitamin D supplementation upon musculoskeletal health in postmenarchal females. J Clin Endocrinol Metab 2010;95(10):4643–51.
[59] El-Hajj Fuleihan G, Nabulsi M, Tamim H, et al. Effect of vitamin D replacement on musculoskeletal parameters in school children: a randomized controlled trial. J Clin Endocrinol Metab 2006;91(2):405–12.
[60] Al-Shaar L, Nabulsi M, Maalouf J, et al. Effect of vitamin D replacement on hip structural geometry in adolescents: a randomized controlled trial. Bone 2013;56(2):296–303.
[61] Soliman AT, Adel A, Wagdy M, et al. Manifestations of severe vitamin D deficiency in adolescents: effects of intramuscular injection of a megadose of cholecalciferol. J Trop Pediatr 2011;57(4):303–6.
[62] Karlsland Åkeson P, Åkesson KE, Lind T, et al. Vitamin D intervention and bone: a randomized clinical trial in fair- and dark-skinned children at Northern Latitudes. J Pediatr Gastroenterol Nutr 2018;67(3):388–94.
[63] Winzenberg T, Powell S, Shaw KA, et al. Effects of vitamin D supplementation on bone density in healthy children: systematic review and meta-analysis. BMJ 2011;342:c7254.

[64] Laing EM, Lewis RD. New concepts in Vitamin D requirements for children and adolescents: a controversy revisited. Front Horm Res 2018;50:42–65.
[65] Hollis BW, Wagner CL. Vitamin D requirements during lactation: high-dose maternal supplementation as therapy to prevent hypovitaminosis D for both the mother and the nursing infant. Am J Clin Nutr 2004;80(6):1752S–8S.
[66] Greer FR, Marshall S. Bone mineral content, serum vitamin D metabolite concentrations, and ultraviolet B light exposure in infants fed human milk with and without vitamin D2 supplements. J Pediatr 1989;114(2):204–12.
[67] Hollis BW, Wagner CL, Howard CR, et al. Maternal versus infant vitamin D supplementation during lactation: a randomized controlled trial. Pediatrics 2015;136(4):625–34.
[68] Manson JE, Cook NR, Lee I-M, et al. Vitamin D supplements and prevention of cancer and cardiovascular disease. N Engl J Med 2019;380(1):33–44.

Advances in Pediatrics 68 (2021) 195–209
ADVANCES IN PEDIATRICS

Pediatric Breast Masses

An Overview of the Subtypes, Workup, Imaging, and Management

Maria E. Knaus, MD[a], Julia E. Grabowksi, MD[b,*]

[a]Center for Surgical Outcomes Research, Abigail Wexner Research Institute, Nationwide Children's Hospital, 700 Children's Drive, Columbus, OH 43205, USA; [b]Division of Pediatric Surgery, Department of Surgery, Ann & Robert H. Lurie Children's Hospital of Chicago, Northwestern University Feinberg School of Medicine, 225 East Chicago Avenue, Chicago, IL 60611, USA

Keywords

• Pediatric breast mass • Adolescent breast mass • Fibroadenoma • Phyllodes tumor • Breast malignancy • Pediatric breast imaging • Secretory breast carcinoma

Key points

- Most breast masses in pediatric and adolescent girls are palpable and may present with discomfort or other symptoms.
- Most pediatric and adolescent breast masses are benign, with fibroadenomas being the most common. Pediatric breast cancer is extremely rare.
- Ultrasound is the primary imaging modality used to assess pediatric breast masses. Mammography and computed tomography scans are not routinely used. MRI has specific indications.
- In low-risk, asymptomatic patients with small, benign-appearing breast masses, observation alone is safe for initial management.

INTRODUCTION

Breast masses affect only approximately 2% to 3% of the pediatric and adolescent female population. The presentation, workup, and management of breast masses in pediatric and adolescent female individuals are distinct from that in adult women. Pediatric patients tend to present with a palpable mass that often causes symptoms of pain, cosmetic concerns, and anxiety. The vast majority of these lesions are benign, with the incidence of breast cancer in female patients aged 21 or younger estimated at 0.02% [1–3]. As such, there has been recent

*Corresponding author. *E-mail address:* JEGrabowski@luriechildrens.org

https://doi.org/10.1016/j.yapd.2021.05.006
0065-3101/21/

literature that recommends observation for most pediatric breast masses without concerning characteristics, such as size, family history of breast cancer, and prior radiation [4–8]. Despite the rarity of malignancy in pediatric and adolescent breast lesions, the presence of a breast mass is often disconcerting to patients, parents, and providers. It is, therefore, critical for all providers to pediatric patients to understand the nuances of pediatric breast masses so as to provide the appropriate care and counseling for these patients and their families. This article reviews the different types of pediatric breast masses, workup and imaging, and the current options for management.

THE SPECTRUM OF PEDIATRIC BREAST MASSES

Cysts

Examples of benign cysts include simple cysts, galactoceles, retroareolar (Montgomery) cysts, and macrocysts or "blue-domed cysts." These cysts tend to be well-circumscribed, freely mobile, and contain sterile fluid. Solitary cysts are more common in children than multiple cysts. Most simple cysts regress on their own, but for those that cause symptoms, the optimal treatment is aspiration [9–11].

Montgomery cysts occur when the glands of Montgomery, located along the areola, become obstructed. It is estimated that up to 60% of patients with Montgomery cysts present with painful inflammation, and the remaining patients present with a painless, retroareolar mass. Treatment of these cysts consists of antibiotics and nonsteroidal anti-inflammatory drugs (NSAIDs) in those patients who present with infection and inflammation. Most of these cysts resolve with conservative management [12].

Fibrocystic changes (formerly known as fibrocystic disease) is the second most common breast lesion in adolescents after fibroadenomas. It is a normal variant of female physiology and though not typically seen in the first decade of life, it affects up to 50% of women of reproductive age. Believed to be due to estrogen and progesterone imbalances, patients may develop lumps, nodules, and cord-like thickening within the breast. These lumps may become tender and larger in relation to the menstrual cycle. Treatment consists of reassurance, a supportive bra, and NSAIDs. Oral contraceptives may help decrease obvious disease in up to 90% of women [10,13]. Anecdotal evidence suggests that evening primrose oil, vitamin E and calcium supplementation, and decreased caffeine intake may be helpful, but there have not been significant data to support these treatments [10].

Neonatal lesions

Neonatal breast hypertrophy is a common, and normal, occurrence in newborn infants during the first week of life. It occurs secondary to high levels of circulating prolactin triggered by a drop in maternal estrogen at the end of pregnancy. It can affect up to 70% to 90% of male and female neonates and resolves on its own. Stimulation or massage of the breast can lead to persistence of the hypertrophy or can lead to *neonatal mastitis* and *abscess*, so observation alone is recommended. In the setting of neonatal mastitis or abscess, intravenous antibiotics are the treatment of choice, with ultrasound-guided aspiration reserved for abscesses. Incision and drainage may be used in larger abscesses or those that continue to progress after aspiration [13–16].

Male lesions

Pubertal gynecomastia can affect up to 64% of all male individuals, and typically occurs approximately 6 months to 1 year after the onset of puberty. It is the most common breast lesion in adolescent male individuals and can be identified by unilateral or bilateral subareolar breast development. Pubertal gynecomastia is benign and usually resolves after 1 to 2 years. The exact cause of it is unknown, as there has not been a clear correlation with an imbalance in sex hormones [9,16,17]. *Pathologic gynecomastia* makes up 2% to 3% of all cases of gynecomastia, and has an identifiable, pathologic cause such as endocrine abnormalities from a variety of etiologies (tumors, hyperthyroidism, testicular trauma, idiopathic); drugs such as spironolactone, anabolic steroids, and marijuana; or idiopathic. If gynecomastia is being considered as the diagnosis, laboratory workup should be pursued, with additional workup pending those results. Ultrasound is indicated if the physical examination is uncertain [16,17]. Gynecomastia can often times be confused with general obesity, as well. Mastectomy may be offered in situations in which there are persistent issues with pain or self-esteem as a result of the gynecomastia [17]. In general, male individuals are also susceptible to development of the lesions that occur in female individuals that are outlined in the following.

Common benign lesions

There are numerous types of lesions that present as a pediatric breast mass, and the overwhelming majority are benign. It has been estimated that more than 90% of all pediatric breast masses are *fibroadenomas*, making them the most common benign breast mass in this population [18,19]. Fibroadenomas present as rubbery, smooth-edged, painless, mobile masses [11]. There can be multiple lesions in one breast, they can be bilateral, and they can also be lobulated [20]. Fibroadenomas typically appear during adolescence, but there have been reports of them occurring in premenarchal female individuals; they are rare in male individuals [13]. They very rarely contain malignancy [4,21]. Fibroadenomas tend to be slow-growing and more than one-third of them may resolve on their own [11,13].

Common fibroadenomas are usually 2 to 5 cm in size [13,22]. If they grow to be more than 5 cm, they are further classified as *giant fibroadenomas*, which account for up to 2% of all fibroadenomas [22]. *Juvenile fibroadenomas* are giant fibroadenomas that occur in young or adolescent female individuals. They are rapidly growing masses, usually larger than 5 to 10 cm, and are characterized by the histologic finding of hypercellular stromal proliferation. These tumors, which may be associated with noticeable, dilated cutaneous veins, are more common in black patients and often occur earlier in adolescence [9,13].

Rare benign lesions

Pseudoangiomatous stromal hyperplasia (PASH) is a benign tumor formed from the proliferation of stromal myofibroblasts. Its histologic characteristics make it appear similar to blood vessels that are surrounded by a dense stroma, thus its name. Given this appearance, it can be confused with angiosarcoma or other vascular tumors but has no known malignant potential. Although its presentation, growth rate, and sonographic appearance can vary, it most commonly mirrors that of a fibroadenoma. It is considered benign but has been known to recur with inadequate margins after excision [11,23].

Tubular adenomas are an uncommon type of benign breast mass. Although typically affecting adult women with an average age of 31, they have been known to affect children [24]. In one series, they accounted for 4% of excised breast lesions in children aged 1 to 19 [4]. A tubular adenoma can be seen in combination with a fibroadenoma, or less commonly, as its own discrete mass. Clinically and on imaging, tubular adenomas can resemble a fibroadenoma, but histologically are differentiated by their scant stromal content. They rarely exceed 5 cm [9,24].

Juvenile papillomatosis (JP) is a proliferative mass that usually gets diagnosed at approximately age 19 [9]. A mobile, well-circumscribed mass anywhere from 3 to 8 cm is typically found in the periphery of the breast. It occurs in both male and female individuals, and there are case reports of JP in male infants [25]. On resection, the mass consists of multiple, small cysts surrounded by a dense stroma, thus giving it its classic "Swiss cheese disease" moniker [9,11,13]. Although JP is a benign condition, it is a marker for an increased risk of breast cancer, requiring long-term surveillance [26–29]. Complete surgical excision is indicated, as JP has been known to recur in cases with incomplete excision [29,30].

Granular cell tumors (GCTs), also known as myoblastomas, are benign masses that occur in both male and female individuals. They account for fewer than 1% of all pediatric breast masses. Despite their benign nature, they often can be confused for malignancy because of their clinical and radiologic findings. They are often fixed, ill-defined, and can cause skin retraction. Like infiltrating ductal carcinoma, GCTs can form cords or projections into the surrounding normal breast parenchyma. An accurate preoperative diagnosis can aid in surgical planning, as GCTs can be treated with wide local excision [9,11].

Vascular lesions of the pediatric breast can be either benign or malignant. Hemangiomas, though rare, are the most common benign vascular tumor in this population. These may be slow or fast growing, and they often involute on their own depending on their histologic subtype [9,16,31]. *Vascular malformations* are another type of vascular lesion. Examples include venous malformations and cystic hygromas. Compared with hemangiomas, these malformations are not discrete masses and may have minimal to no blood flow [11]. Management of vascular lesions may include steroids, sclerotherapy, and surgery. Multidisciplinary clinics involving dermatology, radiology, and surgery are available at many institutions and can often assist in coordinating the treatment of these lesions.

Malignant lesions

Primary breast cancers are rare in pediatric and adolescent patients, with an incidence of 0.02%. Pediatric breast malignancies present with a more advanced stage than adults and tend to be poorly differentiated or undifferentiated. Although pediatric patients tend to undergo less axillary nodal sampling than adults, they have significantly more positive nodes on pathologic examination. Children are less likely to undergo radiation therapy, more likely to receive chemotherapy, and more likely to undergo bilateral mastectomy than a unilateral mastectomy of the affected breast compared with adults [2]. Some series show that pediatric patients have a worse 5-year survival when compared stage-to-stage with adults, whereas other series have shown no overall survival difference [2,32].

Invasive carcinomas are the most common type of breast malignancy in this population, accounting for up to 65% of cases (Table 1) [2,32–34]. *Secretory*

Table 1
Percentage of pediatric malignancy subtypes from recent reviews

Study, year published	Number of patients	Percentage of carcinoma	Percentage of fibroepithelial tumors	Percentage of sarcomas	Percentage of other or NOS malignancies
Richards et al [2], 2017	477	64.8	23.3	8.2	3.8
Gutierrez et al [32], 2008	75	54.7	38.7	6.7	—
Westfal et al [7], 2019; Westfal et al [33], 2019	134	48.5	35.1	14.2	0.8
Xiao et al [34], 2020	270	62.2	22.2	10.4	5.2

According to several recent reviews, carcinoma is the most common breast malignancy in the pediatric and adolescent population, followed by fibroepithelial tumors (phyllodes tumors), and then sarcomas.

Abbreviation: NOS, not otherwise specified.

Data from Richards MK, Goldin AB, Beierle EA, et al. Breast Malignancies in Children: Presentation, Management, and Survival. *Annals of Surgical Oncology.* 2017;24(6):1482-1491.; Gutierrez JC, Housri N, Koniaris LG, Fischer AC, Sola JE. Malignant Breast Cancer in Children: A Review of 75 Patients. *Journal of Surgical Research.* 2008;147(2):182-188.; Westfal ML, Chang DC, Kelleher CM. A population-based analysis of pediatric breast cancer. *Journal of Pediatric Surgery.* 2019;54(1):140-144.; and Xiao Y, Jiang Y, Xiong Y, Ruan S, Huang T. Pediatric Malignant Phyllodes Tumors of the Breast: Characteristics and Outcomes Based on the Surveillance Epidemiology and End Results Database. *Journal of Surgical Research.* 2020;249:205-215.

breast carcinoma is the most common subtype of carcinoma and also accounts for 80% of all primary breast malignancies in children [35]. Secretory carcinoma has a favorable prognosis, with more than a 91% 10-year cause-specific survival [36]. It affects both male and female individuals. It typically presents as a slow-growing, painless mass that may be difficult to differentiate on ultrasound from fibroadenomas. Histologically, it is distinguished by micro-multicystic tumor nodules created by extracellular secretions, separated by bands of connective tissue [9]. Although there are no standardized guidelines for the management of secretory breast carcinoma, Garlick and colleagues [35] recommend simple mastectomy and reconstruction with sentinel lymph node biopsy for pediatric patients, given the higher risk of recurrence with breast-conserving therapy and frequency of axillary node metastases (30%). Although less common in frequency, other subtypes of carcinoma, such as invasive ductal, invasive lobular, anaplastic, inflammatory, and medullary carcinoma, portend a poorer prognosis in the presence of advanced disease given their more aggressive natures [5,11].

Phyllodes tumors were previously known as cystosarcoma phyllodes and are fibroepithelial tumors that can be benign, borderline, or malignant based on their histopathologic features [37]. Although previously thought to be the most common breast malignancy in pediatric patients, newer research shows it is the second most common malignancy (after invasive carcinomas), with phyllodes tumors accounting for 22% to 39% of all pediatric breast malignancies [2,32,34]. Clinically, phyllodes tumors present as rapidly growing masses, usually larger than 6 cm in size on presentation. They can be difficult to differentiate from juvenile and giant fibroadenomas, and a plethora of research has been done in attempts to correctly identify and excise phyllodes tumors while simultaneously observing fibroadenomas. Phyllodes tumors and other fibroepithelial tumors occur more frequently in black children and carry a better prognosis and overall survival than carcinomas and sarcomas [33,34]. To differentiate between a phyllodes tumor and a fibroadenoma, core needle biopsy may be done. However, some phyllodes tumors may appear as fibroadenomas on core needle biopsy, given tumor heterogeneity [38]. Surgical excision with 1-cm margins is the recommended treatment by the National Comprehensive Cancer Network (NCCN). The NCCN guidelines do not recommend axillary staging (axillary dissection or sentinel lymph node biopsy), as the presence of axillary metastases is rare [37,39–42]. Positive margins incur a higher recurrence rate of both benign and malignant phyllodes tumors [43].

Sarcomas, exclusive of phyllodes tumors, consist of 8% to 14% of pediatric breast cancers [2,32,33]. Various subtypes include rhabdomyosarcoma, fibrosarcoma, leiomyosarcoma, and angiosarcoma. Chest wall malignancies, such as Ewing sarcoma and osteosarcoma, can involve the breast. Alveolar rhabdomyosarcoma is the most common soft tissue sarcoma in children and accounts for up to 12% of all pediatric solid malignancies. It has been reported as both a primary and metastatic lesion of the pediatric breast. Prognosis is poor, with reports of long-term survival being approximately 50% in primary breast rhabdomyosarcoma and 15% in metastatic rhabdomyosarcoma to the breast [44–46].

Metastatic malignancies have been reported to occur more frequently than primary breast cancers in children [31]. Rhabdomyosarcoma, leukemia, and lymphoma are the most common malignancies that metastasize to the breast [5,9]. Primary breast lymphomas are exceedingly rare [47,48]. Neuroblastoma, melanoma, renal cell carcinoma, and hepatocellular carcinoma have all been reported to metastasize to the breast [49]. These metastases should be treated according to their primary tumor [50].

Secondary breast cancers occur during their lifetime in up to 40% of female individuals who underwent mantle radiotherapy. Although not often used today, it was a common treatment in children with Hodgkin lymphoma. In patients who receive higher doses of radiation (>40 Gy), their relative risk for developing invasive breast cancer or ductal carcinoma in situ is 10.5 compared with the general population. Breast cancer is diagnosed at a median time of 20 years after mantle radiotherapy, and, in this population of patients, close surveillance and counseling are important [51,52].

WORKUP

History and physical examination

Breast masses generally present as a palpable mass identified by either the patient or primary care provider. The approach to diagnosing a pediatric breast mass starts with a thorough history and physical examination. Important components of the history of present illness and past medical and family history include the following:

- Duration and characteristics of the mass(es), such as change in size and subjective characteristics of the mass (eg, hard, painful)
- Associated symptoms: weight loss, fatigue, fever, skin changes, nipple discharge, lymphadenopathy
- Details regarding menarche (age at first period, regularity of cycles, use of oral contraceptives, history of pregnancy and breastfeeding) and changes or characteristics of the mass with regard to the menstrual cycle
- Prior trauma to the area
- Personal history of malignancy or chest radiation
- Family history of malignancy (particularly breast or ovarian) and genetic syndromes or predispositions

Important components of the physical examination include the following:

- A complete breast examination of both breasts, including examination of all quadrants, the nipple-areolar complex, and the axilla
- Attention to skin changes, nipple retraction, nipple discharge, and inflammatory changes
- Mass position documented using the clock orientation
- Mass characteristics, including size, firmness, mobility, and regularity of borders

- Palpation of axillary, cervical, and supraclavicular lymph nodes
- Documentation of Tanner staging

Imaging

Ultrasound is the first-line imaging modality to assess pediatric breast masses. It avoids the use of ionizing radiation and has high diagnostic sensitivity and specificity when assessing the dense fibroglandular tissues found in younger patients [5,11,53]. Ultrasound has utility in characterizing breast masses and determining their size. It can also help determine which lesions may require biopsy, resection, or observation [54]. Radiologists stress the importance of knowledge of the appearance of the pediatric breast on ultrasound, understanding the clinical context, and appropriate technical aspects while the ultrasound is being obtained [53].

Mammography is rarely used in the pediatric and adolescent population, as it not only delivers ionizing radiation, but also has a low sensitivity in the dense tissue found in pediatric and adolescent breasts. Computed tomography does not have a role in the workup of pediatric breast masses given its radiation burden. MRI may be used to evaluate vascular and lymphatic malformations, chest wall lesions, or to assess lesions that involve multiple anatomic cavities. It may also have a role in the surveillance of high-risk populations, such as those with the BRCA mutation. It can also be useful in surgical planning [11,16,53].

The Breast Imaging-Reporting and Data System (BI-RADS) was developed by the American College of Radiology to standardize the terminology, assessment, reporting, and classification of breast imaging [55]. This system was developed to stratify adult breast lesions according to their likelihood of malignancy based on certain mammogram, ultrasound, and MRI findings (Table 2). Although it is routinely used in the adult population, few studies have examined its applicability to the pediatric and adolescent population, in which the

Table 2
Breast Imaging-Reporting and Data System (BI-RADS) assessment categories and likelihood of malignancy

	Assessment category	Likelihood of cancer
0	Incomplete	Not applicable
1	Negative	Essentially 0%
2	Benign	Essentially 0%
3	Probably benign	>0% to ≤2%
4	Suspicious	4a: Low Suspicion >2% to ≤10% 4b: Moderate suspicion >10% to ≤50% 4c: High suspicion >50% to <95%
5	Highly suggestive of malignancy	≥95%
6	Known biopsy-proven malignancy	Not applicable

BI-RADS categories based off ultrasound findings. Certain categories convey a certain likelihood of cancer.
Data from ACR BI-RADS Atlas, Breast Imaging Reporting and Data System. American College of Radiology; 2013.

risk of malignancy is much lower. In a study reviewing 51 excised pediatric breast masses, the investigators concluded that BI-RADS overestimated the risk of malignancy: there were no malignant masses in the cohort, but 25 masses assigned a BI-RADS 4 (Suspicious) [56]. A designation of BI-RADS 4 confers a 2% to 95% chance of malignancy and typically leads to tissue biopsy [55]. Given the overestimation of malignancy identified by the previously mentioned study, the current BI-RADS system should not be applied to children. Prospective trials including a larger number of pediatric patients are required to make additional inferences.

MANAGEMENT OF A PEDIATRIC BREAST MASS

Although there are established algorithms to manage breast lesions in adult women, clear guidelines for the management of breast masses in the pediatric population are lacking. Breast cancers are extremely rare in children, and this information is important reassurance for families and patients who often present with significant anxiety. However, unlike adult patients who commonly present with lesions detected on surveillance imaging, pediatric patients often present with a solid mass that may be symptomatic. Most published data regarding the surgical management of pediatric breast lesions focuses on pathologic diagnoses and not on symptomatic relief, whereas clinically, surgical decision-making often centers on ameliorating symptoms. Therefore, treatment guidelines based on the risk of malignancy alone may not be appropriate in this population.

There is a growing body of literature that supports observation alone as a safe initial management for small, benign-appearing breast masses in low-risk children [4,5,7]. In a cohort of 37 adolescent female individuals with 45 palpable breast masses evaluated by Jawahar and colleagues, benign phyllodes tumors were 3 of 22 biopsied or excised masses and the remainder were fibroadenomas [57]. A retrospective review of nearly 2000 female pediatric and adolescent patients demonstrated that more than 80% of biopsies and excisions revealed pathology that would have been safe to observe [7]. One study found that costs increased by a factor of 4.5 in pediatric patients who underwent biopsy as a first step rather than ultrasound surveillance ($4491 vs $986) [21]. In addition, a recent analysis of 119 pediatric patients who underwent excision of a breast mass found that almost 1 in 4 patients underwent excision due to patient and family anxiety, rather than pain, growth, or abnormal imaging [4].

Core needle biopsy and fine needle aspiration are the 2 primary ways to obtain an image-guided tissue sample for breast lesions in adults. Although fine needle aspiration has shown reliability in diagnosing some adolescent breast masses and is less invasive, core needle biopsy may better differentiate between fibroadenomas and phyllodes tumors [53,58,59]. These techniques are used in children to varying degrees, depending on hospital resources and provider discretion. Unlike in the adult population, needle-based biopsy techniques in children often require anesthesia. Furthermore, as they may be nondiagnostic in differentiating lesions and do not treat underlying symptoms, they may be less practical in children. Needle biopsy may be of particular use in patients with a concern for a metastatic lesion or with a history of chest radiation.

The "gray area" for pediatric practitioners involves how to manage likely benign breast masses. The decision for observation must be weighed against patient symptoms and the possibility of malignancy, given that fibroadenomas and phyllodes tumors are so similar clinically and radiologically. In the absence of accepted guidelines for the management of pediatric breast masses, several studies have developed evidence-based algorithms for their workup and management in recent years (Table 3).

Gao and colleagues [5] developed criteria for excision to balance the concern for iatrogenic injury to the breast with the risk of malignancy. They classify a probably benign mass on ultrasound as being oval-shaped, having circumscribed margins, and a parallel orientation. If a mass meets these criteria, and is 4 cm or smaller, they advocate for ultrasound follow-up only. However, if the mass shows atypical or malignant features on ultrasound, is rapidly enlarging, is larger than 4 cm, or if the patient has a history of malignancy, mantle radiation, or a genetic mutation or syndrome, then the mass requires biopsy. Malignant features on ultrasound include indistinct, spiculated, or microlobulated margins, an irregular shape, and antiparallel orientation [5].

McLaughlin and colleagues [8] created an algorithm based off the principle that size itself does not predict a pathologic diagnosis. They advocate for initial management of pediatric breast masses based off risk stratification and symptoms. Patients who are high risk (personal or family history of malignancy, risk factors for malignancy) should undergo excision. Symptomatic, low-risk patients can undergo 3-month to 6-month ultrasound follow-up or biopsy, with surgery reserved for indeterminate findings or for the diagnosis of a phyllodes tumor or malignancy. In contrast, asymptomatic patients can undergo continued observation with 3-month to 6-month follow-up. However, if the mass is persistent, doubles in size, or increases in size by more than 2 cm in a 3-month to 6-month period, surgery is recommended [8].

Other studies suggest that benign-appearing masses smaller than 3 to 5 cm can be followed with ultrasound at 3-month to 12-month intervals until mass resolution or age 29 in (1) asymptomatic patients; (2) patients without a history of prior radiation to the breast tissue or family or personal risk factors for malignancy; and (3) masses with a minimal growth rate, although studies vary on limitations on growth from any increase in size to a volume change of 16% a month to a 50% increase in size over 12 months [6,53,57]. With similar approaches, the incidence of biopsy is reduced from 47% to 6% [59–61]. Brownstone and colleagues [22] cite a review of more than 1000 pediatric patients with breast masses performed by Sanders and her colleagues [62]. In this review, the incidence of phyllodes tumors rose to 3.6% in lesions larger than 3 cm compared with an incidence of less than 1% in lesions smaller than 3 cm. This increase in the chance of possible malignancy led both research

Table 3
Management recommendations for benign-appearing pediatric breast masses

Study	Size cutoff for intervention	Growth cutoff for intervention	Ultrasound follow-up	Additional criteria for intervention
Gao et al [5], 2015	>4 cm[b]	Rapidly enlarging[a]	Not specified	Atypical or malignant features on ultrasound, patient history of malignancy, mantle radiation, or genetic mutation/syndrome[b]
Luhar et al [59], 2017	>4 cm[a]	—	3, 6, 12, and 24 mo	Suspicious features on ultrasound, patient history of radiation to breast tissue[a,b]
Jawahar et al [57], 2015	>3 cm[b]	16% volume change per month[a]	Every 6 mo until mass resolution or age 29	Mass must be benign appearing on ultrasound to undergo follow-up only
McLaughlin et al [8], 2018	—	Doubles in size or grows by >2 cm[a]	3–6 mo	Personal or family history of malignancy, risk factors for malignancy, or if mass is persistent[a]
Brownstone et al [22], 2019	>3 cm[a]	—	6, 12, and 24 mo	If patient is symptomatic or mass does not have benign features[a]
Sanders et al [62], 2018	>3 cm[b], >5 cm[a]	Doubles in size[b]	6 and 12 mo	Atypical features on ultrasound, including cystic areas, hyperlobulation, angularity, irregular margins[b]
Omar at al [6], 2018	>5 cm[b]	50% growth[a]	12 and 24 mo	Mass must have features of fibroadenoma on ultrasound to undergo follow-up only
Valeur et al [53], 2015	>5 cm[a,b]	Any growth[a]	6, 12, and 24 mo	Any symptoms (such as pain), patient history of malignancy, mass with irregular shape, angular margins, or shadowing on ultrasound[a]

Various recent publications with recommendation for size cutoffs, growth cutoffs, and other features for excision of a probably benign breast mass, along with recommendations for ultrasound follow-up.

[a]Recommendation for surgical excision.

[b]Recommendation for biopsy.

Data from Gao Y, Saksena MA, Brachtel EF, Termeulen DC, Rafferty EA. How to approach breast lesions in children and adolescents. *European Journal of Radiology.* 2015;84(7):1350-1364; Luhar AP, Chiang M, Langer J, Gupta E, Goodarzian F, Sura A. Improving Pediatric Breast Ultrasound Reporting and Recommendations. *Journal of the American College of Radiology.* 2017;14(11):1451-1454.; Jawahar A, Vade A, Ward K, Okur G, Subbaiah P. Biopsy Versus Conservative Management of Sonographically Benign-Appearing Solid Breast Masses in Adolescents. 2015;34(4):617-625.; McLaughlin CM, Gonzalez-Hernandez J, Bennett M, Piper HG. Pediatric breast masses: an argument for observation. *Journal of Surgical Research.* 2018;228:247-252.; Brownstone ND, Celie KB, Spigland NA, Otterburn DM. Pediatric Breast Fibroadenomas: A Systematic Review and Algorithm for Treatment. *Ann Plast Surg.* 2019;83(5):601-605.; Sanders LM, Sharma P, El Madany M, King AB, Goodman KS, Sanders AE. Clinical breast concerns in low-risk pediatric patients: practice review with proposed recommendations. *Pediatr Radiol.* 2018;48(2):186-195.; Omar L, Gleason MK, Pfeifer CM, Sharma P, Kwon JK. Management of Palpable Pediatric Breast Masses With Ultrasound Characteristics of Fibroadenoma: A More Conservative Approach. *American Journal of Roentgenology.* 2018;212(2):450-455.; Valeur NS, Rahbar H, Chapman T. Ultrasound of pediatric breast masses: what to do with lumps and bumps. *Pediatr Radiol.* 2015;45(11):1584-1599.

teams to recommend either biopsy (Sanders and colleagues [62]) or excision (Brownstone and colleagues [22]) of masses larger than 3 cm.

SUMMARY

Most pediatric and adolescent breast masses are benign. Nine of 10 pediatric breast masses are believed to be fibroadenomas. Breast cancer is extremely rare in children. Primary workup of a breast mass includes a detailed history and physical and possible ultrasound. The differential diagnosis of a pediatric breast mass includes fibrocystic changes, cysts, a fibroadenoma, JP, and malignancies such as secretory breast carcinoma, phyllodes tumors, rhabdomyosarcoma, or metastatic lesions to the breast. In certain cases, core needle biopsy or fine needle aspiration may be indicated to obtain a tissue diagnosis. For small, benign-appearing breast masses in low-risk, asymptomatic patients, observation alone is safe. Several studies have proposed criteria for observation as well as surgical excision of a mass, but there is no consensus guideline. Clinical judgment takes precedence, and providers should have honest discussions with patients and their families.

CLINICS CARE POINTS

- The vast majority of pediatric and adolescent breast masses are benign, with fibroadenomas being the most common lesion. Pediatric breast cancer is extremely rare.
- If indicated, ultrasound is the primary imaging modality used to assess pediatric and adolescent breast masses. The BI-RADS classification system has not been shown to be applicable to the pediatric population.
- The literature tells us that, for most small, benign-appearing breast masses in low-risk, asymptomatic patients, observation alone is safe for initial management. Patients with symptoms may be approached differently.
- There are variable recommendations regarding lesion size and growth characteristics in which a provider should consider surgical excision. In general, lesions 3 to 5 cm in size or those that are growing should be referred to a pediatric surgeon.

Disclosure

The authors have nothing to disclose.

References

[1] Cancer Stat Facts: Female Breast Cancer. Available at: https://seer.cancer.gov/statfacts/html/breast.html. Accessed October 22, 2020.

[2] Richards MK, Goldin AB, Beierle EA, et al. Breast malignancies in children: presentation, management, and survival. Ann Surg Oncol 2017;24(6):1482–91.

[3] Neinstein LS, Atkinson J, Diament M. Prevalence and longitudinal study of breast masses in adolescents. J Adolesc Health 1993;14(4):277–81.

[4] Knell J, Koning JL, Grabowski JE. Analysis of surgically excised breast masses in 119 pediatric patients. Pediatr Surg Int 2016;32(1):93–6.
[5] Gao Y, Saksena MA, Brachtel EF, et al. How to approach breast lesions in children and adolescents. Eur J Radiol 2015;84(7):1350–64.
[6] Omar L, Gleason MK, Pfeifer CM, et al. Management of palpable pediatric breast masses with ultrasound characteristics of fibroadenoma: a more conservative approach. AJR Am J Roentgenol 2018;212(2):450–5.
[7] Westfal ML, Perez NP, Hung YC, et al. Pathologic discordance to clinical management decisions suggests overtreatment in pediatric benign breast disease. Breast Cancer Res Treat 2019;176(1):101–8.
[8] McLaughlin CM, Gonzalez-Hernandez J, Bennett M, et al. Pediatric breast masses: an argument for observation. J Surg Res 2018;228:247–52.
[9] Stocker JT, Dehner LP, Coffin C. The breast. In: Pediatric pathology. 2nd edition. Philadelphia: Lippincott, Williams, & Wilkins; 2001. p. 993–1015.
[10] Greydanus DE, Matytsina L, Gains M. Breast disorders in children and adolescents. Prim Care Clin Off Pract 2006;33(2):455–502.
[11] Chung EM, Cube R, Hall GJ, et al. From the archives of the AFIP: breast masses in children and adolescents: radiologic-pathologic correlation. Radiographics 2009;29(3):907–31.
[12] Huneeus A, Schilling A, Horvath E, et al. Retroareolar cysts in the adolescent. J Pediatr Adolesc Gynecol 2003;16(1):45–9.
[13] De Silva NK, Brandt ML. Disorders of the breast in children and adolescents, Part 2: breast masses. J Pediatr Adolesc Gynecol 2006;19(6):415–8.
[14] De Silva NK, Brandt ML. Disorders of the breast in children and adolescents, Part 1: Disorders of growth and infections of the breast. J Pediatr Adolesc Gynecol 2006;19(5):345–9.
[15] Masoodi T, Mufti GN, Bhat JI, et al. Neonatal mastitis: a clinico-microbiological study. J Neonatal Surg 2014;3(1):2.
[16] Kaneda HJ, Mack J, Kasales CJ, et al. Pediatric and adolescent breast masses: a review of pathophysiology, imaging, diagnosis, and treatment. AJR Am J Roentgenol 2013;200(2):W204–12.
[17] West KW, Rescorla FJ, Scherer LR 3rd, et al. Diagnosis and treatment of symptomatic breast masses in the pediatric population. J Pediatr Surg 1995;30(2):182–6 [discussion: 186–7].
[18] Sanchez R, Ladino-Torres MF, Bernat JA, et al. Breast fibroadenomas in the pediatric population: common and uncommon sonographic findings. Pediatr Radiol 2010;40(10):1681–9.
[19] Breast Disorders: Pediatric Surgery NaT. APSA; 2018. Available at: https://www.pedsurglibrary.com/apsa/view/Pediatric-Surgery-NaT/829149/all/Breast_Disorders. Accessed October 26, 2020.
[20] Fallat ME, Ignacio RC Jr. Breast disorders in children and adolescents. J Pediatr Adolesc Gynecol 2008;21(6):311–6.
[21] Englert EG, Ares G, Henricks A, et al. Analysis of factors predicting surgical intervention and associated costs in pediatric breast masses: a single center study. Pediatr Surg Int 2018;34(6):679–85.
[22] Brownstone ND, Celie KB, Spigland NA, et al. Pediatric breast fibroadenomas: a systematic review and algorithm for treatment. Ann Plast Surg 2019;83(5):601–5.
[23] Shehata BM, Fishman I, Collings MH, et al. Pseudoangiomatous stromal hyperplasia of the breast in pediatric patients: an underrecognized entity. Pediatr Dev Pathol 2009;12(6):450–4.
[24] Irshad A, Ackerman SJ, Pope TL, et al. Rare breast lesions: correlation of imaging and histologic features with WHO classification. Radiographics 2008;28(5):1399–414.
[25] Rice HE, Acosta A, Brown RL, et al. Juvenile papillomatosis of the breast in male infants: two case reports. Pediatr Surg Int 2000;16(1–2):104–6.

[26] Sedloev T, Bassarova A, Angelov K, et al. Combination of juvenile papillomatosis, juvenile fibroadenoma and intraductal carcinoma of the breast in a 15-year-old girl. Anticancer Res 2015;35(9):5027–9.
[27] Viswanathan K, McMillen B, Cheng E, et al. Juvenile papillomatosis (swiss-cheese disease) of breast in an adult male with sequential diagnoses of ipsilateral intraductal, invasive, and widely metastatic carcinoma: a case report and review of the disease in males. Int J Surg Pathol 2017;25(6):536–42.
[28] Rosen PP, Lyngholm B, Kinne DW, et al. Juvenile papillomatosis of the breast and family history of breast carcinoma. Cancer 1982;49(12):2591–5.
[29] Peter Rosen P, Kimmel M. Juvenile papillomatosis of the breast: a follow-up study of 41 patients having biopsies before 1979. Am J Clin Pathol 1990;93(5):599–603.
[30] Cheng E, D'Alfonso T, Patel A, et al. Mammary juvenile papillomatosis ("Swiss cheese" disease): study of 121 cases reiterates need for long-term follow-up. Breast J 2018;24(6): 1136–7.
[31] Pettinato G, Manivel JC, Kelly DR, et al. Lesions of the breast in children exclusive of typical fibroadenoma and gynecomastia. A clinicopathologic study of 113 cases. Pathol Annu 1989;24(Pt 2):296–328.
[32] Gutierrez JC, Housri N, Koniaris LG, et al. Malignant breast cancer in children: a review of 75 patients. J Surg Res 2008;147(2):182–8.
[33] Westfal ML, Chang DC, Kelleher CM. A population-based analysis of pediatric breast cancer. J Pediatr Surg 2019;54(1):140–4.
[34] Xiao Y, Jiang Y, Xiong Y, et al. Pediatric malignant phyllodes tumors of the breast: characteristics and outcomes based on the surveillance epidemiology and end results database. J Surg Res 2020;249:205–15.
[35] Garlick JW, Olson KA, Downs-Kelly E, et al. Secretory breast carcinoma in an 8-year-old girl: a case report and literature review. Breast J 2018;24(6):1055–61.
[36] Horowitz DP, Sharma CS, Connolly E, et al. Secretory carcinoma of the breast: results from the survival, epidemiology and end results database. Breast 2012;21(3):350–3.
[37] Leraas HJ, Rosenberger LH, Ren Y, et al. Pediatric phyllodes tumors: a review of the National Cancer Data Base and adherence to NCCN guidelines for phyllodes tumor treatment. J Pediatr Surg 2018;53(6):1123–8.
[38] Lee AH, Hodi Z, Ellis IO, et al. Histological features useful in the distinction of phyllodes tumour and fibroadenoma on needle core biopsy of the breast. Histopathology 2007;51(3):336–44.
[39] Gradishar WJ, Moran MS, Abraham J, et al. Clinical practice guidelines in oncology: breast cancer. Plymouth Meeting (PA): National Comprehensive Cancer Network; 2020. Available at: https://www.nccn.org/professionals/physician_gls/pdf/breast.pdf. Accessed November 9, 2020.
[40] Gullett NP, Rizzo M, Johnstone PA. National surgical patterns of care for primary surgery and axillary staging of phyllodes tumors. Breast J 2009;15(1):41–4.
[41] Cheng S-P, Chang Y-C, Liu T-P, et al. Phyllodes tumor of the breast: the challenge persists. World J Surg 2006;30(8):1414–21.
[42] Ben hassouna J, Damak T, Gamoudi A, et al. Phyllodes tumors of the breast: a case series of 106 patients. Am J Surg 2006;192(2):141–7.
[43] Rajan PB, Cranor ML, Rosen PP. Cystosarcoma phyllodes in adolescent girls and young women: a study of 45 patients. Am J Surg Pathol 1998;22(1):64–9.
[44] Hays DM, Donaldson SS, Shimada H, et al. Primary and metastatic rhabdomyosarcoma in the breast: neoplasms of adolescent females, a report from the Intergroup Rhabdomyosarcoma Study. Med Pediatr Oncol 1997;29(3):181–9.
[45] Binokay F, Soyupak SK, Inal M, et al. Primary and metastatic rhabdomyosarcoma in the breast: report of two pediatric cases. Eur J Radiol 2003;48(3):282–4.
[46] Pareekutty NM, Bhagat M, Vora T, et al. Rhabdomyosarcoma of the breast: report of two cases with the review of literature. J Indian Assoc Pediatr Surg 2016;21(2):81–3.

[47] Cao YB, Wang SS, Huang HQ, et al. [Primary breast lymphoma–a report of 27 cases with literature review]. Ai Zheng 2007;26(1):84–9.
[48] Ishizuka Y, Horimoto Y, Fujimura J, et al. Primary breast non-Hodgkin's lymphoma in a 14-year-old girl: a case report. Surg Case Rep 2020;6(1):87.
[49] Chateil JF, Arboucalot F, Pérel Y, et al. Breast metastases in adolescent girls: US findings. Pediatr Radiol 1998;28(11):832–5.
[50] Kennedy RD, Boughey JC. Management of pediatric and adolescent breast masses. Semin Plast Surg 2013;27(1):19–22.
[51] Travis LB, Hill D, Dores GM, et al. Cumulative absolute breast cancer risk for young women treated for Hodgkin lymphoma. J Natl Cancer Inst 2005;97(19):1428–37.
[52] Gold DG, Neglia JP, Dusenbery KE. Second neoplasms after megavoltage radiation for pediatric tumors. Cancer 2003;97(10):2588–96.
[53] Valeur NS, Rahbar H, Chapman T. Ultrasound of pediatric breast masses: what to do with lumps and bumps. Pediatr Radiol 2015;45(11):1584–99 [quiz: 1581–3].
[54] Stavros AT, Thickman D, Rapp CL, et al. Solid breast nodules: use of sonography to distinguish between benign and malignant lesions. Radiology 1995;196(1):123–34.
[55] D'Orsi CJ, Sickles EA, Mendelson EB, et al. ACR BI-RADS® Atlas, Breast Imaging Reporting and Data System. Reston (VA): American College of Radiology; 2013.
[56] Koning JL, Davenport KP, Poole PS, et al. Breast Imaging-Reporting and Data System (BI-RADS) classification in 51 excised palpable pediatric breast masses. J Pediatr Surg 2015;50(10):1746–50.
[57] Jawahar A, Vade A, Ward K, et al. Biopsy versus conservative management of sonographically benign-appearing solid breast masses in adolescents. J Ultrasound Med 2015;34(4): 617–25.
[58] Pacinda SJ, Ramzy I. Fine-needle aspiration of breast masses. J Adolesc Health 1998;23(1): 3–6.
[59] Luhar AP, Chiang M, Langer J, et al. Improving pediatric breast ultrasound reporting and recommendations. J Am Coll Radiol 2017;14(11):1451–4.
[60] Gordon PB, Gagnon FA, Lanzkowsky L. Solid breast masses diagnosed as fibroadenoma at fine-needle aspiration biopsy: acceptable rates of growth at long-term follow-up. Radiology 2003;229(1):233–8.
[61] Jacklin RK, Ridgway PF, Ziprin P, et al. Optimising preoperative diagnosis in phyllodes tumour of the breast. J Clin Pathol 2006;59(5):454–9.
[62] Sanders LM, Sharma P, El Madany M, et al. Clinical breast concerns in low-risk pediatric patients: practice review with proposed recommendations. Pediatr Radiol 2018;48(2): 186–95.

Advances in Pediatrics 68 (2021) 211–225

ADVANCES IN PEDIATRICS

Pituitary Tumors in Children

Craig A. Alter, MD[a,c,*], Karuna V. Shekdar, MD[b,c], Laurie E. Cohen, MD[d,e]

[a]Division of Endocrinology, The Children's Hospital of Philadelphia, 34th and Civic Center Boulevard, Philadelphia, PA 19104, USA; [b]Division of Radiology, The Children's Hospital of Philadelphia, 34th and Civic Center Boulevard, Philadelphia, PA 19104, USA; [c]Raymond and Ruth Perelman School of Medicine at the University of Pennsylvania, Philadelphia, PA, USA; [d]Division of Endocrinology, Boston Children's Hospital, 300 Longwood Avenue, Boston, MA 02115, USA; [e]Harvard Medical School, Boston, MA, USA

Keywords

• Craniopharyngioma • Microadenoma • Pars intermedia cyst • Pituitary adenoma • Prolactinoma • Rathke cleft cyst

Key points

- Pituitary tumors or cysts are common findings in pediatric brain scans.
- Findings should prompt questions relating to potential pituitary hormone deficiencies or excesses, as well as to any visual concerns.
- A pituitary focused MRI differs from a brain MRI by having thinner slices and may include the administration of the intravenous contrast agent gadolinium.
- Clinical correlation should focus on hormones in the pituitary: thyrotropin, also known as thyroid-stimulating hormone, adrenocorticotropin, luteinizing hormone, follicle-stimulating hormone, prolactin, growth hormone, and vasopressin, also known as antidiuretic hormone.

INTRODUCTION

Pituitary tumors and cysts are common findings on pediatric brain scans. In 1 study, they were detected in 57% of children [1]. They may be discovered incidentally during an evaluation for headaches or developmental delays, or they may be found when imaging the pituitary and hypothalamus after a new diagnosis of growth hormone (GH) deficiency or precocious puberty, although usually the MRI scan is normal in those settings. There are other times where a pituitary tumor is suspected clinically, such as in an adolescent with headaches,

*Corresponding author. *E-mail address:* alterc@email.chop.edu

https://doi.org/10.1016/j.yapd.2021.05.007
0065-3101/21/

delayed or arrested puberty, and galactorrhea (prolactinoma). In this article, the authors describe the clinical significance of various abnormalities found and whether further investigation or treatment is required. However, first, it is important to understand the various radiologic methods of scanning the region of the pituitary, because not all the methods offer equal precision.

PITUITARY IMAGING

Imaging evaluation of the pituitary gland and the sella turcica, where it sits, is typically performed using MRI. MRI offers multiplanar imaging with excellent anatomic resolution and also has the advantage of absence of ionizing radiation. However, an MRI examination is usually longer than a computed tomography study. The longer duration of the MRI study may require the use of sedation in younger children or in claustrophobic patients. A computed tomography study is usually shorter, but with the disadvantages of use of ionizing radiation and inferior resolution to MRI.

When requesting an MRI to evaluate the hypothalamic–pituitary area, a pituitary protocol should be requested, which provides thin slices through the area to provide visualization and a detailed evaluation of the pituitary gland and the surrounding structures, such as the cavernous sinuses, the traversing cranial nerves III to VI, the cavernous segment of the internal carotid artery, and the optic chiasm. Imaging is obtained in at least 2 orthogonal planes, that is, the sagittal and coronal planes. With increasing concern for gadolinium deposition in the brain, the use of contrast enhancement is limited to the evaluation of pituitary mass lesions. For certain indications, it is necessary to image the entire brain. For example, certain tumors (ie, germinomas) may disseminate and require imaging of the brain and spine, and some developmental pituitary anomalies can be associated with other midline congenital defects.

Normal MRI appearance of the pituitary gland

The pituitary gland is located in the sella turcica, a fossa in the sphenoid bone within the central skull base (Fig. 1). The pituitary gland consists of 2 lobes, the anterior pituitary (adenohypophysis) and the posterior pituitary (neurohypophysis). The adenohypophysis is isointense to the brain parenchyma, and the neurohypophysis is brighter or hyperintense compared with the brain parenchyma on T1-weighted images. The T1 hyperintensity of the neurohypophysis is attributed to the protein hormone granules within. It is important to identify the presence and location of the T1 hyperintensity ("bright spot") of the neurohypophysis. The bright spot may be found in an ectopic location when there is a pituitary developmental abnormality, or it may be absent if there is vasopressin, also known as antidiuretic hormone, deficiency owing to mass effect or infiltration from space-occupying lesions.

The appearance of the pituitary gland depends on the age of the patient. The neonatal pituitary gland is diffusely enlarged and T1 hyperintense owing to the influence of the maternal hormones. A prepubertal pituitary gland shows a concave superior contour. During puberty, there is physiologic enlargement

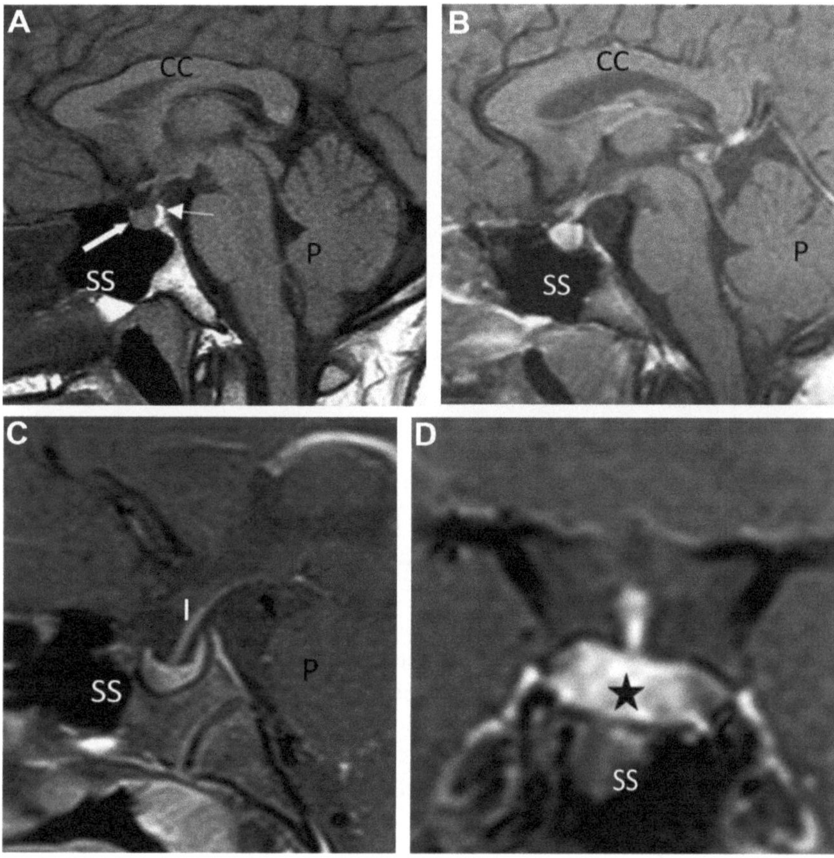

Fig. 1. Normal appearance of pituitary gland on MRI. (*A*) Precontrast T1 sagittal in a 13-year-old pubertal girl. Thick white arrow, anterior pituitary; thin white arrow, bright posterior pituitary. (*B*) Postcontrast T1 sagittal image with homogenous enhancement of pituitary gland. (*C*) Postcontrast T1 sagittal image in a prepubertal 7-year-old boy with concave superior contour of enhancing pituitary gland. (*D*) Postcontrast coronal T1 image with a normal enhancing pituitary gland (*) and enhancing infundibulum/pituitary stalk. CC, corpus callosum; P, pons; SS, sphenoid sinus; I, infundibulum or pituitary stalk.

or hyperplasia of the pituitary gland, which can impart a convex superior contour to the gland [2].

The pituitary stalk is the inferior continuation of the hypothalamus inserting to the superior aspect of the pituitary gland in the midline. The pituitary stalk is broader superiorly and gradually tapers inferiorly [3].

A normal pituitary gland enhances diffusely and homogeneously after the administration of intravenous gadolinium. There is also enhancement of the pituitary stalk, but the hypothalamus does not show any enhancement. Many focal lesions of the pituitary gland, such as microadenomas, are hypoenhancing and stand out in contrast with the surrounding enhancing pituitary gland. Other pituitary and

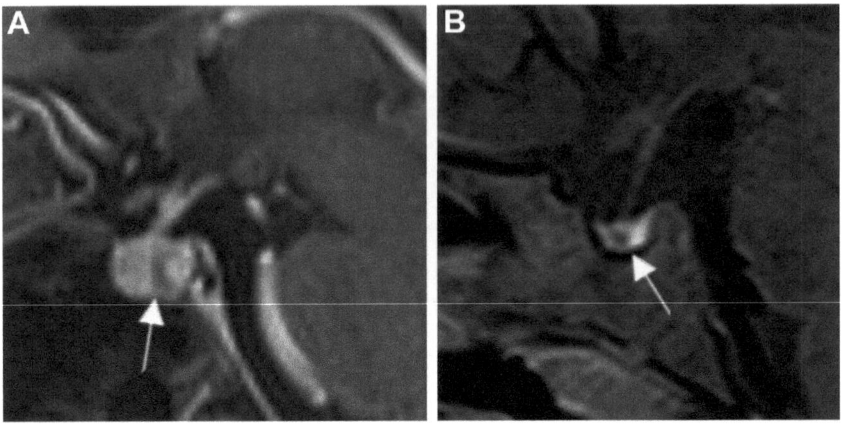

Fig. 2. Pars intermedia cyst. Postcontrast T1 sagittal MRI of 2 different patients showing small nonenhancing cyst (*white arrows*) less then 3 mm in size, between the anterior and posterior pituitary gland consistent with pars intermedia cyst. In both patients, this finding was incidental.

suprasellar mass lesions, such as meningiomas, craniopharyngiomas (CPs), and germinomas, can show increased enhancement after contrast administration.

The optic chiasm is located immediately superior to the pituitary stalk. Sellar and suprasellar mass lesions can cause elevation or compression of the optic chiasm and may result in visual field defects.

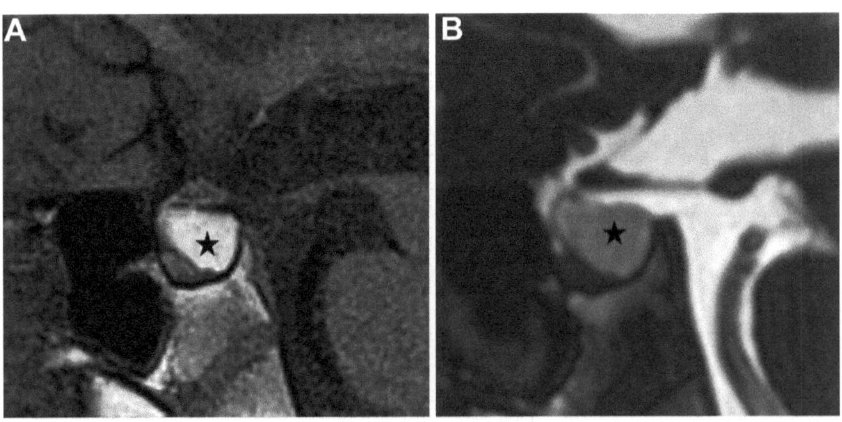

Fig. 3. Rathke cleft cyst. (*A*) Noncontrast T1 sagittal image showing an 11-mm bright signal pituitary cyst (*) with suprasellar extension. (*B*). Heavily T2-weighted image showing an intermediate signal cyst (*) causing anterior displacement of the pituitary stalk. The patient underwent fenestration to decompress the cyst, which was confirmed to be a Rathke cleft cyst.

The interpretation of any MRI study of the pituitary gland includes assessment of the size of the gland, the presence and location of the T1 bright spot of the neurohypophysis, evaluation of the pituitary stalk, and enhancement pattern. Additional findings to look for include the presence of cysts or mass lesions and calcifications. Attention must be paid to the structures adjacent to the pituitary gland, which include the cavernous sinuses and traversing structures and the optic chiasm. In every case of a suprasellar mass lesion or pituitary stalk enlargement, the pineal region should be evaluated carefully for presence of a mass lesion.

The characteristic imaging features are described along with specific pathologic entities.

PITUITARY CYSTS

Pars intermedia cysts (Fig. 2) form within the pituitary gland along the posterior margin of the Rathke pouch (precursor of the anterior pituitary gland). These lesions are typically asymptomatic and measure less than 3 mm. The classic configuration is of a flattened cystic cavity broadest in the coronal plane, located at the junction of anterior and posterior lobes.

Rathke cleft cysts (Fig. 3) are incidental pituitary cysts that arise from the nonobliterated intrasellar lumen of Rathke pouch. When Rathke cleft cysts are large, they become symptomatic, because of the exerted mass effect. In many instances, pars intermedia cysts may be difficult to distinguish from pure Rathke cleft cysts. Many pars intermedia cysts that are greater than 3 mm are considered Rathke cleft cysts on imaging [1,4].

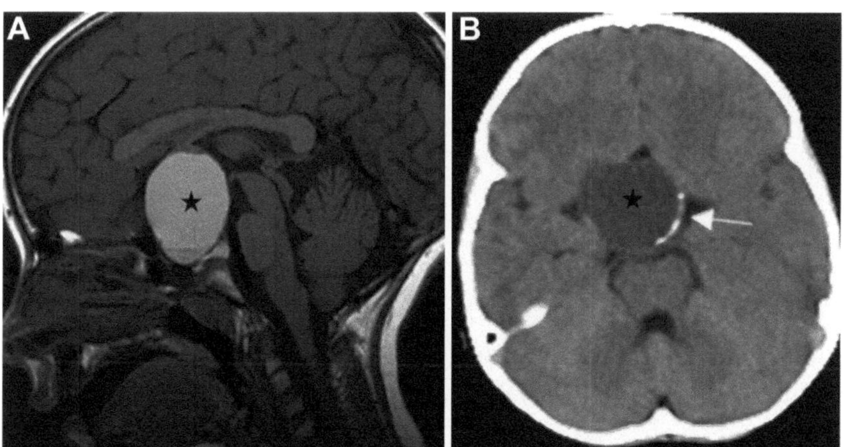

Fig. 4. CP in a 6-year-old boy. (*A*) MRI showing cystic suprasellar mass with (*) bright signal on a noncontrast T1 sagittal image. (*B*) A computed tomography scan of same patient shows the cystic mass with peripheral calcification (*white arrow*).

PITUITARY TUMORS

Craniopharyngioma

CPs (Fig. 4) account for 1.2% to 4.6% of all central nervous system tumors [5] and about 6% of pediatric brain tumors [6]. There are 2 peaks of incidence: in childhood at age 5 to 14 years and in adulthood at age 50 to 74 years of age [7]. Childhood CP almost always have an adamantinomatous pathology [8] with finger-like projections that extend into the surrounding structures causing tissue damage and gliosis [9], may be cystic, and may have calcifications (see Fig. 4B) [10]. Ninety-five percent of adamantinomatous craniopharyngioma have activating mutations in exon 3 of the *CTNNB1* gene, which encodes beta-catenin, leading to overactivation of the WNT/beta-catenin pathway [8]. Adult CP may have a papillary (14%–50%) [9] or adamantinomatous pathology. Papillary CP are usually well-circumscribed with less frequent infiltration of the surrounding tissue, as well as rarely present with calcifications [11]. Of papillary CP, 81% to 100% have a BRAF-activating mutation V600E [8].

CPs are thought to arise from the neoplastic transformation of ectopic embryonal remnants along the hypophyseal duct through which the Rathke pouch migrates to form the anterior pituitary gland [12,13]. Because they arise along the hypophyseal duct, they may be located in an infradiaphragmatic location (below the dura mater through which the pituitary stalk passes) and/or a suprasellar location above the pituitary gland to the floor of third ventricle [14]. Although they are benign histologically, they can cause significant morbidity, because they are located close to and can invade the pituitary gland and its stalk, the hypothalamus, the optic nerves and chiasm, and the Circle of Willis [15,16]. When infradiaphragmatic, they are more likely to present with pituitary hormone deficiencies, and when suprasellar, they are more likely to

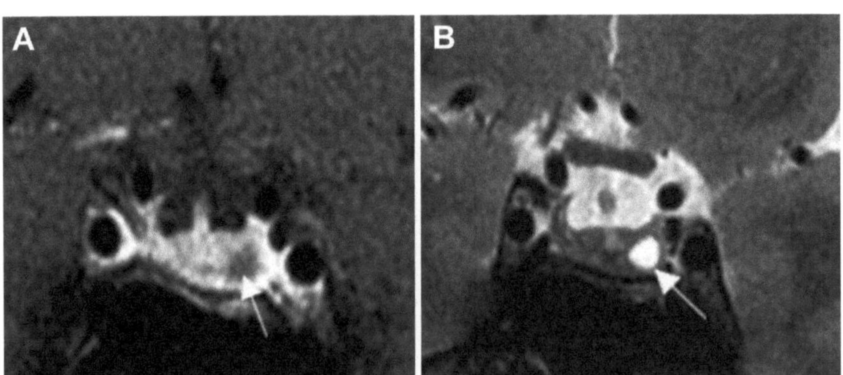

Fig. 5. Pituitary microadenoma on MRI. (*A*) Postcontrast T1 coronal image with nonenhancing microadenoma (*white arrow*). (*B*) T2 coronal image further defines the bright microadenoma (*white arrow*).

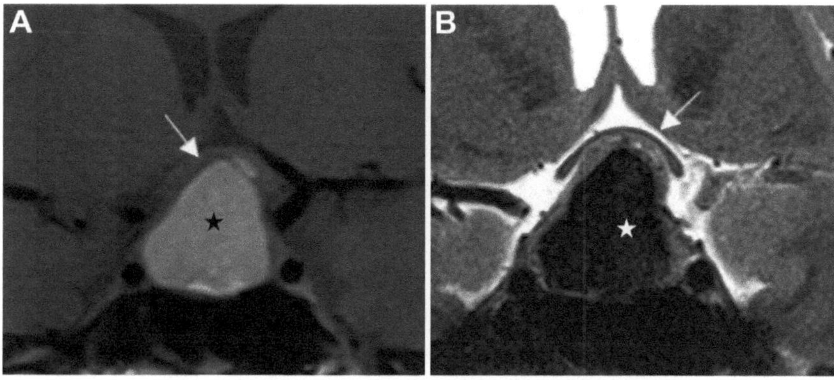

Fig. 6. A 16-year-old girl with a macroadenoma-prolactinoma on MRI. (*A*) Macroadenoma on noncontrast T1 coronal image with hemorrhage within (*). (*B*) T2 coronal image with dark signal of hemorrhage within. Note superior displacement of the optic chiasm (*thin white arrow*).

present with hypothalamic dysfunction and signs of increased intracranial pressure [14,17].

Major morbidity also occurs during surgical resection of the CP with injury to the surrounding structures, as well as owing to scarring and reactive changes after resection and radiation therapy. These complications include hypopituitarism, hypothalamic (morbid) obesity, visual and neurologic deficits, cerebrovascular disease, seizures, decreased cognitive function, and impairments in social and emotional functioning [5,8]. CP also frequently recur, often within the first 3 years [16], although the overall survival rate of childhood CP is high at 87% to 95% [10].

Pituitary adenoma

When the MRI reveals an adenoma, it may be classified as functional (hormone secreting) or nonfunctional. The most common functional adenoma is a prolactinoma, followed by adrenocorticotropic hormone secreting, GH-secreting, and rarely, thyroid-stimulating hormone secreting [18]. An adenoma with its longest dimension of less than 1 cm is termed a microadenoma (Fig. 5), 1 to 4 cm a macroadenoma, and above 4 cm, a giant adenoma [19]. Prolactinomas (Fig. 6) result in a serum prolactin of greater than 100 ng/mL and typically more than 300 ng/mL, and as high as several thousand nanograms per milliliter. When the prolactin is increased but less than 100 ng/mL, the mass may not be a true prolactinoma but a nonfunctioning adenoma with concomitant pituitary stalk compression. Of note, certain medications, such as antipsychotics, can cause hyperprolactinemia with levels that are typically less than 100 ng/mL, although on rare reports they can be greater than 200 ng/mL [20], and in those individuals, an adenoma incidentally found may be nonfunctional.

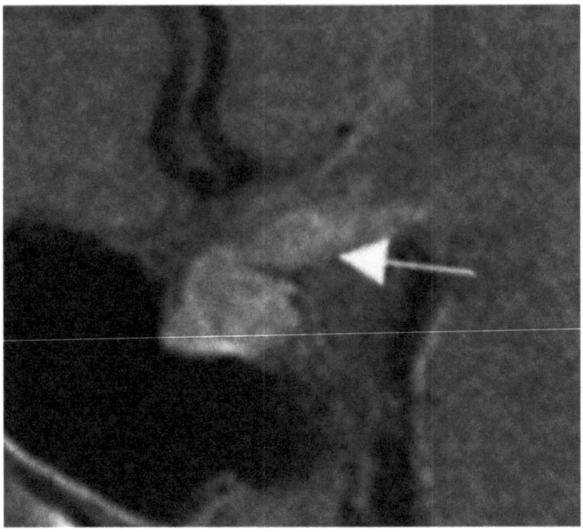

Fig. 7. Suprasellar germinoma. Postcontrast T1 sagittal MRI showing nodular thickening and enhancement (*white arrow*) in the suprasellar region, which was proven to be a germinoma.

Hypothalamic hamartoma

Individuals with central precocious puberty or gelastic (laughing) seizures may have a hypothalamic hamartoma, which is a malformation in the hypothalamus that has a similar appearance to normal brain tissue. These lesions do not typically enlarge once discovered [21].

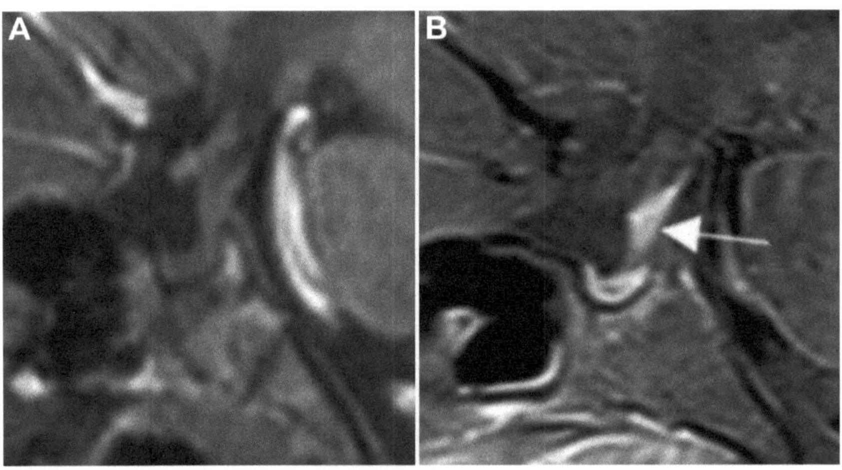

Fig. 8. Langerhans cell histiocytosis. (*A*) Noncontrast T1 sagittal image showing the absence of the normal bright spot of the neurohypophysis. (*B*) Postcontrast T1 sagittal image of the same patient showing a thickened pituitary stalk (*white arrow*).

Optic pathway glioma

Optic pathway gliomas grow in the region of the pituitary; however, they are not part of the pituitary; they may involve the hypothalamus. They may be associated with neurofibromatosis type 1, in which case they may wax and wane [22].

Pituitary stalk thickening

In addition to nonvisualization of the posterior pituitary bright spot (which can be a nonspecific finding), individuals presenting with diabetes insipidus (DI) may also have a thickened pituitary stalk, which suggests an infiltrative process. The most common diagnoses that are associated with pituitary stalk thickening in children are hypophysitis (inflammation of the pituitary gland), germ cell tumors (Fig. 7), and Langerhans cell histiocytosis (Fig. 8). When the stalk is thickened, follow-up scans are recommended every 3 months for the first year and then the interval is gradually increased. If the pituitary stalk is not thickened, follow-up scans should still be done, because there can be a progression of disease, especially of a germ cell tumor; progression is generally seen by 6 months but can occur years later [23].

Germ cell tumors include germinomas (pure germ cell tumors), as well as non–germinomatous germ cell tumors such as teratoma, yolk sac tumor, and embryonal carcinoma. A small percentage of those with germ cell tumors have the tumor markers alpha-fetoprotein and/or human chorionic gonadotropin in the serum and/or cerebrospinal fluid, and both the blood and the cerebrospinal fluid should be evaluated. Clues for Langerhans cell histiocytosis may include associated skin lesions; skeletal survey should also be done to

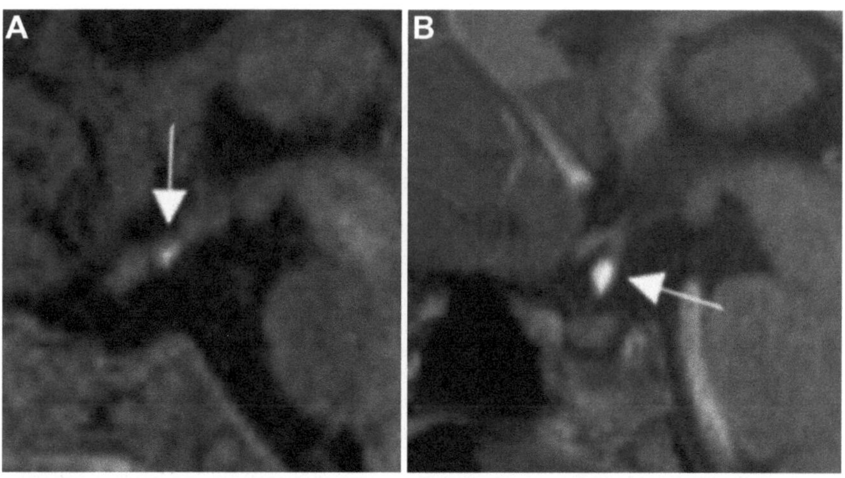

Fig. 9. Ectopic posterior pituitary (EPP). Two different patients with T1 MRI showing an ectopic location of bright signal of posterior pituitary (*white arrow*). (*A*) The ectopic posterior pituitary is anterior to the tuber cinereum. (*B*) The ectopic posterior pituitary is along the pituitary infundibulum.

look for associated bone lesions. After DI, GH deficiency is the most common pituitary hormone deficit [24].

Hypophysitis is generally due to autoimmune destruction of the pituitary. Hypophysitis may be associated with both anterior and posterior pituitary deficits. Idiopathic DI is presumed likely due to hypophysitis. Caution must be used, because germ cell tumors and hypophysitis have similar presentations with lymphocytic infiltration [25].

OTHER STRUCTURAL NONTUMOROUS FINDINGS IN THE PITUITARY AND HYPOTHALAMIC REGION

Ectopic posterior pituitary

As mentioned elsewhere in this article, the posterior pituitary appears bright on the noncontrast MRI T1 image (Fig. 9). An ectopic bright spot located either on the pituitary stalk or above the stalk suggests a developmental abnormality. When this entity is discovered, the diagnosis of a GH deficiency is strengthened, especially if there is an associated thin or interrupted pituitary stalk. The presence of an ectopic posterior pituitary conveys a risk for additional anterior pituitary hormone deficiencies, but not usually DI. An ectopic posterior pituitary may also be found incidentally on MRI [26].

Optic nerve hypoplasia, hypopituitarism, and septo-optic dysplasia

Septo-optic dysplasia is a congenital malformation where there is small pituitary, underdevelopment of the optic nerves, and absence of midline brain structures such as the septum pellucidum and corpus callosum. Occasionally, there are further midline structural problems such as cleft lip and palate. Developmental delay may be seen. A child may present at birth with hypoglycemia (from GH and cortisol deficiency), and with a small phallus if male (from GH deficiency and hypogonadism). Nystagmus may be another clue noted after a few months of life [27].

Empty sella syndrome

An MRI may reveal a flattening of the pituitary owing to filling of the sella turcica with cerebrospinal fluid. It can be idiopathic or secondary to a tumor, increased intracranial pressure, or head trauma. If found, an investigation for other pituitary hormone deficiencies is recommended, but typically returns normal [28].

EVALUATION OF THE CHILD WITH A PITUITARY MASS

Physical examination

As with most endocrinological concerns, the physical examination focuses on the growth pattern. A child with poor growth with maintenance of weight (which can result in frank obesity) suggests GH deficiency and/or hypothyroidism. Although poor weight gain generally argues against endocrine dysfunction, infants with GH deficiency with or without other pituitary hormone deficiencies may have poor feeding and failure to thrive [29]. Likewise, patients with a germ cell tumor and DI can present with poor growth and poor weight

Table 1
Assessment of pituitary hormone competency

Hormone	Laboratory tests
Thyroid-stimulating hormone	Free T4 and thyroid-stimulating hormone
Adrenocorticotropic hormone	7:30–8:00 AM cortisol for deficiency; 24-hour urinary free cortisol and creatinine, or midnight salivary cortisol if concern for excess
Luteinizing hormone, follicle-stimulating hormone	Morning luteinizing hormone, follicle-stimulating hormone, estradiol (girls), testosterone (boys, free testosterone level if obese)
GH	Insulin-like growth factor I with or without insulin-like growth factor binding protein 3 (random GH if GH excess is suspected)
Prolactin	Prolactin
Antidiuretic hormone	Fasting electrolytes, serum and urine osmolality Water deprivation study may be needed
Oxytocin	Not currently measured

gain (unpublished data). Poor growth with excessive weight gain suggests glucocorticoid excess.

The pubertal stage should be assessed. Pubic hair staging is insufficient, because it may be age appropriate owing to adrenal androgen production despite inappropriately small testicles in a boy or absent breast development in a girl with hypogonadotropic hypogonadism. Germ cell tumors, if human chorionic gonadotropin producing, may present with precocious puberty in boys with phallus enlargement and pubic hair development out of proportion to mild testicular enlargement, because human chorionic gonadotropin can stimulate the testosterone-producing Leydig cells of the testes. If excessive height growth is present suggestive of GH excess, then jaw protrusion and teeth gapping should be assessed.

Congenital disease may be associated with midline defects and/or nystagmus. An assessment of visual fields revealing bitemporal hemianopsia and a funduscopic examination revealing hypoplastic optic disks suggests a mass effect on the optic chiasm and nerves. A papular rash mimicking eczema or seborrheic dermatitis can be a sign of Langerhans cell histiocytosis [30].

Testing

When there is a mass discovered in the sella turcica, laboratory studies are needed to evaluate pituitary function. When a small cyst of the pituitary is discovered incidentally without additional clinical concerns, such as a pars intermedia cyst, no evaluation is mandated.

A typical pituitary assessment consists of obtaining a 7:30 to 8:00 AM serum sample. Water can be continued unless DI is being investigated, in which case the patient should be nil per os for as long as they can generally go without drinking and for at least 4 hours. We recommend (Table 1):

- Prolactin (only test necessary in patient with a pituitary microadenoma and no clinical findings) [31,32].
- Thyroid axis: thyroid-stimulating hormone, free T4 (or total T4 with a T3 resin uptake to calculate a free thyroxine index)
- Adrenal axis: cortisol and adrenocorticotropic hormone (if evaluating for central adrenal insufficiency; this is not the evaluation for the cortisol excess of Cushing syndrome, which includes either a 24-hour urine collection for free cortisol and creatinine, or midnight salivary cortisol levels)
- GH axis: insulin-like growth factor I with or without insulin-like growth factor binding protein 3; and if gigantism is suspected, a random GH, hemoglobin A1c, and glucose
- Pubertal axis: ultrasensitive or pediatric luteinizing hormone, follicle-stimulating hormone, estradiol (girls), testosterone (boys; free testosterone level only if obese) for those under 6 months or of pubertal age
- DI: If polyuria and polydipsia, chemistry panel with electrolytes, calcium, serum osmolality, and urinalysis with osmolality after a period of not drinking (note that hypercalcemia and hypokalemia can cause nephrogenic DI)
- A bone age (radiograph of the left hand and wrist).

TREATMENT

Pituitary tumor and cyst treatment

The goal of treatment is to alleviate headaches, preserve or protect vision, and restore normal pituitary function. If there is mass effect on the brain or optic nerves, then neurosurgical intervention may be needed, except in the case of prolactinoma. This operation should be done at a center with experience at endoscopic endonasal pituitary surgery. If there is hydrocephalus, the surgeon may place a ventriculoperitoneal shunt. CPs are typically treated with surgery. Cysts may be followed to see if there is progression to decide if removal is necessary. As mentioned previously, small, under 3 mm, pars intermedia cysts do not need to be treated.

Prolactinoma is treated with just medication in most instances. Cabergoline and bromocriptine are oral dopamine agonists that effectively decrease both prolactin levels and the size of the tumor. Cabergoline has a longer half-life and is the drug of choice. These medicines may cause nausea and abdominal discomfort, but are usually well-tolerated. Surgery is rarely needed, but is considered when there is a large mass effect on the optic nerves (although that can still typically be treated with medication), medication intolerance, or medication resistance.

Hormone replacement

Hormone replacement can be complex and is typically managed by a pediatric endocrinologist. Levothyroxine is administered similarly as in a child with primary hypothyroidism; however, the thyroid-stimulating hormone cannot be used to monitor the dosage. The goal is typically to maintain the free T4 level in the upper one-half of the normal range. Adrenal hormone daily replacement is usually administered at lower doses than needed to treat someone with primary adrenal insufficiency or congenital adrenal hyperplasia. The family must be taught stress dosing of steroids (at doses similar to that of primary adrenal insufficiency). Typically, a family is given injectable hydrocortisone for emergencies. Mineralocorticoid replacement is unnecessary because the physiologic pathway for aldosterone release involves the renin–angiotensin system, rather than adrenocorticotropic hormone.

GH is administered subcutaneously, most commonly at night. Currently, several companies are developing weekly GH preparations. GH is usually well-tolerated, although there are rare adverse effects of pseudotumor cerebri and slipped capital femoral epiphysis. A mild increase in blood glucose is often seen, but is not clinically significant, unless the patient has an underlying risk for type 2 diabetes mellitus.

Replacement of pubertal hormones includes estrogen administration to girls and testosterone to boys once they are of pubertal age. For girls, estrogen is available in skin patch formulation or oral preparations. The dose is gradually increased every 3 to 6 months. For boys, testosterone is most commonly given by intramuscular injections, initially about every 4 weeks. There are topical preparations, although the patch form may cause irritation and the gel form may expose family members and contacts. Some clinicians prescribe weekly subcutaneous injection, although that method is not approved by the US Food and Drug Administration.

The treatment of DI requires knowledge of the fluid balance of intake and output. The management of DI where the child has lost the ability to detect thirst is a complicated and difficult situation. Desmopressin is a long-acting version of vasopressin with long half-life and a lower ability to constrict blood vessels. Preparations include oral tablets (and outside of the United States, sublingual) and inhalation via nasal spray or a rhinal tube. Some families prefer a combination of these therapies. The nasal form has more rapid onset but less ability to modify dosing, whereas the tablets are easier to transport but take longer to show effect. The rhinal tube allows for lower dose increments, but is complicated to administer.

The other posterior pituitary hormone, oxytocin, is not typically replaced, although its therapeutic benefits are being studied by various groups.

SUMMARY

There are several congenital abnormalities of the pituitary gland with prenatal onset that can result in pituitary hormone deficiencies. These abnormalities include the ectopic posterior pituitary with an absent or thin pituitary stalk and septo-optic dysplasia. MRI of the brain may detect a pituitary cyst or tumor incidentally. The discovery of a cyst measuring less than or equal to 3 mm between the anterior and posterior lobes (pars intermedia cyst) requires no follow-up under most circumstances. If an MRI shows a concern in the pituitary, evaluation involves a careful history for evidence of pituitary hormone deficiencies, including DI, or for hormone excesses, such as hyperprolactinemia. A careful review of the growth chart and questions relating to general well-being are paramount in interpreting laboratory studies. Any delay or arrest in pubertal development is important to assess. When a suspected pituitary abnormality is the primary reason for the MRI, the MRI is best ordered as a pituitary protocol, where the slices are thinner in the pituitary and hypothalamic regions; gadolinium contrast should be administered if there is concern for a pituitary microadenoma.

CLINICS CARE POINTS

- When there is a concern of a pituitary lesion, a specific MRI of the hypothalamic–pituitary region should be requested
- Cysts less than 3 mm between the anterior and posterior pituitary lobes are benign and do not cause endocrine or mass abnormalities (pars intermedia cysts)
- Prolactinomas usually result in a serum prolactin of greater than 100 ng/mL and typically above 300 ng/mL, and as high as several thousand nanograms per milliliter.
- Pituitary stalk (infundibulum) thickening suggests an infiltrative process with the most common diagnoses: hypophysitis, germ cell tumors, and Langerhans cell histiocytosis.
- Congenital hypopituitarism may present at birth with hypoglycemia, and in males, also a small phallus.
- A comprehensive pituitary serum assessment consists of an 8:00 AM cortisol, adrenocorticotropic hormone, prolactin, free T4, thyroid-stimulating hormone, insulin-like growth factor I with or without insulin-like growth factor binding protein 3, and in those less than 5 months of age or of pubertal age, luteinizing hormone, follicle-stimulating hormone, estradiol/testosterone, and electrolytes.

DISCLOSURE

The authors have no relevant financial disclosures.

References

[1] Mahdi ES, Webb RL, Whitehead MT. Prevalence of pituitary cysts in children using modern magnetic resonance imaging techniques. Pediatr Radiol 2019;49:1781–7.
[2] Tien RD, Kucharczyk J, Bessette J, et al. MR imaging of the pituitary gland in infants and children: changes in size, shape, and MR signal with growth and development. AJR Am J Roentgenol 1992;158:1151–4.
[3] Sari S, Sari E, Akgun V, et al. Measures of pituitary gland and stalk: from neonate to adolescence. J Pediatr Endocrinol Metab 2014;27:1071–6.
[4] Gunes A, Ozbal Gunes S. The neuroimaging features of Rathke's cleft cysts in children with endocrine-related diseases. Diagn Interv Radiol 2020;26:61–7.
[5] Erfurth EM. Diagnosis, background, and treatment of hypothalamic damage in craniopharyngioma. Neuroendocrinology 2020;110:767–79.
[6] Craniopharyngioma – Childhood Statistics. Available at: https://www.cancer.net/cancer-types/craniopharyngioma-childhood/statistics. Accessed April 11, 2020.
[7] Muller HL, Merchant TE, Puget S, et al. New outlook on the diagnosis, treatment and follow-up of childhood-onset craniopharyngioma. Nat Rev Endocrinol 2017;13:299–312.

[8] Muller HL. Management of endocrine disease: childhood-onset craniopharyngioma: state of the art of care in 2018. Eur J Endocrinol 2019;180:R159–74.
[9] Gump JM, Donson AM, Birks DK, et al. Identification of targets for rational pharmacological therapy in childhood craniopharyngioma. Acta Neuropathol Commun 2015;3:30.
[10] Muller HL. The diagnosis and treatment of craniopharyngioma. Neuroendocrinology 2020;110:753–66.
[11] Zoicas F, Schofl C. Craniopharyngioma in adults. Front Endocrinol (Lausanne) 2012;3:46.
[12] Pascual JM, Rosdolsky M, Prieto R, et al. Jakob Erdheim (1874-1937): father of hypophyseal-duct tumors (craniopharyngiomas). Virchows Arch 2015;467:459–69.
[13] Muller HL, Merchant TE, Warmuth-Metz M, et al. Craniopharyngioma. Nat Rev Dis Primers 2019;5:75.
[14] Castro-Dufourny I, Carrasco R, Prieto R, et al. The infundibulo-tuberal syndrome caused by craniopharyngiomas: clinicopathological evidence from an historical French cohort (1705-1973). Pituitary 2015;18:642–57.
[15] Zacharia BE, Bruce SS, Goldstein H, et al. Incidence, treatment and survival of patients with craniopharyngioma in the surveillance, epidemiology and end results program. Neuro Oncol 2012;14:1070–8.
[16] Bao Y, Pan J, Qi ST, et al. Origin of craniopharyngiomas: implications for growth pattern, clinical characteristics, and outcomes of tumor recurrence. J Neurosurg 2016;125(1):24–32.
[17] Pan J, Qi S, Liu Y, et al. Growth patterns of craniopharyngiomas: clinical analysis of 226 patients. J Neurosurg Pediatr 2015;17(4):418–33.
[18] Zhang N, Zhou P, Meng Y, et al. A retrospective review of 34 cases of pediatric pituitary adenoma. Childs Nerv Syst 2017;33:1961–7.
[19] Russ S, Shafiq I. Pituitary adenoma. Treasure Island (FL): StatPearls; 2020.
[20] Molitch ME. Nonfunctioning pituitary tumors and pituitary incidentalomas. Endocrinol Metab Clin North Am 2008;37:151–71, xi.
[21] Cristobal A, Vorona G, Ritter A, et al. Pre- and postnatal MR imaging of an asymptomatic giant hypothalamic hamartoma. Radiol Case Rep 2020;15:1250–5.
[22] Siwa A, Autrata R, Vejmelkova K, et al. Neurofibromatosis type 1 and optic pathway glioma. Cesk Slov Oftalmol 2019;75:200–8.
[23] Robison NJ, Prabhu SP, Sun P, et al. Predictors of neoplastic disease in children with isolated pituitary stalk thickening. Pediatr Blood Cancer 2013;60:1630–5.
[24] Donadieu J, Rolon MA, Pion I, et al. Incidence of growth hormone deficiency in pediatric-onset Langerhans cell histiocytosis: efficacy and safety of growth hormone treatment. J Clin Endocrinol Metab 2004;89:604–9.
[25] Di Iorgi N, Allegri AE, Napoli F, et al. Central diabetes insipidus in children and young adults: etiological diagnosis and long-term outcome of idiopathic cases. J Clin Endocrinol Metab 2014;99:1264–72.
[26] Ybarra M, Hafiz R, Robinson ME, et al. A new imaging entity consistent with partial ectopic posterior pituitary gland: report of six cases. Pediatr Radiol 2020;50:107–15.
[27] Webb EA, Dattani MT. Septo-optic dysplasia. Eur J Hum Genet 2010;18:393–7.
[28] Lenz AM, Root AW. Empty sella syndrome. Pediatr Endocrinol Rev 2012;9:710–5.
[29] Herber SM, Milner RDG. Growth hormone deficiency presenting under age 2 years. Arch Dis Child 1984;59:557–60.
[30] Leung AKC, Lam JM, Leong KF. Childhood Langerhans cell histiocytosis: a disease with many faces. World J Pediatr 2019;15:536–45.
[31] Freda PU, Beckers AM, Katznelson L, et al. Pituitary incidentaloma: an endocrine society clinical practice guideline. J Clin Endocrinol Metab 2011;96:894–904.
[32] Thaker VV, Lage AE, Kumari G, et al. Clinical course of nonfunctional pituitary microadenoma in children: a single-center experience. J Clin Endocrinol Metab 2019;104:5906–12.

Advances in Pediatrics 68 (2021) 227–244

ADVANCES IN PEDIATRICS

Adrenal Tumors in Childhood

John S. Fuqua, MD

Indiana University School of Medicine, 705 Riley Hospital Drive, Room 5960, Indianapolis, IN 46202, USA

Keywords

• Adrenocortical tumor • Virilization • Cushing syndrome • Pheochromocytoma • Paraganglioma

Key points

- Adrenocortical tumors are rare in children and usually present with virilization before age 5 years. They may also present as Cushing syndrome or with mixed effects.
- Germline mutations in oncogenes occur in children with adrenocortical tumors, including TP53, which causes Li-Fraumeni syndrome.
- Pheochromocytoma and paraganglioma are catecholamine-secreting tumors arising from chromaffin cells and usually present with hypertension.
- More than 50% of children with pheochromocytoma and paragangliomas have mutations in oncogenes putting them at risk for other malignancies, with the most common gene being VHL leading to von Hippel-Lindau syndrome.
- Treatment of adrenocortical tumors and pheochromocytoma/paraganglioma is surgical. Appropriate preoperative and postoperative management is critical to prevent morbidity.

INTRODUCTION

Adrenal neoplasms are rare in the pediatric population. However, they may be malignant, and they typically manifest with concerning symptoms and signs that may be life altering. Higher-stage malignant adrenal tumors carry poor prognoses. In the last decade, more has been learned about the genetic underpinnings of these lesions, which should lead to improved diagnosis and management decisions. This article focuses primarily on adrenocortical tumors and pheochromocytoma, with limited discussion of nodular adrenocortical disease.

E-mail address: jsfuqua@iu.edu

https://doi.org/10.1016/j.yapd.2021.05.015

EMBRYOLOGY AND EARLY DEVELOPMENT OF THE ADRENAL GLAND

The fetal adrenal cortex develops from celomic epithelial precursors on the urogenital ridge between 4 and 6 weeks' gestation. By 7 to 8 weeks' gestation, the fetal adrenal cortex develops 2 zones: the fetal zone and the definitive zone [1]. The fetal zone represents 80% to 90% of the cortical volume and secretes cortisol under the influence of adrenocorticotropic hormone, but the principal product is DHEA-S (dehydroepiandrosterone sulfate), which undergoes conversion to estrogens in the placenta. By late gestation, the definitive zone has begun differentiation into the zona glomerulosa and the zona fasciculata. The adrenal medulla develops from neural crest–derived chromaffin cells that migrate ventrally to approach the cortical precursors under the influence of neuropilins [2]. Late in the first trimester, the chromaffin cells imbed into the cortical mass and become enveloped, but a structurally complete medulla does not form until after birth. At birth, the fetal adrenal is nearly as large as the kidney because of the large fetal zone. However, the fetal zone rapidly involutes as the adult cortex develops in the first few months. The zona reticularis does not develop until later in childhood.

ADRENOCORTICAL TUMORS

Presentation

Pediatric adrenocortical tumors (ACTs) were first described in 1865 [3]. They are rare, comprising only 0.2% of all childhood malignancies, and it is estimated that there are only 25 cases diagnosed per year in the United States [4]. The International Pediatric Adrenocortical Tumors Registry (IPACTR) is hosted by St. Jude Hospital, and, based on these data, the worldwide annual incidence is thought to be 0.3 to 0.38 cases per million children less than age 15 years [5]. Interestingly, the southern region of Brazil has a 10-fold to 15-fold higher rate of disease, which may be because of a founder effect [6]. Across the lifespan, there is a bimodal distribution of cases, with a peak at about 3.8 years and a second peak occurring in the range of 30 to 50 years old. Most pediatric ACTs occur in children less than 5 years old. There is a female predisposition, with a female/male ratio of 1.7:1 in those less than 3 years old, increasing to 6.2:1 in the teenage years [7]. The reason for the young age at presentation is not fully understood but is in part related to the increased prevalence of oncogene mutations in pediatric ACT. In addition, it is thought that pediatric ACTs develop in the regressing fetal adrenal zone because of the early age at first manifestation, the occasional detection of an ACT in neonates, and the predominance of androgen-secreting tumors in childhood [1].

Pediatric adrenocortical tumors are functional in 90% of cases. An analysis of 254 patients with ACTs by the IPACTR showed that 55% presented with isolated virilization, whereas only 5.5% had isolated Cushing syndrome. Those with a mixed virilizing/Cushing phenotype comprised an additional 29%, and there were a few patients with elements of hyperaldosteronism. Isolated aldosterone excess (Conn syndrome) occurred in only 2 children [7]. Patients presenting with isolated Cushing syndrome tended to be older, with a median age of 12.6 years. Feminizing adrenal tumors are very rare.

As a result of the secretory nature of ACTs, the most common signs include rapid penile or clitoral enlargement, sexual hair growth, hirsutism, acne, and increased height velocity (Fig. 1). These signs may be mixed with cushingoid features, such as rapid weight gain or moon facies (Fig. 2A, B). In mixed presentations, the growth suppression from hypercortisolism may limit the growth acceleration from hyperandrogenism. Patients may complain of abdominal pain. The high prevalence of functioning tumors leads to a short time to diagnosis, with approximately two-thirds of patients diagnosed within 6 months of the first signs [7].

Laboratory studies are consistent with the endocrine pathophysiology [5]. Serum concentrations of testosterone, androstenedione, and particularly DHEA-S are often significantly increased. Estradiol, 17-hydroxyprogesterone, and 11-deoxycortisol levels may be increased. Measures of cortisol secretion may be abnormal, including lack of suppression in response to dexamethasone and increased 24-hour urinary cortisol and midnight salivary cortisol levels. If there is concern for adrenal medullary disease, plasma free metanephrines should be assessed (discussed later in relation to pheochromocytoma). Imaging studies are critical to establish the extent of disease, such as tumor location, size, invasion of local structures, and the presence of tumor thrombus in the inferior vena cava. The most common locations of distant metastases are the liver and lungs, so chest imaging is required in addition to abdominal imaging [8]. Kidney, brain, and bone metastases occur less often, and bone or central nervous system imaging is not routinely required in the absence of clinical suspicion. For abdominal imaging, the choice of computed tomography (CT) versus MRI may be based on local preference, [9] although MRI does not require radiation exposure. Imaging of the chest is best done by CT.

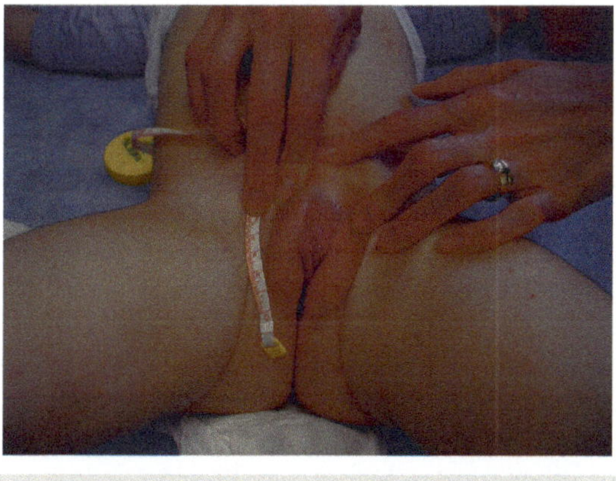

Fig. 1. Genitalia of a 2-year-old girl with an ACT. Note clitoromegaly, rugation, and pigmentation of the labia majora, and pubic hair.

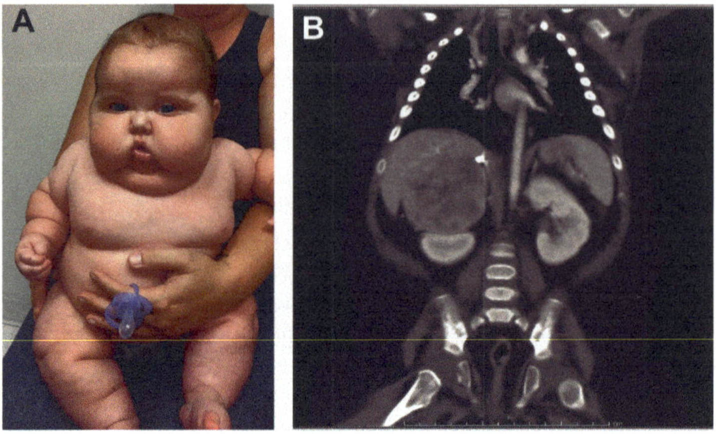

Fig. 2. (*A*) A 1-year-old boy with Cushing syndrome caused by an ACT. No virilization was present. (*B*) Coronal reconstruction of computed tomography imaging showing a right ACT measuring 5.6 cm in diameter with punctate calcifications.

Molecular pathogenesis and association with malignancy syndromes

Adrenocortical tumors occur more commonly in inherited malignancy syndromes such as Li-Fraumeni syndrome, Beckwith-Wiedemann syndrome, and familial adenomatous polyposis (FAP, Gardner syndrome), although a minority of children with ACT have one of these syndromes [10].

Li and Fraumeni [11] first reported an autosomal dominantly inherited association of soft tissue sarcomas and breast carcinoma in 1969. Affected families were found to carry germline mutations in the TP53 gene, encoding the tumor suppressor p53. This protein regulates genes controlling the cell cycle as well as apoptosis, DNA repair, and senescence, and somatic inactivation of p53 or members of its pathway are extremely common in malignant tumors, including ACTs. In families with Li-Fraumeni syndrome, cancers of the breast, brain, and adrenal as well as sarcomas comprise 80% of malignancies. Approximately 10% of patients with germline mutations in TP53 syndrome have adrenocortical cancer [12]. In contrast, 64% to 71% of children enrolled in the IPACTR (in which patients from Brazil are over-represented) have mutations in TP53 but were not from families recognized as having Li-Fraumeni syndrome [10,13]. Findings such as this have led to the concept that the onset of cancers seen in affected families may vary depending on the specific TP53 mutation. A good example of this concept is the experience in southern Brazil, where the incidence of ACT is 10 to 15 times higher than in most parts of the world. Among unrelated children with ACT in this region, 78% to 98% carry the R337H mutation in exon 10 of TP53 [14,15]. However, the mutation has low penetrance, especially in the first few decades of life. From 10% to 15% of individuals carrying the R337H mutation develop ACT [15]. Although the occurrence of other tumors before age 30 years is low in people with the R337H mutation, the lifetime risk of tumors and the tumor types are similar to those seen in classic Li-Fraumeni syndrome [6].

Familial adenomatous polyposis (FAP) is an autosomal dominantly inherited condition in which affected patients have hundreds to thousands of colon polyps, increased risk for colon cancer, thyroid tumors, and ACTs. Mutations in the adenomatous polyposis coli (APC) gene have been identified as the cause of FAP and adrenocortical tumorigenesis [16]. The APC gene is involved in the WNT/β-catenin pathway. In the absence of WNT binding to the frizzled receptor, β-catenin is degraded by a complex of binding proteins, including APC, axin, and glycogen synthase kinase 3β. On WNT binding, the degradation complex is dispersed, and β-catenin accumulates, migrates to the nucleus, and activates target genes regulating the cell cycle and cell adhesion [17]. Disruption of the degradation complex by mutations in APC allow unregulated β-catenin accumulation, leading to tumorigenesis. Somatic mutations in the WNT/β-catenin pathway occur in 38% of adrenal adenomas and 85% of adrenal carcinomas and have also been implicated in numerous other cancers, including colon, gastric, and hepatocellular carcinomas [18]. MicroRNAs may also interact with the WNT/β-catenin pathway. MicroRNAs are short RNA strands that bind to messenger RNA (mRNA) and repress translation or increase degradation of mRNA. MicroRNAs play important roles in cell proliferation, differentiation, and apoptosis. MicroRNA449 has been found to play a role in nodular adrenal disease, acting through inhibition of WNT/β-catenin pathway genes. Elements of this pathway are potential therapeutic targets [19].

Abnormalities in the insulinlike growth factor (IGF) system are also involved in ACT development. Beckwith-Wiedemann syndrome (BWS) is caused by abnormal imprinting at chromosome 11p15, a locus including the IGF2 gene, leading to IGF2 overexpression. Adrenocortical tumors have been found in 7% of individuals with BWS [20]. In addition, in ACTs from pediatric patients without BWS, overexpression of both IGF2 and the gene for its receptor, IGF1R, have been found to be particularly prevalent [21]. Overexpression of IGF1R may be mediated by downregulation of microRNA mir100 [22]. Analysis of tumor tissue has shown that loss of heterozygosity at chromosome 11p leading to overexpression of IGF2 is an early event in tumor development [23], and inhibition of the IGF1 receptor may be a treatment strategy [24].

Grading and staging of adrenocortical tumors

Differentiation between a benign adrenocortical adenoma and adrenocortical carcinoma may be difficult. In adults, pathologists frequently use the Weiss criteria to grade tumors [25]. This strategy is based on a series of histologic features, including nuclear grade; mitotic rate; atypical mitoses; percentage of clear cells; microscopic necrosis; and venous, sinusoidal, and capsular invasion. The presence of 3 or more of these findings is highly correlated to recurrence or metastasis. However, children with ACTs have better prognoses than adults with similar histopathologic findings, with grade IV tumors per Weiss criteria correlating well with prognosis in adults but not in children [26]. This difference has led to the adoption of a grading system put forth by Wieneke and colleagues [27]. This system includes 11 items and puts more weight on tumor size and local invasion in addition to measures of cellular atypia. The scoring yielded 3 categories: (1) patients with up to 2 criteria had a benign long-term clinical outcome; (2) those with 3 criteria were indeterminate for malignancy; and (3) tumors meeting 4 or more criteria were characterized as malignant and those patients had poor outcomes. Other investigators have validated this system [28].

In general, benign adrenocortical adenomas tend to weigh less than 200 g, are well defined and spherically shaped, with no invasion into local structures. On histology, they resemble the normal zona fasciculata or reticularis. Adrenocortical carcinomas are more likely to be larger with marked lobulation and large areas of necrosis or hemorrhage. Microscopic examination reveals larger cells that are arranged in alveolar clusters, with eosinophilic cytoplasm [29].

The MacFarlane/Sullivan staging system was proposed in 1958, modified in 1978, and is based on series of patients ranging from neonates to age 69 years old [30]. Several newer staging systems based exclusively on childhood data have been proposed in the last 25 years. These systems have variably incorporated tumor size, degree of residual tumor, normalization of hormone levels postoperatively, and the presence of distal metastases. Using the staging criteria proposed by Sandrini and colleagues [10,31] in 1997 and modified by others (Table 1), an analysis of 58 Brazilian children showed greater than 90% long-term survival for stage 1. Survival rates for stages 2 and 3 were intermediate, but were significantly lower at 52% and 25%, respectively. Virtually none of the patients with stage 4 disease survived. The IPACTR, working through the Children's Oncology Group, has proposed a similar staging system that incorporates spread to retroperitoneal lymph nodes [10].

Estimates of the overall survival rate for children with adrenocortical tumors vary widely, ranging from 46% to 74% [5,29]. In addition to disease stage, favorable factors important in the prognosis include age less than 3 years and the

Table 1
Staging strategy for adrenocortical tumor in children

Stage	Criteria
I	Completely resected, small tumors (<100 g and <200 cm^3) with normal postoperative hormone levels
II	Completely resected large tumors ($\geq$100 g or $\geq$200 cm^3) with normal postoperative hormone levels
III	Unresectable; Gross or microscopic residual disease Tumor spillage Stage I and II tumors with hormone levels that fail to normalize after surgery Retroperitoneal lymph node involvement
IV	Distant metastases

From Ribeiro RC, Pinto EM, Zambetti GP, Rodriguez-Galindo C. The International Pediatric Adrenocortical Tumor Registry initiative: contributions to clinical, biological, and treatment advances in pediatric adrenocortical tumors. Mol Cell Endocrinol. 2012 Mar 31;351(1):37-43. https://doi.org/10.1016/j.mce.2011.10.015.

presence of virilization at diagnosis [7]. Factors associated with decreased survival include glucocorticoid secretion and an increased Ki67-labeling index [5].

Treatment

Surgical removal of the tumor is the mainstay of treatment, with the goal of a complete microscopic resection. Malignant ACTs tend to be locally invasive and adhere to surrounding structures. As a result, en bloc resection of kidney, liver segments, or portions of the pancreas may be needed. Selection of a laparoscopic versus open procedure is controversial, with some studies showing poorer prognosis with a laparoscopic approach [32]. Some investigators suggest that laparoscopic adrenalectomy is acceptable if there is no local invasion noted in the staging evaluation [5]. Tumors typically have a thin capsule and are friable and easily ruptured. Intraoperative tumor spillage worsens the long-term prognosis, and having an experienced surgeon is thus important. The role of retroperitoneal lymph node dissection is not established in children, but it may improve the prognosis in adults [33]. All ACTs should be considered malignant at the time of surgery [5].

Because of the extreme rarity of ACTs in children, the role of chemotherapy is not well studied. It is recommended in children with intraoperative tumor spillage, residual disease, or in those with local or distant metastases. This recommendation differs from that in adults, in whom chemotherapy is used earlier because of higher recurrence rates [5]. The most studied medication is mitotane, which inhibits steroidogenesis and is antiproliferative and adrenolytic, leading to apoptosis of the zona fasciculata and zona reticularis. The prognosis is better when serum mitotane concentrations exceed 14 mg/L for at least 6 months, which can be attained by daily dosing of 4 g/m^2 of body surface area [34,35]. Mitotane toxicity may limit dosing and commonly takes the form of abdominal pain, vomiting, and diarrhea. Neurotoxicity may lead to lethargy, ataxia, depression, and vertigo and is most often seen when serum concentrations exceed 20 mg/L [29]. Because it inhibits steroidogenesis, patients receiving mitotane require glucocorticoid and mineralocorticoid replacement. Mitotane induces hepatic cytochrome P450 3A4, which accelerates glucocorticoid clearance. Thus, patients may require higher doses to avoid symptoms of adrenal insufficiency [36]. Combination chemotherapy including cisplatin, etoposide, and doxorubicin along with mitotane has been shown to improve survival in adults, but it has not been systematically studied in children [37]. Adrenocortical tumors have been considered to be radioresistant, so radiation therapy has not traditionally been used. However, it is useful as palliative therapy in adults with refractory disease [34]. Routine radiation therapy in children is not recommended because of the potential for secondary malignancies, especially in those with TP53 mutations [5].

PRIMARY BILATERAL ADRENAL HYPERPLASIAS

This group of nodular adrenal diseases comprises 10% of primary adrenal causes of Cushing syndrome [38]. It is divided into micronodular forms, which tend to affect children and young adults, and macronodular hyperplasia, which occurs more commonly in older adults. Micronodular bilateral adrenal hyperplasia includes the subgroups of primary pigmented nodular adrenal disease (PPNAD) and isolated micronodular adrenal disease (iMAD) [39].

Primary pigmented nodular adrenal disease

PPNAD typically presents with Cushing syndrome in the second, third, and fourth decades and is more frequent in women. Cushing syndrome caused by PPNAD tends to be mild and may be cyclical [40]. Between 50% and 80% of patients with PPNAD have Carney complex, whereas about 60% of those with Carney complex ultimately develop PPNAD [41,42]. Carney complex is a rare multiple neoplasia syndrome. Common features include multiple skin lentigines, blue nevi, PPNAD, myxomas of the skin and heart, large clear cell Sertoli cell tumors of the testes, thyroid nodules and carcinoma, acromegaly, and psammomatous melanotic schwannomas. Carney complex is most often caused by mutations in the PRKAR1A gene, encoding a regulatory subunit of protein kinase A. Other genes in the protein kinase A (PKA) pathway may also carry mutations, such as genes encoding the PKA catalytic subunits or phosphodiesterases [19]. Patients with Cushing syndrome associated with Carney complex may have a paradoxic increase in cortisol production in response to dexamethasone, arising from overexpression of glucocorticoid receptors on adrenocortical cells and acting through a PKA-mediated mechanism [43]. Small adrenal nodules may be seen on high-resolution CT scans, appearing as hypodense, round, and well-delineated lesions [42]. Cushing syndrome caused by nodular adrenal disease is usually treated with bilateral adrenalectomy, although more limited surgery may be effective. Histology shows multiple 1-mm to 4-mm nodules with brown, black, yellow, or red pigmentation, with internodular adrenal atrophy [44]. Patients with Carney complex require surveillance for other manifestations. Recommendations include annual echocardiography and ultrasonography of the thyroid and testes as well as annual measurement of urinary free cortisol and IGF1. In children and adolescents, growth and puberty should also be monitored [42].

Isolated micronodular adrenocortical disease

iMAD is a subset of micronodular bilateral adrenal hyperplasia. Like PPNAD, it leads to Cushing syndrome, but it is not associated with other nonadrenal disorders. iMAD usually presents in infancy and childhood and usually occurs earlier than PPNAD. It also tends to cause mild to moderate Cushing syndrome that may be cyclical [40,45]. On histology, nodules are less than 10 mm in size and are not grossly pigmented. There is no internodular adrenal atrophy. iMAD is caused by mutations in PDE11A and PDE8B, both of which encode phosphodiesterases, leading to cellular accumulation of cyclic AMP, aberrant signal transduction, and tumorigenesis [45,46]. As in cases of PPNAD, iMAD is usually treated with bilateral adrenalectomy [38].

Primary bilateral macronodular adrenal hyperplasia

Primary bilateral macronodular adrenal hyperplasia (PBMAH) most commonly presents with Cushing syndrome in older adults, aged 40 to 60 years

[45]. It may develop slowly with a long period of subclinical hypercortisolism and milder Cushing syndrome that may require decades to be detected [45,47]. As with micronodular adrenal hyperplasia, patients with PBMAH may have a paradoxic increase in cortisol secretion in response to dexamethasone. Interestingly, aberrant expression of G-protein-coupled receptors commonly leads to activation of the cAMP/PKA pathway and stimulation of tumor growth by ligands other than ACTH, including the gastric inhibitory polypeptide (GIP) receptor, adrenergic receptors, and the V1a vasopressin receptor [48]. Although mutations in FAP and multiple endocrine neoplasia type 1 (MEN1) may lead to PBMAH, abnormalities in ARMC5 are the most common cause, occurring in 40% of cases [49]. PBMAH may also rarely occur in McCune-Albright syndrome, in which case it may present as early as the first year of life [47].

PHEOCHROMOCYTOMA/PARAGANGLIOMA

Presentation

Pheochromocytomas and paragangliomas (PPGL) are neuroendocrine tumors derived from chromaffin tissue of the adrenal medulla or extra-adrenal sympathetic ganglia in the thorax, abdomen, and pelvis. PPGL secrete catecholamines, which lead to most of the presenting symptoms. Paragangliomas (PGLs) located in the head and neck are derived from parasympathetic nervous tissue and are usually nonfunctional. Although the mean age at diagnosis is 51 ± 16 years, PPGL can occur at any age. The overall annual incidence is 0.46 per 100,000, but about 10% to 20% occur in the childhood population, giving an incidence rate of 0.2 to 0.5 per million children [50,51]. The median age at diagnosis in children is about 13 years, and about 75% of PPGL in children are pheochromocytomas (PHEOs).

Symptoms of PPGL include headache, tachycardia, diaphoresis, and pallor. Less common are asthenia, weight loss, abdominal pain, fever, and seizures. Hypertension is seen in most patients. In a recent Italian cooperative study, 19 out of 20 symptomatic patients with PHEO and 15 out of 22 with PGL presented with hypertension [52]. Hypertension may be severe and can be associated with hypertensive cardiomyopathy. In a study of a large number of children referred for evaluation of hypertension, 1.7% had a PPGL [53]. Because there is a high prevalence of predisposing germline mutations, many patients are found to have PPGL on prospective screening studies if they have a family history of PPGL or associated syndromes. PPGL are rarely biochemically silent, and most of those not identified on screening present with catecholamine-related symptoms.

Evaluation

PPGL are more commonly associated with heritable germline mutations than any other cancer type [54]. Thus, genetic testing is a key component of the evaluation for any patient with confirmed PPGL, especially children. Testing also allows for potential diagnosis in asymptomatic relatives. Patients with PPGL may have a family history consistent with a known predisposing syndrome, such as von Hippel-Lindau (VHL), multiple endocrine neoplasia type 2

(MEN2), and neurofibromatosis type 1 (NF1). In addition, genetic testing identifies those with mutations in the genes encoding components of succinate dehydrogenase (collectively known as SDHx), who have a high risk of metastases. The likelihood of a germline mutation is especially high in cases of multifocal tumors, extra-adrenal tumors, and when there are known metastases. Decision algorithms have been published [55] with the goal of optimizing genetic testing, but the advancement of testing technology has made the use of gene panels faster and more cost-efficient.

The major diagnostic approach to PPGL is measurement of plasma free metanephrine levels or 24-hour urinary metanephrine levels, including both metanephrine and normetanephrine. Their measurement is preferred to catecholamines because metanephrines are specific for chromaffin tissue versus sympathetic nervous tissue and because chromaffin tissue releases metanephrines continually, as opposed to the episodic release of catecholamines [55]. PPGL that occur in the setting of MEN2 and NF1 typically produce both metanephrine and normetanephrine, whereas PPGL associated with VHL or SDHx mutations lack the enzymatic machinery to produce metanephrine. Tumors caused by SDHx mutations also produce 3-methoxytyramine, a metabolite of dopamine (Fig. 3). Measurement of 3-methoxytyramine may aid in the evaluation of these tumors, but it is not widely available clinically [56]. Biochemical testing is more commonly abnormal in cases of PHEO than in PGL. In a recent retrospective study, 91% of patients with childhood PHEO had abnormal biochemical testing compared with 43% of patients with PGL [52]. Typically, levels are increased at least 2-fold the upper level of normal [57,58], and levels of either metanephrine or normetanephrine greater than 3 times the upper limit of normal are rarely false-positives. Increase of both metabolites is also uncommonly a false-positive [55]. Some PPGL are biochemically silent, particularly PGL of the head and neck. Chromogranin A may be a useful tumor marker in these cases. It is recommended to confirm PPGL biochemically before moving to imaging studies.

Numerous medications and dietary substances are well known to interfere with assays of metanephrines. Many of these are listed in Table 2. Avoiding intake of dietary interferences for 3 days is usually sufficient. An additional important factor to consider is patient posture. Reference intervals for metanephrines are established following a 30-minute recumbent period. Drawing blood while the patient is seated in a chair may increase the frequency of falsely abnormal test results 2.8-fold [59].

After establishing the biochemical diagnosis of a PPGL, imaging is required for localization (Fig. 4). CT is recommended as the first-line imaging modality because of its higher resolution (5 mm). However, MRI may be a better option in children because it avoids radiation exposure [55], which is particularly true in this population, many of whom are at high risk for other malignancies. In children and adolescents, most PHEOs are unilateral, with 10% being bilateral at diagnosis. PGLs are unifocal at diagnosis in 83% of children, and 71% are located in the abdomen. Most of the rest are roughly equally distributed between the pelvis and mediastinum, with a small number in the head and

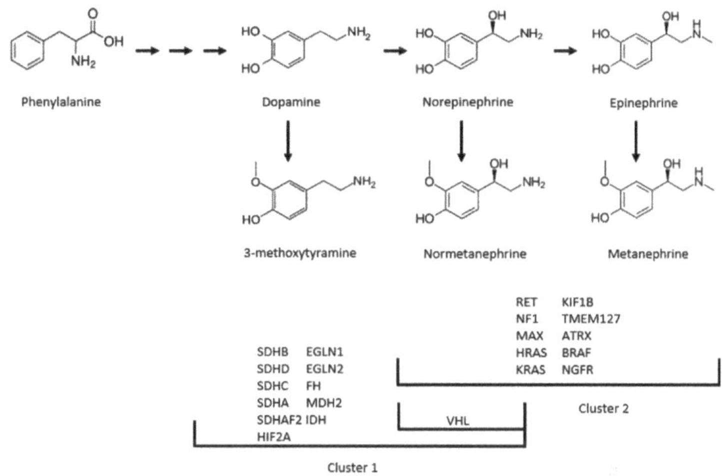

Fig. 3. Dopamine, norepinephrine, and epinephrine are metabolized by the enzyme catechol-O-methyltransferase to 3-methoxytyramine, normetanephrine, and metanephrine, respectively. Germline mutations in genes that lead to PPGL are in 2 clusters. PPGL in patients with mutations in cluster 1 genes are noradrenergic and dopaminergic and produce normetanephrine along with 3-methoxytyramine, with the exception of PPGL in VHL syndrome, which only produce normetanephrine. Tumors resulting from cluster 2 mutations are adrenergic and produce metanephrine, with or without cosecretion of normetanephrine. A third cluster comprises genes that undergo somatic mutations, including MAML3 and CSDE1. ATRX, alpha-thalassemia/mental retardation syndrome, X-linked; BRAF, BRAF protooncogene; CSDE1, cold shock domain–containing E1; EGLN1, Egl-9 prolyl hydroxylase 1; EGLN2, Egl-9 prolyl hydroxylase 2; FH, fumarate hydratase; HIF2A, hypoxia inducible factor 2 alpha; HRAS, HRAS protooncogene; IDH, isocitrate dehydrogenase; KIF1B, kinesin family member 1B; KRAS, KRAS protooncogene; MAML3, mastermindlike transcriptional coactivator 3; MAX, Myc-associated factor X; MDH2, malate dehydrogenase; NF1, neurofibromatosis type 1; NGFR, nerve growth factor receptor; RET, rearranged during transfection; SDHA, succinate dehydrogenase subunit A; SDHAF2, succinate dehydrogenase complex assembly factor 2; SDHB, succinate dehydrogenase subunit B; SDHC, succinate dehydrogenase subunit C; SDHD, succinate dehydrogenase subunit D; TMEM127, transmembrane protein 127; VHL, VHL tumor suppressor; WNT, Wingless/Int-1.

neck [51,52]. There is a high rate of metachronous development of bilateral or multifocal disease in patients with germline mutations. Malignancy in PPGL is defined by the presence of metastatic disease rather than by histologic examination. Although the presence of metastases at diagnosis is uncommon in children (14% in a national French database), all PPGL should be considered as potentially malignant and evaluated accordingly [51,60]. Risk factors for malignant disease include tumor size greater than 5 to 6 cm, extra-adrenal locations, noradrenergic/dopaminergic biochemistry, mutation in SDHB or SDHA, multiple tumor locations, and age less than 20 years [58]. The most common sites of metastatic disease are bone, lung, lymph nodes, and liver.

Multiple functional imaging modalities assist in the evaluation for metastatic disease. These modalities include ^{123}I-MIBG (metaiodobenzylguanidine)

Table 2
Medications and dietary substances that interfere with biochemical testing for pheochromocytomas and paragangliomas

Dietary substances	Medications
Eggs	Acetaminophen
Bananas	Selective serotonin reuptake inhibitors
Cheese	Methamphetamine
Nuts	Tricyclic antidepressants
Chocolate	Buspirone
Vanilla	Sulfasalazine
Caffeine	Cocaine
Black tea	Ephedrine
Nicotine	Monoamine oxidase inhibitors
Alcohol	Methyldopa
—	Levodopa

scintigraphy or single-photon emission CT, ^{18}F-fluorodeoxyglucose–PET/CT, ^{18}F-FDOPA–PET/CT (fluoro-3,4-dihydroxyphenylalnine-PET/CT), and ^{68}Ga-DOTA-SSA (dodecanetetraacetic acid-somatostatin analog) scintigraphy or PET/CT, and recommendations vary on which is best. The best modality may depend on whether a germline mutation is present and which gene is mutated [55]. Current recommendations are to use ^{68}Ga-DOTA-SSA PET/

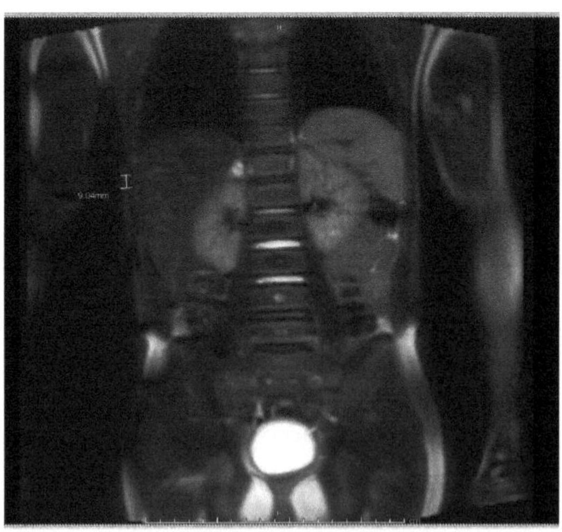

Fig. 4. MRI from a 7-year-old boy with a VHL mutation showing a 1.1-cm diameter T2-hyperintense, contrast-enhancing mass in the right adrenal consistent with a pheochromocytoma.

CT or scintigraphy for any PGL or for PHEO associated with SDHx mutations and ^{18}F-FDOPA PET/CT or scintigraphy for PHEO not associated with SDHx mutations [58,61,62].

Molecular pathogenesis

Germline mutations are extraordinarily common in patients with PPGL, and there are now greater than 20 known susceptibility genes (see Fig. 3). Mutations in SDHB, SDHC, SDHD, VHL, RET, and NF1 are particularly common. Overall, it is estimated that 40% to 50% of all patients with PPGL carry such a mutation. In the pediatric population, germline mutations seem to be even more common, with estimates ranging from 50% to 70% [51,52,54]. The most common mutated gene in children with PHEO is VHL, and the most common in PGL is SDHB.

Genetic studies have identified 3 clusters of genes that lead to PPGL through related mechanisms (see Fig. 3) [63]. Genes involved in the pseudohypoxic tumorigenic pathway comprise cluster 1. These genes include VHL and the SDHx genes. Abnormalities in this cluster interfere with oxidative phosphorylation by Krebs cycle enzymes, leading to accumulation of metabolites that increase hypoxia inducible factor-α (HIF-α), which promotes tumor formation [58,63]. Cluster 1 mutations tend to cause aggressive and often metastatic tumors that are more often extra-adrenal in location (except for VHL-associated tumors). Cluster 1 tumors are usually dopaminergic and noradrenergic, and biochemical testing reveals normal metanephrine levels but increases in levels of normetanephrine and 3-methoxytyramine. The exception to this is VHL-associated tumors, which are primarily noradrenergic and do not tend to secrete dopamine. Cluster 2 genes include RET, NF1, and others. Mutations in these genes cause activation of multiple kinase signaling pathways that promote cell proliferation, survival, and angiogenesis, including phosphoinositide 3-kinase (PI3K)/protein kinase B (AKT), mammalian target of rapamycin (mTOR), and RAS/RAF/extracellular signal-regulated kinase (ERK) [58]. Cluster 2 tumors tend to be less aggressive, metastasize less frequently, and are more likely to be located in the adrenals. These tumors are adrenergic and may also be noradrenergic. Therefore, biochemical testing shows increased levels of metanephrine, with or without increased normetanephrine. Cluster 3 genes are involved in the WNT signaling pathways acting through β-catenin and are associated with aggressive tumor behavior. Cluster 3 gene mutations are exclusively somatic [62]. An understanding of the molecular cause of PPGL may lead to personalized therapies [63].

Treatment

Surgery of localized tumors is the only curative option. Complete resection is more likely in cases of PHEO than in PGL (>90% vs 50%–75%) [51,52]. Patients undergoing surgery are at high risk for hypertensive crises, and mortality is high unless adequate preoperative preparation occurs. Current recommendations are to establish α-adrenergic blockade for 10 to 14 days at gradually increasing doses to control blood pressure [50]. Blockade of α-adrenergic receptors leads to vasodilation with lowering of blood pressure and increased potential for orthostasis. Thus, recommendations also include increased fluid and sodium intake. Commonly used α-adrenergic blockers include phenoxybenzamine and doxazosin. After 3 to 4 days of α-blockade, β-adrenergic blockers can be started to control tachycardia. β-Blockade should not be started before α-blockade, because unopposed β-blockade removes β_2-adrenergic receptor–mediated vasodilation and permits severe vasoconstriction from α_1 receptor stimulation.

Several medications can cause hypertensive crises in patients with untreated PPGL via a variety of mechanisms. These medications include (1) sympathomimetic drugs, such as amphetamine and methylphenidate; (2) opioids, such as morphine; (3) tricyclic antidepressants, such as imipramine; (4) serotonin reuptake inhibitors, such as fluoxetine; and (5) corticosteroids, such as hydrocortisone and dexamethasone [50].

A laparoscopic surgical approach is preferable for small (<6 cm) and noninvasive PHEOs. Open procedures are appropriate for large PHEOs and PGLs so as to optimize tumor resection and to avoid tumor rupture [55]. Variable PGL tumor locations may necessitate multiple specialist involvement, including otolaryngology, cardiovascular surgery, and interventional radiology. Cortical-sparing partial adrenalectomy should be considered in cases of bilateral PHEO or if a PHEO develops in the contralateral gland after prior adrenalectomy, with the goal of preventing postoperative adrenal insufficiency. Partial adrenalectomy successfully prevents glucocorticoid deficiency in 80% to 90% of cases. However, partial adrenalectomy increases the recurrence risk when medullary remnants are left behind [64].

Postoperatively, patients are at increased risk for both hypertension and hypotension as well as hypoglycemia. Glucocorticoids are required in patients rendered surgically adrenally insufficient. If partial adrenalectomy is performed, patients should be monitored for adrenal insufficiency.

In patients with metastases or recurrences that are not amenable to surgical resection, traditional chemotherapy has included cyclophosphamide, vincristine, and dacarbazine. Although this regimen may lead to symptomatic improvement, it is not clear whether there is an increase in overall survival [62]. Alternative treatments for patients with nonresectable disease include radiofrequency ablation, tumor embolization, or peptide receptor radionuclide therapy with ^{131}I-MIBG for those with uptake on scintigraphy or with ^{177}Lu-DOTATATE (dodecanetetraacetic acid-tyr3-octreotate) [65]. Mutation cluster-specific approaches that are under study include HIF-α, vascular endothelial growth factor, and tyrosine kinase inhibitors for cluster 1 mutations and mTOR inhibitors for mutations in cluster 2, as well as other novel approaches [62,65].

Outcomes

Repeat biochemical testing for PPGL is recommended 2 to 4 weeks after surgery to demonstrate a biochemical cure and should be repeated annually thereafter [55]. Given the high rate of germline mutations, metachronous disease, recurrences, and metastases are common. As an example, in a group of children with PPGL after a median follow-up period of 53 months, 8 out of 81 patients had a new PPGL, 8 out of 81 had a local relapse, and 10 out of 81 had a metastatic relapse [51]. In a similar study conducted in children during the same time frame, 6 out of 28 patients with PHEO had a new tumor or relapse after a mean follow up of 59 months. For those with a PGL, 4 out of 22 had a recurrence after a mean of 52 months [52]. Thus, late recurrences are common, and the 5-year event-free survival rate has been estimated at 61%. Nevertheless, overall survival in the pediatric age range is good. In a review of 9 pediatric studies published over the past 15 years, the reported mortality was 4% [51]. At this time, there are no pediatric-specific guidelines for treatment of PPGL. With the higher prevalence of germline mutations and other differences between the adult and pediatric populations, such guidelines could help improve the care of children with PPGL.

CLINICS CARE POINTS

- The most common signs of pediatric adrenocortical tumors include rapid penile or clitoral enlargement, sexual hair growth, hirsutism, acne, and increased height velocity.
- In cases of mixed androgen- and cortisol-secreting adrenocortical tumors, growth suppression from hypercortisolemia may limit the growth acceleration from hyperandrogenemia.
- In addition to low disease stage, favorable factors in the prognosis of pediatric adrenocortical tumors include age < 3 years and the presence of virilization.
- Symptoms of pheochromocytoma and paraganglioma include headache, tachycardia, diaphoresis, and pallor. Hypertension is seen in most patients and is a common presenting complaint.
- Pheochromocytomas and paragangliomas are more commonly associated with heritable germline mutations than any other cancer type, and genetic testing is a key component of the evaluation.
- The biochemical evaluation of pheochromocytoma and paraganglioma includes plasma free metanephrines or 24-hour urinary metanephrines. Levels of either metanephrine or normetanephrine > 3 times the upper limit of normal are rarely false positives.

Disclosure

The author has no commercial of financial conflicts of interest related to this topic.

References

[1] Ishimoto H, Jaffe RB. Development and function of the human fetal adrenal cortex: a key component in the feto-placental unit. Endocr Rev 2011;32(3):317–55.
[2] Imai A, Kurihara Y. Endogenous infection in mice with streptozotocin-induced diabetes. A feature of bacterial translocation. Can J Microbiol 1984;30(11):1344–8.
[3] Ogle JW. Unusually large mass of carcinomatous deposit in one of the suprarenal capsules of a child. Trans Pathol Soc Lond 1865;16:250.

[4] Faria AM, Almeida MQ. Differences in the molecular mechanisms of adrenocortical tumorigenesis between children and adults. Mol Cell Endocrinol 2012;351(1):52–7.
[5] Brondani VB, Fragoso M. Pediatric adrenocortical tumor - review and management update. Curr Opin Endocrinol Diabetes Obes 2020;27(3):177–86.
[6] Garritano S, Gemignani F, Palmero EI, et al. Detailed haplotype analysis at the TP53 locus in p.R337H mutation carriers in the population of Southern Brazil: evidence for a founder effect. Hum Mutat 2010;31(2):143–50.
[7] Michalkiewicz E, Sandrini R, Figueiredo B, et al. Clinical and outcome characteristics of children with adrenocortical tumors: a report from the International Pediatric Adrenocortical Tumor Registry. J Clin Oncol 2004;22(5):838–45.
[8] Gupta N, Rivera M, Novotny P, et al. Adrenocortical carcinoma in children: a clinicopathological analysis of 41 patients at the Mayo Clinic from 1950 to 2017. Horm Res Paediatr 2018;90(1):8–18.
[9] Ilias I, Sahdev A, Reznek RH, et al. The optimal imaging of adrenal tumours: a comparison of different methods. Endocr Relat Cancer 2007;14(3):587–99.
[10] Ribeiro RC, Pinto EM, Zambetti GP, et al. The international pediatric adrenocortical tumor registry initiative: contributions to clinical, biological, and treatment advances in pediatric adrenocortical tumors. Mol Cell Endocrinol 2012;351(1):37–43.
[11] Li FP, Fraumeni JF Jr. Soft-tissue sarcomas, breast cancer, and other neoplasms. A familial syndrome? Ann Intern Med 1969;71(4):747–52.
[12] Gonzalez KD, Noltner KA, Buzin CH, et al. Beyond Li Fraumeni syndrome: clinical characteristics of families with p53 germline mutations. J Clin Oncol 2009;27(8):1250–6.
[13] Varley JM, McGown G, Thorncroft M, et al. Are there low-penetrance TP53 Alleles? evidence from childhood adrenocortical tumors. Am J Hum Genet 1999;65(4):995–1006.
[14] Latronico AC, Pinto EM, Domenice S, et al. An inherited mutation outside the highly conserved DNA-binding domain of the p53 tumor suppressor protein in children and adults with sporadic adrenocortical tumors. J Clin Endocrinol Metab 2001;86(10):4970–3.
[15] Ribeiro RC, Sandrini F, Figueiredo B, et al. An inherited p53 mutation that contributes in a tissue-specific manner to pediatric adrenal cortical carcinoma. Proc Natl Acad Sci U S A 2001;98(16):9330–5.
[16] Gaujoux S, Pinson S, Gimenez-Roqueplo AP, et al. Inactivation of the APC gene is constant in adrenocortical tumors from patients with familial adenomatous polyposis but not frequent in sporadic adrenocortical cancers. Clin Cancer Res 2010;16(21):5133–41.
[17] Rattis FM, Voermans C, Reya T. Wnt signaling in the stem cell niche. Curr Opin Hematol 2004;11(2):88–94.
[18] Tissier F, Cavard C, Groussin L, et al. Mutations of beta-catenin in adrenocortical tumors: activation of the Wnt signaling pathway is a frequent event in both benign and malignant adrenocortical tumors. Cancer Res 2005;65(17):7622–7.
[19] Rauschecker M, Stratakis CA. Molecular genetics of adrenocortical tumor formation and potential pharmacologic targets. Minerva Endocrinol 2012;37(2):133–9.
[20] Lapunzina P. Risk of tumorigenesis in overgrowth syndromes: a comprehensive review. Am J Med Genet C Semin Med Genet 2005;137C(1):53–71.
[21] Peixoto Lira RC, Fedatto PF, Marco Antonio DS, et al. IGF2 and IGF1R in pediatric adrenocortical tumors: roles in metastasis and steroidogenesis. Endocr Relat Cancer 2016;23(6):481–93.
[22] Doghman M, El Wakil A, Cardinaud B, et al. Regulation of insulin-like growth factor-mammalian target of rapamycin signaling by microRNA in childhood adrenocortical tumors. Cancer Res 2010;70(11):4666–75.
[23] Pinto EM, Chen X, Easton J, et al. Genomic landscape of paediatric adrenocortical tumours. Nat Commun 2015;6:6302.
[24] De Martino MC, van Koetsveld PM, Feelders RA, et al. IGF and mTOR pathway expression and in vitro effects of linsitinib and mTOR inhibitors in adrenocortical cancer. Endocrine 2019;64(3):673–84.

[25] Weiss LM. Comparative histologic study of 43 metastasizing and nonmetastasizing adrenocortical tumors. Am J Surg Pathol 1984;8(3):163–9.
[26] Mendonca BB, Lucon AM, Menezes CA, et al. Clinical, hormonal and pathological findings in a comparative study of adrenocortical neoplasms in childhood and adulthood. J Urol 1995;154(6):2004–9.
[27] Wieneke JA, Thompson LD, Heffess CS. Adrenal cortical neoplasms in the pediatric population: a clinicopathologic and immunophenotypic analysis of 83 patients. Am J Surg Pathol 2003;27(7):867–81.
[28] Chatterjee G, DasGupta S, Mukherjee G, et al. Usefulness of Wieneke criteria in assessing morphologic characteristics of adrenocortical tumors in children. Pediatr Surg Int 2015;31(6):563–71.
[29] Rodriguez-Galindo C, Figueiredo BC, Zambetti GP, et al. Biology, clinical characteristics, and management of adrenocortical tumors in children. Pediatr Blood Cancer 2005;45(3):265–73.
[30] Sullivan M, Boileau M, Hodges CV. Adrenal cortical carcinoma. J Urol 1978;120(6): 660–5.
[31] Sandrini R, Ribeiro RC, DeLacerda L. Childhood adrenocortical tumors. J Clin Endocrinol Metab 1997;82(7):2027–31.
[32] Mihai R. Diagnosis, treatment and outcome of adrenocortical cancer. Br J Surg 2015;102(4):291–306.
[33] Reibetanz J, Jurowich C, Erdogan I, et al. Impact of lymphadenectomy on the oncologic outcome of patients with adrenocortical carcinoma. Ann Surg 2012;255(2):363–9.
[34] Ho J, Turkbey B, Edgerly M, et al. Role of radiotherapy in adrenocortical carcinoma. Cancer J 2013;19(4):288–94.
[35] Redlich A, Boxberger N, Strugala D, et al. Systemic treatment of adrenocortical carcinoma in children: data from the German GPOH-MET 97 trial. Klin Padiatr 2012;224(6):366–71.
[36] Chortis V, Taylor AE, Schneider P, et al. Mitotane therapy in adrenocortical cancer induces CYP3A4 and inhibits 5alpha-reductase, explaining the need for personalized glucocorticoid and androgen replacement. J Clin Endocrinol Metab 2013;98(1):161–71.
[37] Pinto EM, Zambetti GP, Rodriguez-Galindo C. Pediatric adrenocortical tumours. Best Pract Res Clin Endocrinol Metab 2020;34(3):101448.
[38] Lodish M, Stratakis CA. A genetic and molecular update on adrenocortical causes of Cushing syndrome. Nat Rev Endocrinol 2016;12(5):255–62.
[39] Almeida MQ, Stratakis CA. Carney complex and other conditions associated with micronodular adrenal hyperplasias. Best Pract Res Clin Endocrinol Metab 2010;24(6):907–14.
[40] Gunther DF, Bourdeau I, Matyakhina L, et al. Cyclical Cushing syndrome presenting in infancy: an early form of primary pigmented nodular adrenocortical disease, or a new entity? J Clin Endocrinol Metab 2004;89(7):3173–82.
[41] Bertherat J, Horvath A, Groussin L, et al. Mutations in regulatory subunit type 1A of cyclic adenosine 5′-monophosphate-dependent protein kinase (PRKAR1A): phenotype analysis in 353 patients and 80 different genotypes. J Clin Endocrinol Metab 2009;94(6): 2085–91.
[42] Kamilaris CDC, Faucz FR, Voutetakis A, et al. Carney complex. Exp Clin Endocrinol Diabetes 2019;127(2–03):156–64.
[43] Louiset E, Stratakis CA, Perraudin V, et al. The paradoxical increase in cortisol secretion induced by dexamethasone in primary pigmented nodular adrenocortical disease involves a glucocorticoid receptor-mediated effect of dexamethasone on protein kinase A catalytic subunits. J Clin Endocrinol Metab 2009;94(7):2406–13.
[44] Lowe KM, Young WF Jr, Lyssikatos C, et al. Cushing syndrome in carney complex: clinical, pathologic, and molecular genetic findings in the 17 affected Mayo Clinic patients. Am J Surg Pathol 2017;41(2):171–81.
[45] Bourdeau I, Parisien-La Salle S, Lacroix A. Adrenocortical hyperplasia: a multifaceted disease. Best Pract Res Clin Endocrinol Metab 2020;34(3):101386.

[46] Lodish M. Genetics of adrenocortical development and tumors. Endocrinol Metab Clin North Am 2017;46(2):419–33.
[47] Carney JA, Young WF, Stratakis CA. Primary bimorphic adrenocortical disease: cause of hypercortisolism in McCune-Albright syndrome. Am J Surg Pathol 2011;35(9):1311–26.
[48] Vassiliadi DA, Tsagarakis S. Diagnosis and management of primary bilateral macronodular adrenal hyperplasia. Endocr Relat Cancer 2019;26(10):R567–81.
[49] Stratakis CA, Berthon A. Molecular mechanisms of ARMC5 mutations in adrenal pathophysiology. Curr Opin Endocr Metab Res 2019;8:104–11.
[50] Berends AMA, Buitenwerf E, de Krijger RR, et al. Incidence of pheochromocytoma and sympathetic paraganglioma in the Netherlands: a nationwide study and systematic review. Eur J Intern Med 2018;51:68–73.
[51] de Tersant M, Genere L, Freycon C, et al. Pheochromocytoma and Paraganglioma in children and adolescents: experience of the French Society of Pediatric Oncology (SFCE). J Endocr Soc 2020;4(5):bvaa039.
[52] Virgone C, Andreetta M, Avanzini S, et al. Pheochromocytomas and paragangliomas in children: data from the Italian Cooperative Study (TREP). Pediatr Blood Cancer 2020;67(8):e28332.
[53] Wyszynska T, Cichocka E, Wieteska-Klimczak A, et al. A single pediatric center experience with 1025 children with hypertension. Acta Paediatr 1992;81(3):244–6.
[54] Bausch B, Wellner U, Bausch D, et al. Long-term prognosis of patients with pediatric pheochromocytoma. Endocr Relat Cancer 2014;21(1):17–25.
[55] Lenders JW, Duh QY, Eisenhofer G, et al. Pheochromocytoma and paraganglioma: an endocrine society clinical practice guideline. J Clin Endocrinol Metab 2014;99(6): 1915–42.
[56] Rao D, Peitzsch M, Prejbisz A, et al. Plasma methoxytyramine: clinical utility with metanephrines for diagnosis of pheochromocytoma and paraganglioma. Eur J Endocrinol 2017;177(2):103–13.
[57] Lenders JWM, Kerstens MN, Amar L, et al. Genetics, diagnosis, management and future directions of research of phaeochromocytoma and paraganglioma: a position statement and consensus of the Working Group on Endocrine Hypertension of the European Society of Hypertension. J Hypertens 2020;38(8):1443–56.
[58] Nolting S, Ullrich M, Pietzsch J, et al. Current management of pheochromocytoma/paraganglioma: a guide for the practicing clinician in the era of precision medicine. Cancers (Basel) 2019;11(10):1505.
[59] Lenders JW, Willemsen JJ, Eisenhofer G, et al. Is supine rest necessary before blood sampling for plasma metanephrines? Clin Chem 2007;53(2):352–4.
[60] Pacak K, Eisenhofer G, Tischler AS. Phaeochromocytoma - advances through science, collaboration and spreading the word. Nat Rev Endocrinol 2020;16(11):621–2.
[61] Han S, Suh CH, Woo S, et al. Performance of (68)Ga-DOTA-conjugated somatostatin receptor-targeting peptide PET in detection of pheochromocytoma and paraganglioma: a systematic review and metaanalysis. J Nucl Med 2019;60(3):369–76.
[62] Ilanchezhian M, Jha A, Pacak K, et al. Emerging treatments for advanced/metastatic pheochromocytoma and paraganglioma. Curr Treat Options Oncol 2020;21(11):85.
[63] Jochmanova I, Pacak K. Genomic landscape of pheochromocytoma and paraganglioma. Trends Cancer 2018;4(1):6–9.
[64] Grubbs EG, Rich TA, Ng C, et al. Long-term outcomes of surgical treatment for hereditary pheochromocytoma. J Am Coll Surg 2013;216(2):280–9.
[65] Mercado-Asis LB, Wolf KI, Jochmanova I, et al. Pheochromocytoma: a genetic and diagnostic update. Endocr Pract 2018;24(1):78–90.

Advances in Pediatrics 68 (2021) 245–259

ADVANCES IN PEDIATRICS

Advances in the Surgical Management of Esophageal Atresia

Alexis N. Bowder, MD, Dave R. Lal, MD, MPH[1,*]

Division of Pediatric Surgery, Department of Surgery, Medical College of Wisconsin, 999 North 92nd Street, Suite 320, Milwaukee, WI 53226, USA

Keywords

• Esophageal atresia (EA) • Tracheoesophageal fistula (TEF)
• Tracheoesophageal repair

Key points

- Esophageal atresia (EA) is frequently diagnosed after birth in infants with feeding intolerance and increased oral secretions.
- Patients with EA commonly have other associated congenital anomalies (VACTERL [vertebral, anorectal, cardiac, tracheoesophageal fistula, renal, and limb/radial anomalies]) that need to be investigated.
- Despite a reduction in mortality to less than 10%, most patients undergoing EA/tracheoesophageal fistula repair experience at least 1 complication.
- Wide variation in perioperative care and lack of evidence-based guidelines contribute to a persistently high rate of postoperative morbidity.
- Adults that have undergone EA repair as infants report equivalent health-related quality of life to those in the general population.

INTRODUCTION

Incidence

The incidence of esophageal atresia (EA) with or without a tracheoesophageal fistula (TEF) has remained stable over time. The estimated worldwide incidence of EA is 1 in every 3500 live births, with 70% to 90% having an

[1]Present address: 3615 North 87th Street. Milwaukee. WI 53222.

*Corresponding author. Division of Pediatric Surgery, Department of Surgery, Medical College of Wisconsin, 999 North 92nd Street, Suite 320, Milwaukee, WI 53226, USA. *E-mail address:* Dlal@chw.org

https://doi.org/10.1016/j.yapd.2021.05.004
0065-3101/21/

associated TEF [1]. However, there is geographic variability, with incidence ranging from 1 in 2440 live births in Finland to 1 in 4500 births in Australia and the United States [2–4]. Approximately one-third of infants with EA are born prematurely, presumably because of the resulting polyhydramnios from the inability to swallow amniotic fluid. In recent studies, the mean gestation age was 36.5 weeks, with 38% of patients born between 30 and 36 weeks' estimated gestational age [5].

Cause/pathogenesis

Abnormalities in the embryonic development of the foregut lead to EA. The precise mechanism remains ill-defined and likely involves a combination of familial, genetic, environmental, and biomechanical factors. Several studies have explored familial cases of EA and, based on this literature, it is estimated that siblings of an affected child have a 0.5% to 2% risk of EA and the risk to a child of an affected parent is approximately 3% to 4% [6]. Prenatal factors associated with EA include advanced maternal age and gestational diabetes [7].

Ten percent of patients with EA have an associated genetic syndrome such as trisomy 13, 18, or 21 [7]. In addition, increased rates of EA/TEF are seen in patients with single-gene disorders, including Feingold syndrome (N-MYC), anophthalmia-esophageal-genital syndrome (SOX-2), and CHARGE (coloboma, heart defects, choanal atresia, retarded growth and development, genital malformations and ear anomalies) syndrome (CDH7) [7].

The embryologic insults that cause EA commonly affect other organ systems. Nearly 70% of patients with EA have at least 1 associated congenital anomaly [8]. The acronym VACTERL (vertebral, anorectal [imperforate anus, anal atresia], cardiac, TEF, renal, and limb/radial anomalies) is used to describe the most common defects. The most common anomaly is congenital heart disease, which is present in more than a third of patients [8] (Table 1).

Prenatal and postnatal diagnosis

Maternal polyhydramnios, a dilated upper esophageal pouch (pouch sign), with either a small or absent stomach bubble are the hallmark prenatal ultrasonography findings suggestive of EA [9]. The predictive value of these prenatal ultrasonography findings is estimated to be around 10% to 40% [8,10,11]. A recent study performed at 11 pediatric surgery institutions in the United States found that only 13% of 396 infants with EA anomalies were diagnosed in the prenatal period [8]. MRI has been found to be more sensitive and specific in the prenatal diagnosis of EA [12].

After birth, infants with excessive drooling and feeding intolerance (typically choking) should undergo further testing to evaluate for EA. The simplest method to diagnose EA is by attempting to place an orogastric tube into the stomach. The diagnosis is confirmed when a tube cannot be passed 10 cm from the gums, or there is no return of gastric contents. Note that smaller-caliber tubes are prone to curling in the upper esophagus, giving a false sense of esophageal continuity. For that reason, a 10-French or larger tube is preferred.

Table 1
Incidence of associated anomalies in a retrospective 11-institution study of 396 patients with esophageal atresia

Anomaly	Number of cases (%)
Congenital heart disease	**137 (35%)**
Ventricular septal defect	74 (19%)
Atrial septal defect	49 (12%)
Musculoskeletal	**129 (33%)**
Vertebral abnormality	88 (22%)
Limb abnormality	54 (14%)
Genitourinary	**119 (30%)**
Renal abnormality	92 (23%)
Genital/urinary abnormality	12 (3%)
Intestinal	79 (20%)
Imperforate anus	**47 (12%)**
Atresia	23 (6%)
Cloaca	9 (2%)
Intracranial/cranial facial	**65 (16%)**
Craniofacial abnormality	34 (9%)
Chromosomal	**43 (11%)**
Trisomy 21	8 (2%)

Incidence of associated anomalies (n = 396).

Data from: Lal DR, Gadepalli SK, Downard CD, et al. Perioperative management and outcomes of esophageal atresia and tracheoesophageal fistula. *J Pediatr Surg.* 2017;52(8):1245-1251. https://doi.org/10.1016/j.jpedsurg.2016.11.046.

After the diagnosis of EA is established, the next step is to determine whether a TEF is present, the length of the esophageal gap (distance between the proximal and distal esophageal ends), and to assess for additional anomalies (VACTERL). A radiograph of the chest confirms that the orogastric tube stops short of the stomach. Patients with a TEF have gas in their stomachs and intestines within 24 hours of life. Infants with pure EA, without a distal TEF, have no gastric or intestinal gas.

In patients with EA/TEF, the esophageal gap length can be estimated by placing downward pressure on the orogastric tube, thereby stretching the blind-ending esophagus, while a chest radiograph is obtained. The esophageal gap length can be estimated by measuring the distance from the end of the orogastric tube in the proximal esophagus to the carina (surrogate for the most common proximal extent of the TEF/distal esophagus). Some surgeons obtain a pouchogram to further evaluate the size of the proximal pouch and the presence of a proximal fistula. This test is done by injecting 1 to 2 mL of radiopaque contrast under fluoroscopy through a catheter placed in the proximal pouch with the patient upright. It is important that isotonic, absorbable contrast be used for this study in case of contrast aspiration.

In patients with EA and no distal TEF, estimation of the distal esophageal length requires access to the stomach via a gastrostomy tube. A guidewire, endoscope, or metal probe can be inserted retrograde through the gastrostomy and advanced into the distal pouch under fluoroscopy. If possible, endoscopic intubation of the distal pouch is preferred because a blindly placed probe can indent the diaphragm in a similar manner to a short distal pouch. The gap length is definitively determined by measuring the distance between the 2 esophageal ends with the use of a radiopaque ruler (see Fig. 2A, B).

Patients with isolated TEF (no EA) typically present outside the newborn period with cyanosis, coughing, choking with feeds, recurrent aspirations, and pneumonias. They require further evaluation with a contrast study and frequently endoscopy to verify the diagnosis. Once the EA or EA/TEF diagnosis is confirmed, the radiographs should be reviewed for vertebral and rib anomalies.

Classification

The first classification system for EA/TEF was described by Vogt [13] in 1929 and subsequently modified by Ladd and Gross [14,15]. For clarity and uniformity, the current preference is to describe the anatomic abnormality instead of relying on historical classification systems. However, because of the persistent use of the Gross classification, both the anatomic description and Gross classification are shown in Fig. 1 and discussed later. By far the most common type of EA/TEF is a proximal EA with distal TEF (Gross type C), which occurs in 86% of cases [8]. Imaging findings include the presence of distal intestinal gas (stomach and bowel). The second most common anatomic type is EA without a TEF (Gross type A or pure EA), which is seen in 8% of patients [8]. Plain

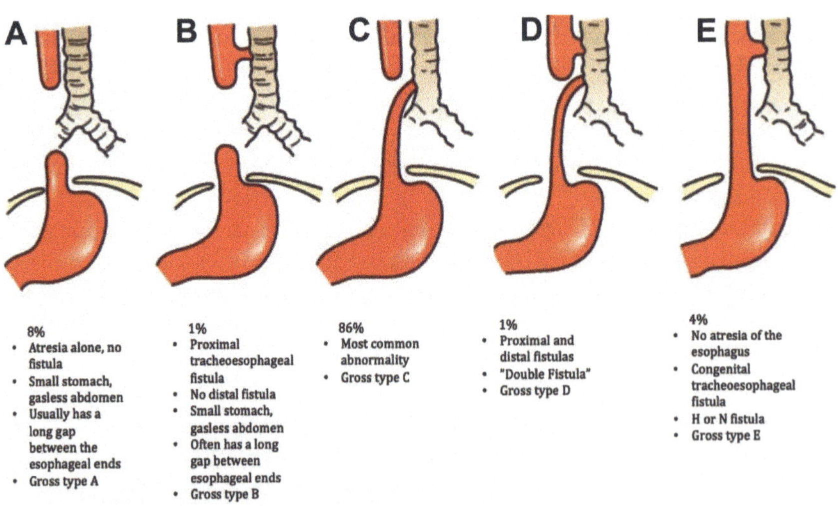

Fig. 1. The anatomic and Gross classifications of EA with and without TEFs. A) Gross type A B) Gross type B, C) Gross type C D) Gross type D and E) Gross Type E (*Adapted from* Sabiston Textbook of Surgery: The Biological Basis of Modern Surgical Practice, 20e > Chapter 66. Pediatric Surgery.)

films in isolated EA show no gastric or intestinal gas, and a prenatal diagnosis is more common in infants with pure EA compared with those with EA/TEF [8]. Isolated TEF without EA (Gross type E, H type) occurs in 4% of patients [8]. Because of the intact esophagus, these patients present later in the newborn period with choking/cyanosis during feeds, aspiration, and recurrent pneumonias [16]. The TEF can be difficult to diagnose and missed with fluoroscopic studies. Double endoscopy (bronchoscopy and esophagoscopy) with attempts at cannulation of the fistula via bronchoscopy and injection of methylene blue into the esophagus with visualization of the dye in the trachea have been recommended for definitive diagnosis [17]. Other rare types (1%) include EA with proximal TEF (Gross type B) and EA with both a proximal and distal TEF (Gross type D). Type B patients have no distal gas on plain films and type D do.

Patients with EA can be further classified by gap length. As the gap length increases, repair becomes more challenging and may not be feasible. Long-gap EA (LGEA) is a commonly used term but does not have an agreed-on definition by pediatric surgeons [18]. Measurements that qualify a patient as having LGEA are based on the gap distance measured either by vertebral bodies (range, >2–4) or in centimeters (range, >2–5 cm) [18]. When and how this measurement occurs is also varied across the literature. The measurement can occur intraoperatively with active stretching of the two esophageal ends or in their passive, resting state. Recent guidelines from the American Pediatric Surgical Association (APSA) recommend that, in patients with isolated EA, esophageal gap measurement should occur at least 2 weeks after gastrostomy creation. The gap-measuring procedure should be performed with fluoroscopy, in the operating room, while dynamically stretching the two esophageal ends as previously described [18] (Fig. 2A, B).

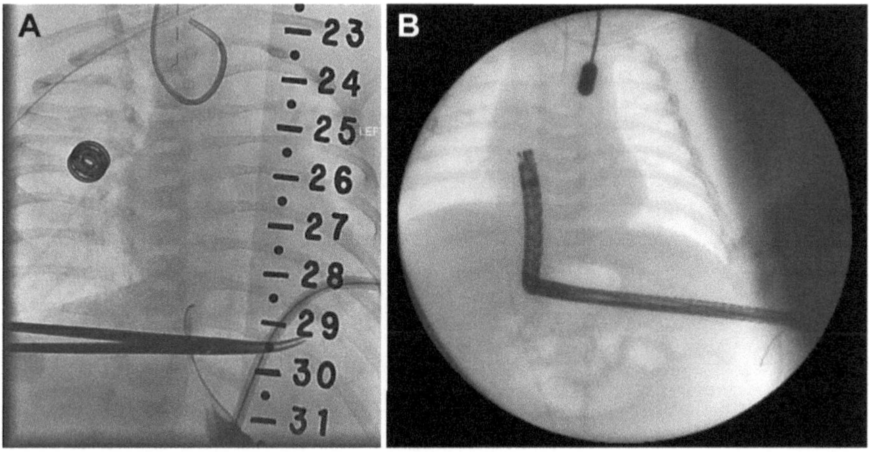

Fig. 2. Fluoroscopic measurement of a patient with long-gap EA with a radiopaque ruler present and flexible wire in the distal esophagus (A) and endoscope in the distal esophagus (B).

Preoperative work-up

Additional congenital anomalies occur in nearly 70% of patients with EA [8]. Therefore, patients should undergo evaluation for these anomalies before surgery. A preoperative echocardiogram is necessary to exclude congenital heart disease and to determine the side of the aortic arch. Five percent of patients with EA have a right-sided arch, which may complicate exposure during the repair [19]. In addition, patients with EA can have other vascular anomalies, including double aortic arch, circumflex aorta, and/or aberrant right subclavian arteries, which, if suspected, can be further evaluated with a computed tomography angiogram or cardiac MRI [8,20,21].

Other commonly associated anomalies include those of the musculoskeletal system, genitourinary tract, intestine, spine, and craniofacial locations (see Table 1). The presence of musculoskeletal anomalies should be evaluated with plain radiographs, and common findings include hemivertebrae, butterfly or fused vertebrae, rib abnormalities, and caudal regression [1]. Renal ultrasonography is used to evaluate for the presence, location, and ascent of the kidneys and help identify genitourinary anomalies, which are present in up to 30% of patients with EA [8]. Intestinal anomalies include atresia, pyloric stenosis, and anorectal malformations. Duodenal atresia has been reported in 2% to 5% of patients and should be suspected if a double bubble is seen on initial abdominal plain films [22]. To evaluate for anorectal malformations, a physical examination of the anus and confirmation of patency should be part of the initial assessment [23]. In addition, MRI or ultrasonography of the spine should be performed before age 1 year to evaluate for both tethered cord and cord lipomas [24].

Preoperative management

Before the 1940s, all infants with EA died shortly after birth. In 1941, Cameron Haight performed the first successful surgical repair of EA in an infant [3]. Over the ensuing 70-plus years, advances in surgery, anesthesia, neonatology, nutrition, and ventilation have resulted in survival rates greater than 90% for infants with EA born in high-income countries [5,8]. Associated anomalies, chiefly complex congenital heart disease, are now responsible for most deaths in infants with EA [8]. Thus, after a diagnosis of EA is made in a newborn, surgical repair is deferred (typically 24–48 hours) until a work-up can be completed to identify associated anomalies. During this preoperative period, it is necessary to drain the proximal pouch to prevent aspiration, as well as to minimize both agitation and positive pressure ventilation to prevent abdominal distension and respiratory compromise.

The most critical issues for patients with EA/TEF in the preoperative period are aspiration of upper pouch secretions, abdominal distension, and reflux of gastric acid leading to a combination of pneumonitis and respiratory compromise. To minimize the risk of aspiration, patients with EA/TEF should be placed in a semiupright or prone position with an elevated head. The patient must be nil by mouth and an orogastric tube positioned in the upper esophageal pouch and set to suction to decompress the pouch. Agitation, crying, and positive pressure ventilation (PPV) should be avoided if possible because they can lead to progressive gastric and abdominal distension resulting in decreasing diaphragmatic excursion and worsening respiratory mechanics.

Emergent maneuvers in the preoperative period

Newborns with EA/TEF can develop severe respiratory distress caused by aspiration, prematurity, or other issues requiring PPV. If the TEF is large, air during PPV may preferentially flow into the gastrointestinal tract, resulting in progressive gastric distension and, in extreme cases, abdominal compartment syndrome and gastric rupture [25]. Maneuvers to decrease the amount of air passing through the fistula include the use of high-frequency oscillatory ventilation; placement of the endotracheal tube distal to the fistula (at the carina or in the right main stem bronchus), which is difficult to maintain in newborns; obstructing the fistula with a Fogarty catheter; temporarily obstructing the distal esophagus with a ligature or Foley catheter; or placing a gastrostomy tube and attaching it to a Pleur-evac on water seal, which decreases gastric distension but often does not solve the ventilation difficulties [26]. If the stomach becomes massively dilated leading to abdominal compartment syndrome, emergent decompression with a needle or placement of a gastrostomy tube can be lifesaving. If these maneuvers fail to improve oxygenation and ventilation, emergent thoracotomy with transpleural ligation and division of the TEF is definitive [27,28].

SURGICAL MANAGEMENT

Open repair

Open surgical repair of EA/TEF is approached through a right posterolateral thoracotomy in patients with a left-sided aortic arch. A curvilinear skin incision is made below the lower border of the scapula and extends from the paravertebral region posteriorly to the anterior axillary line. Traditionally, subcutaneous tissues and chest wall muscles are divided to elevate the scapula over the fourth intercostal space. Many surgeons now prefer a muscle-sparing technique that spreads rather than divides the serratus anterior and latissimus dorsi muscles, in an attempt to decrease postoperative pain and the long-term morbidity of chest wall and spinal deformities [29].

Once the fourth intercostal space is identified, the intercostal muscles are divided, and the chest is entered via an extrapleural or transpleural approach. With the extrapleural technique, the parietal pleura is meticulously dissected off the chest wall and kept intact surrounding the lung. If a postoperative anastomotic leak develops, the lung is protected by the pleura, and the risk of empyema is substantially less than with a transpleural approach. Advocates for the transpleural approach argue that operative times are less and, with current antibiotic regimens, the risk of postoperative empyema is minimal [1].

With either technique, dissection continues in the posterior mediastinum, and the azygos vein is identified. The azygos vein is an important landmark because the distal TEF is frequently located nearby. The azygos vein is traditionally ligated, although some advocate its preservation [30]. Next, the tracheoesophageal fistula is ligated and divided, leaving 1 to 2 mm of the esophagus on the tracheal side to minimize the risk of a tracheal stricture. The proximal pouch is then mobilized off the posterior trachea and its mediastinal attachments until it can be brought down to the distal esophagus without tension. During this dissection, the presence of a proximal fistula is excluded and the vagus nerve preserved. Frequently, the distal esophagus must also be mobilized to obtain sufficient length to span the esophageal gap.

A primary end-to-end esophageal anastomosis is created after the blind end of the proximal pouch is removed and the distal esophagus edges freshened. The anastomosis is performed with a single layer of absorbable sutures. During the creation of the anastomosis, a small orogastric or nasogastric tube is commonly passed into the stomach to ensure the patency of the distal esophagus and prevent inadvertent suture placement while performing the anastomosis. The catheter may be removed at the end of the operation, or, if it is left in place postoperatively, it is referred to as a transanastomotic (TA) tube. The purpose of a TA tube is to allow decompression of the stomach in the postoperative period and allow for gastric feeds while the infant is nil by mouth, although, as discussed later, the presence of a TA tube may be associated with increased stricture rate [8]. Before closure, a chest tube or closed suction drain is frequently placed in case an anastomotic leak develops.

Surgical approach in patients with a right-sided aortic arch

Approximately 5% of infants with EA/TEF have a right-sided aortic arch (RAA), which can complicate exposure and repair of the EA/TEF [19,20,31,32]. Controversy exists regarding the optimal side to perform a thoracotomy for repair of the EA/TEF in patients with an RAA. A recent multi-institutional retrospective study reported feasibility and safety with repair from either a right or left thoracotomy (no difference in anastomotic leak, recurrent fistula, esophageal dehiscence, or recurrent laryngeal nerve injury) [19]. However, there was a trend toward decreased anastomotic strictures when using a left thoracotomy compared with a right thoracotomy (0% vs 50%, $P = .29$) [19].

Safety of thoracoscopic repair of esophageal atresia/ tracheoesophageal fistula

Almost 60 years after the first successful open repair for EA, the thoracoscopic approach for surgical repair of EA/TEF was reported [33]. Several studies have since explored the safety and efficacy of the thoracoscopic technique. In 2008, a case-controlled matched study found no difference in operative time, postoperative leak, and postoperative stricture between open versus thoracoscopic repair of EA/TEF [34] Allal and colleagues [35] showed that patients undergoing thoracoscopic repair required less postoperative analgesia compared with their open counterparts. In 2011, Szavay and colleagues [36] retrospectively reviewed outcomes and found no difference in the time to extubation or early complication rates between open and thoracoscopic repairs. Recognizing that small sample sizes were a significant limitation to these early studies, Borruto and colleagues [37] performed a meta-analysis that included 166 patients (66 thoracoscopic, 97 open) and found no significant difference in stricture rates or anastomotic leaks between the two procedures. In addition, a large multi-institutional study with 396 patients with EA/TEF found no difference in postoperative stricture rate between open (N = 366) and thoracoscopic repair (N = 33) [8].

Reported advantages of the thoracoscopic technique include improved visualization and decreased risk of scoliosis and chest wall deformities. The combination of magnification and high-definition optics allows improved visualization of the proximal pouch and TEF [38]. In addition, others have reported improved functional and aesthetic outcomes after thoracoscopic repair, including a decrease in winged scapula, thoracic scoliosis, and asymmetry of the thoracic wall compared with patients undergoing a thoracotomy [37–39].

Critics of the thoracoscopic approach point out longer operative times, a steep learning curve with initially high conversion to open rates, and increased acidosis from prolonged insufflation of carbon dioxide. Szavay and colleagues [36] reported significantly longer operative time with the thoracoscopic approach compared with an open technique (141 minutes vs 106 minutes, respectively). Thoracoscopic conversion to open rates has been reported to be as high as 32% [40]. Studies exploring neonates undergoing thoracoscopic procedures, including EA repair, have found the use of a CO_2 pneumothorax can lead to severe acidosis and decreased regional cerebral oxygen saturation [41,42]. The long-term effect of this acidosis and decreased cerebral perfusion on the developing brain is unknown.

Surgical management of long-gap esophageal atresia

Just as the definition and measurement of LGEA vary widely across the literature, so does the preferred method for surgical management. Options include delayed primary repair, esophageal myotomy, partial gastric mobilization, esophageal lengthening/traction, gastric tube, gastric transposition, colon/jejunal interposition, and primary thoracoscopic repair [18]. A recent survey of pediatric surgeons in the United States found that respondents preferred the use of staged traction of the native esophagus followed closely by gastric transposition for LGEA repair [18].

Most surgeons would agree that preservation of the native esophagus is preferable if feasible. Therefore, in a suggested algorithm created by APSA, delayed primary repair was advocated. In this approach, the infant undergoes gastrostomy tube placement and waiting (several weeks to months) for somatic growth of the esophageal ends to allow the potential of primary repair [18].

If primary esophageal anastomosis is not technically feasible, esophageal lengthening by staged traction is another option to preserve the native esophagus [18]. Foker and colleagues [43] first described this technique, which uses traction sutures on both the proximal and distal esophageal ends, which exit through the chest wall. These external traction sutures are pulled in opposite directions, inducing gradual esophageal growth and ultimately the potential for primary esophageal repair.

When primary anastomosis is not attainable, esophageal replacement with gastric, jejunal [44], or colonic transposition is necessary. The optimal conduit for an esophageal replacement remains controversial, with none being clearly superior. Institutional, surgeon, and regional preferences typically dictate conduit choice. In general, colonic transpositions are associated with anastomotic leaks, strictures, and progressive intrathoracic dilation and redundancy of the colon conduit, whereas gastric transposition is associated with anastomotic leaks, early reflux, and strictures. Multiple studies have found equivalent outcomes between gastric and colonic transposition with no difference in postoperative mortality, anastomotic complication, and graft loss [45–47]. A recent National Surgical Quality Improvement Project–Pediatric (NSQIP-P) database study from 2012 to 2018 also reported no difference in outcomes between gastric and colonic transposition. However, postoperative morbidity was common, with 52% of patients undergoing either procedure developing a complication. Furthermore, nearly 20% required reoperation within the first 30 days, and death occurred in 3% [47].

Historically, esophageal replacement has been performed in an open fashion, but advances in surgical technique and equipment have allowed minimally invasive gastric and colonic transpositions [48,49]. Advocates of the minimally invasive approach cite improved visualization and safety, especially during the posterior mediastinal dissection, which is frequently performed blindly with the open technique. Robust data comparing open with minimally invasive esophageal replacement are lacking, but single-institution case reports show safety, feasibility, and comparable outcomes [48,49].

Complications/outcomes

Since the first successful surgical repair of EA/TEF, mortality has decreased to less than 10%, but postoperative morbidity remains high at more than 60%. The most common complications include anastomotic stricture (>40%), anastomotic leak (~20%), vocal cord dysfunction (~7%), and recurrent fistula (~5%) [8]. Table 2 shows postoperative complications and length of stay stratified by EA type reported by The Midwest Pediatric Surgery Consortium (MWPSC). Multiple investigators have identified significant variation in the perioperative care of patients with EA/TEF as a contributing factor to their persistently high morbidity. The perioperative care of patients with EA/TEF is primarily guided by surgical training and experience as opposed to evidence-based guidelines.

To explore specific factors associated with morbidity, identify best practices, and standardize care, the MWPSC performed a retrospective study of infants with proximal EA and distal TEF (Gross type C) undergoing repair at 11 academic Children's Hospitals in the United States. The use of a TA tube was associated with an increase in anastomotic stricture formation (odds ratio

Table 2
Postoperative complications and length of stay by type

	All types (n = 396)	Type C (n = 335)	Type A (pure EA) (n = 27)	Types B and D (n = 16)	Type E (H type) (n = 18)
Mortality[a]	29 (7.5%)	26 (7.9%)	2 (7.4%)	1 (6.3%)	0
Overall morbidity	245 (61.9%)	210(60%)	21 (77.8%)	13(81.3%)	10 (55.6%)
Anastomotic stricture[b]	165 (42.5%)	143 (43.6%)	14(51.9%)	7 (46.7%)	1 (5.6%)
Anastomotic leak	89 (22.9%)	67 (20.4%)	11 (40.7%)	7 (46.7%)	4 (22.2%)
Vocal cord dysfunction (paralysis/paresis)	26 (6.7%)	15 (4.6%)	3(11.1%)	3(20%)	5 (27.8%)
Recurrent fistula	19 (4.9%)	17(5.2%)	1 (3.7%)	0	1 (5.6%)
Surgical site infection[c]	9 (2.3%)	6(1.8%)	1 (3.7%)	1 (6.7%)	1 (5.6%)
Postoperative shock[c]	27 (6.9%)	23 (7.0%)	3(11.1%)	1 (6.7%)	0
Postoperative sepsis[c]	26 (6.7%)	21 (6.4%)	4(14.8%)	0	1 (5.6%)
Postoperative MSOF[c]	14 (3.6%)	13 (4.0%)	1 (3.7%)	0	0
Chylothorax[c]	9 (2.6%)	9 (3.1%)	0	0	0
Complete esophageal dehiscence	9 (2.3%)	6(1.8%)	1 (3.7%)	2(13.3%)	0
LOS (d), median (IQR)[d]	36(20–81)	32(19–60)	126(94–167)	142(38–178)	44 (24–77)

Postoperative complications and outcomes. Missing values were excluded from the analysis.
Abbreviations: IQR, interquartile range; LOS, length of stay; MSOF, multiple system organ failure.
[a]Defined as requiring intervention within 1 year of establishing continuity.
[b]Defined as complication occurring within 30 days of the operative procedure.
[c]LOS excludes patients who died.
Adapted from Lal DR, Gadepalli SK, Downard CD, et al. Perioperative management and outcomes of esophageal atresia and tracheoesophageal fistula. *J Pediatr Surg.* 2017;52(8):1245-1251. https://doi.org/10.1016/j.jpedsurg.2016.11.046.

[OR], 2.2; $P = .01$); acid suppression use did not alter the incidence of stricture, leak, or pneumonia ($P > .1$); and the placement of prosthetic material between the esophageal and tracheal suture line was associated with an increase in anastomotic leak (OR, 4.7; $P < .001$) [50]. Additional findings included no benefit in extending prophylactic antibiotics beyond 24 hours or obtaining a postoperative esophagram later than day 5.

The use of TA tubes remains common practice, with an international survey of pediatric surgeons reporting that 83% use in EA repair [8,50,51]. In addition to the data from the MWPSC, a large single-institution study and a meta-analysis of 4 retrospective studies (455 patients) found the use of a TA tube was associated with a significantly increased risk of stricture (relative risk, 1.83, $P < .0005$) [52,53]. Despite these studies, TA tube use remains common, with many surgeons citing the ability to start enteral feeds earlier with the tube and avoidance of total parenteral nutrition. The MWPSC performed a prospective trial and found no benefit to TA tubes in patients with EA compared with those without TA tubes. Specifically, there was no difference in time to full feeds between groups, and an inverse correlation was found between TA tubes and stricture rate over time [54]. The continued use of TA tubes highlights the challenge in transitioning data from clinical studies into clinical practice and overcoming the resistance among surgeons to make shifts in surgical practice based on available evidence.

Long-term outcomes in patients undergoing EA repair continue to evolve as the first patients to survive repair are entering their sixth decade of life. Increased rates of dysphagia, esophageal dysmotility, gastroesophageal reflux, and Barrett esophagus have all been reported. Because of these observations, lifelong surveillance endoscopy with multistaged biopsies is recommended every 5 to 10 years [18]. Other long-term morbidities include nutrition/growth deficiencies and skeletal abnormalities (chest wall and scoliosis). Despite the long-term effects after EA repair, studies have found patients report their overall health-related quality of life equivalent to matched controls in the general population up to 38 years after EA repair [55,56].

SUMMARY

EA with or without TEF is a congenital anomaly diagnosed either prenatally or shortly after birth. Infants with EA have feeding intolerance and increased oral secretions. The diagnosis of EA can be confirmed by the inability to pass an orogastric tube into the stomach, and the presence of intestinal air on radiograph confirms that a distal TEF is present. Before surgical repair, patients with EA should undergo a cardiac echocardiogram to exclude congenital heart disease and to determine the side of the aortic arch. Other recommended imaging studies include renal ultrasonography, radiographs to look for skeletal abnormalities, and MRI/ultrasonography of the spine. Considerable variation exists in the surgical technique and perioperative care of patients with EA, primarily caused by a lack of evidence-based guidelines and, when present, a delay/resistance among surgeons to adopt data from clinical studies. This variation in care is thought to be responsible for a postoperative complication rate of more than 60%, with the most common being anastomotic strictures. Multiple investigators have reported an association between the use of TA tubes and anastomotic strictures; however, their use remains common. Further research is needed to improve outcomes and decrease morbidity in patients with EA.

CLINICS CARE POINTS

- Preoperatively, all infants with EA/TEF require an echocardiogram to determine the side of the aortic arch and exclude congenital heart disease, which is present in more than a third of patients.
- Before repair, patients with EA/TEF should have an orogastric tube placed in the upper esophageal pouch and the infant placed in a semiupright position with an elevated head to minimize the risk of aspiration.

- In patients with EA/TEF awaiting repair that develop severe respiratory distress, emergent thoracotomy with transpleural ligation and division of the TEF can be lifesaving.
- Preservation of the native esophagus via primary repair is preferred for LGEA. If not technically feasible, options include esophageal lengthening (Foker procedure) or esophageal replacement.
- Anastomotic strictures occur in greater than 40% of patients and are associated with the placement of TA tubes after EA repair.

Disclosure

The authors have nothing to disclose.

References

[1] Congenital Anomalies of the Esophagus- ClinicalKey. Available at: https://www-clinicalkey-com.proxy.lib.mcw.edu/#!/content/book/3-s2.0-B9780323072557000696. Accessed November 22, 2020.
[2] Gastro-intestinal atresias in Finland in 1970-79, indicating time-place clustering. | Journal of Epidemiology & Community Health. Available at: https://jech.bmj.com/content/42/3/257.short. Accessed November 22, 2020.
[3] Haight C. Congenital atresia of the esophagus with tracheoesophageal fistula: reconstruction of esophageal continuity by primary anastomosis. Ann Surg 1944;120(4):623–52.
[4] Myers NA. Oesophageal atresia: the epitome of modern surgery. Ann R Coll Surg Engl 1974;54(6):277–87.
[5] Sfeir R, Bonnard A, Khen-Dunlop N, et al. Esophageal atresia: data from a national cohort. J Pediatr Surg 2013;48(8):1664–9.
[6] Pletcher BA, Friedes JS, Breg WR, et al. Familial occurrence of esophageal atresia with and without tracheoesophagel fistula: report of two unusual kindreds. Am J Med Genet 1991;39(4):380–4.
[7] Shaw-Smith C. Oesophageal atresia, tracheo-oesophageal fistula, and the VACTERL association: review of genetics and epidemiology. J Med Genet 2006;43(7):545–54.
[8] Lal DR, Gadepalli SK, Downard CD, et al. Perioperative management and outcomes of esophageal atresia and tracheoesophageal fistula. J Pediatr Surg 2017;52(8):1245–51.
[9] Farrant P. The antenatal diagnosis of oesophageal atresia by ultrasound. Br J Radiol 1980;53(636):1202–3.
[10] Prenatal diagnosis of esophageal atresia. J Pediatr Surg 1995;30(9):1258–63.
[11] Sparey C, Jawaheer G, Barrett AM, et al. Esophageal atresia in the northern region congenital anomaly survey, 1985-1997: prenatal diagnosis and outcome. Am J Obstet Gynecol 2000;182(2):427–31.
[12] Ethun CG, Fallon SC, Cassady CI, et al. Fetal MRI improves diagnostic accuracy in patients referred to a fetal center for suspected esophageal atresia. J Pediatr Surg 2014;49(5):712–5.
[13] Vogt EC. Congenital atresia of the esophagus. Am J Roentgenol 1929;22:463.
[14] Ladd WE. The surgical treatment of esophageal atresia and tracheoesophageal fistulas. N Engl J Med 1944;230:265.
[15] Gross RE. The Surgery of Infancy and Childhood. Philadelphia: WB Saunders; 1953.
[16] Fallon SC, Langer JC, St Peter SD, et al. Congenital H-type tracheoesophageal fistula: a multicenter review of outcomes in a rare disease. J Pediatr Surg 2017;52(11):1711–4.
[17] Karnak İ, Şenocak ME, Hiçsönmez A, et al. The diagnosis and treatment of H-type tracheoesophageal fistula. J Pediatr Surg 1997;32(12):1670–4.

[18] Baird R, Lal DR, Ricca RL, et al. Management of long gap esophageal atresia: a systematic review and evidence-based guidelines from the APSA Outcomes and Evidence Based Practice Committee. J Pediatr Surg 2019;54(4):675–87.
[19] Lal DR, Gadepalli SK, Downard CD, et al. Infants with esophageal atresia and right aortic arch: characteristics and outcomes from the Midwest Pediatric Surgery Consortium. J Pediatr Surg 2019;54(4):688–92.
[20] Berthet S, Tenisch E, Miron MC, et al. Vascular anomalies associated with esophageal atresia and tracheoesophageal fistula. J Pediatr 2015;166(5):1140–4.e2.
[21] Nasr A, McNamara PJ, Mertens L, et al. Is routine preoperative 2-dimensional echocardiography necessary for infants with esophageal atresia, omphalocele, or anorectal malformations? J Pediatr Surg 2010;45(5):876–9.
[22] McDuffie LA, Wakeman D, Warner BW. Diagnosis of esophageal atresia with tracheoesophageal fistula: is there a need for gastrointestinal contrast? J Pediatr 2010;156(5):852.
[23] Quan L, Smith DW. The VATER association. Vertebral defects, anal atresia, T-E fistula with esophageal atresia, Radial and Renal dysplasia: a spectrum of associated defects. J Pediatr 1973;82(1):104–7.
[24] Van den Hondel D, Sloots C, de Jong TH, et al. Screening and treatment of tethered spinal cord in anorectal malformation patients. Eur J Pediatr Surg 2016;26(1):22–8.
[25] Jones TB, Kirchner SG, Lee FA, et al. Stomach rupture associated with esophageal atresia, tracheoesophageal fistula, and ventilatory assistance. AJR Am J Roentgenol 1980;134(4): 675–7.
[26] Filston HC, Chitwood WR, Schkolne B, et al. The fogarty balloon catheter as an aid to management of the infant with esophageal atresia and tracheoesophageal fistula complicated by severe RDS or pneumonia. J Pediatr Surg 1982;17(2):149–51.
[27] Holmes SJK, Kiely EM, Spitz L. Tracheo-oesophageal fistula and the respiratory distress syndrome. Pediatr Surg Int 1987;2(1):16–8.
[28] Malone PS, Kiely EM, Brain AJ, et al. Tracheo-oesophageal fistula and pre-operative mechanical ventilation. Aust N Z J Surg 1990;60(7):525–7.
[29] Taguchi TT, Nagata K, Kinoshita Y, et al. The utility of muscle sparing axillar skin crease incision for pediatric thoracic surgery. Pediatr Surg Int 2012;28(3):239–44.
[30] Sharma S, Sinha SK, Rawat JD, et al. Azygos vein preservation in primary repair of esophageal atresia with tracheoesophageal fistula. Pediatr Surg Int 2007;23(12):1215–8.
[31] Bicakci U, Tander B, Ariturk E, et al. The right-sided aortic arch in children with esophageal atresia and tracheo-esophageal fistula: a repair through the right thoracotomy. Pediatr Surg Int 2009;25(5):423–5.
[32] Harrison MR, Hanson BA, Mahour GH, et al. The significance of right aortic arch in repair of esophageal atresia and tracheoesophageal fistula. J Pediatr Surg 1977;12(6):861–9.
[33] Lobe TE, et al. Thoracoscopic repair of esophageal atresia in an infant: a surgical first. Pediatric endosurgery & innovative techniques 1999;3(3):141–8. Available at. https://www.liebertpub.com/doi/abs/10.1089/pei.1999.3.141.
[34] Al Tokhais T, Zamakhshary M, Aldekhayel S, et al. Thoracoscopic repair of tracheoesophageal fistulas: a case–control matched study. J Pediatr Surg 2008;43(5):805–9.
[35] Allal H, Pérez-Bertólez S, Maillet O, et al. Estudio comparativo de toracoscopia versus toracotomía en atresia esofágica. Cir Pediatr 2009;22(4):177–80.
[36] Szavay PO, Zundel S, Blumenstock G, et al. Perioperative outcome of patients with esophageal atresia and tracheo-esophageal fistula undergoing open versus thoracoscopic surgery. J Laparoendosc Adv Surg Tech 2011;21(5):439–43.
[37] Borruto FA, Impellizzeri P, Montalto AS, et al. Thoracoscopy versus thoracotomy for esophageal atresia repair: review of the literature and meta-analysis. Eur J Pediatr Surg 2012;22(6):415–9.
[38] Holcomb GW, Rothenberg SS, Bax KMA, et al. Thoracoscopic repair of esophageal atresia and tracheoesophageal fistula. Ann Surg 2005;242(3):422–30.

[39] Rothenberg SS. Thoracoscopic repair of esophageal atresia and tracheo-esophageal fistula. Semin Pediatr Surg 2005;14(1):2–7.
[40] Esophageal Atresia and Tracheoesophageal Fistula. Available at: https://www.pedsurglibrary.com/apsa/view/Pediatric-Surgery-NaT/829035/all/Esophageal_Atresia_and_-Tracheoesophageal_Fistula?refer=true. Accessed November 22, 2020.
[41] Costerus S, Vlot J, van Rosmalen J, et al. Effects of neonatal thoracoscopic surgery on tissue oxygenation: a pilot study on (neuro-) monitoring and outcomes. Eur J Pediatr Surg 2019;29(2):166–72.
[42] Neunhoeffer F, Warmann SW, Hofbeck M, et al. Elevated intrathoracic CO2 pressure during thoracoscopic surgery decreases regional cerebral oxygen saturation in neonates and infants-A pilot study. Paediatr Anaesth 2017;27(7):752–9.
[43] Foker JE, Kendall Krosch TC, Catton K, et al. Long-gap esophageal atresia treated by growth induction: the biological potential and early follow-up results. Semin Pediatr Surg 2009;18(1):23–9.
[44] Foker JE, Linden BC, Boyle EM, et al. Development of a true primary repair for the full spectrum of esophageal atresia. Ann Surg 1997;226(4):533–43.
[45] Bradshaw CJ, Sloan K, Morandi A, et al. Outcomes of esophageal replacement: gastric pull-up and colonic interposition procedures. Eur J Pediatr Surg 2018;28(1):22–9.
[46] Gallo G, Zwaveling S, Groen H, et al. Long-gap esophageal atresia: a meta-analysis of jejunal interposition, colon interposition, and gastric pull-up. Eur J Pediatr Surg 2012;22(6): 420–5.
[47] Bludevich BM, Kauffman JD, Smithers CJ, et al. 30-day outcomes following esophageal replacement in children: a national surgical quality improvement project pediatric analysis. J Surg Res 2020;255:549–55.
[48] Juza RM, Arca MJ, Densmore JC, et al. Laparoscopic-assisted transhiatal gastric transposition for long gap esophageal atresia in an infant. J Pediatr Surg 2010;45(7):1534–7.
[49] Esteves E, Sousa-Filho HB, Watanabe S, et al. Laparoscopically assisted esophagectomy and colon interposition for esophageal replacement in children: preliminary results of a novel technique. J Pediatr Surg 2010;45(5):1053–60.
[50] Lal DR, Gadepalli SK, Downard CD, et al. Challenging surgical dogma in the management of proximal esophageal atresia with distal tracheoesophageal fistula: outcomes from the Midwest Pediatric Surgery Consortium. J Pediatr Surg 2018;53(7):1267–72.
[51] Zani A, Eaton S, Hoellwarth M, et al. International survey on the management of esophageal atresia. Eur J Pediatr Surg 2014;24(1):3–8.
[52] Wang C, Feng L, Li Y, et al. What is the impact of the use of transanastomotic feeding tube on patients with esophageal atresia: a systematic review and meta-analysis. BMC Pediatr 2018;18(1):385.
[53] Fusco JC, Calisto JL, Gaines BA, et al. A large single-institution review of tracheoesophageal fistulae with evaluation of the use of transanastomotic feeding tubes. J Pediatr Surg 2017; https://doi.org/10.1016/j.jpedsurg.2017.10.026.
[54] Bence CM, Rymeski B, Gadepalli S, et al. Clinical outcomes following implementation of a management bundle for esophageal atresia with distal tracheoesophageal fistula. J Pediatr Surg 2020; https://doi.org/10.1016/j.jpedsurg.2020.09.049.
[55] Dellenmark-Blom M, Chaplin JE, Gatzinsky V, et al. Health-related quality of life among children, young people and adults with esophageal atresia: a review of the literature and recommendations for future research. Qual Life Res 2015;24(10):2433–45.
[56] Dingemann C, Meyer A, Kircher G, et al. Long-term health-related quality of life after complex and/or complicated esophageal atresia in adults and children registered in a German patient support group. J Pediatr Surg 2014;49(4):631–8.

Advances in Pediatrics 68 (2021) 261–281

ADVANCES IN PEDIATRICS

Trends in Pediatric Recreational Drug Use and Ingestions

Raymen R. Assaf, MA, MD, MPH[a,b,*],
Kelly D. Young, MD, MS[a,b]

[a]Pediatric Emergency Medicine, Department of Emergency Medicine, Harbor-UCLA Medical Center, 1000 West Carson Street, Box 21, Torrance, CA 90502, USA; [b]David Geffen School of Medicine at UCLA, Los Angeles, CA, USA

Keywords

• Toxidrome • Recreational drug use • Drug abuse • Adolescent • Ingestion

Key points

- Adolescent recreational and polysubstance drug use are widespread, substances are easily accessible, and current popular drugs used are constantly evolving.
- Adolescent substance use initiation is particularly concerning because of impacts on neurocognitive and social development, as well as the likelihood of future polysubstance and persistent drug use.
- Clinical presentations may vary widely based on the amount and concentration ingested as well as host factors, and clinicians may be unfamiliar with novel substances used.
- Rather than specific antidotes, emergency-based management is largely focused on key supportive measures essential in patient stabilization following any toxic exposure.

INTRODUCTION

"Classic" toxidromes are a cornerstone of emergency medical education (Table 1), yet a heterogeneous cluster of less understood recreational drug use among youth is rapidly emerging. Poisoning incidents in youth ages 15 to 19 years in the United States doubled from 2000 to 2009, and is now among the leading causes of death in adolescence [1,2]. In infants and toddlers, the increase in

The authors have nothing to disclose.
Funding source. Dr K.D. Young: NIH/NHLBI UO1AI116400.

*Corresponding author. *E-mail address:* rassaf@dhs.lacounty.gov

https://doi.org/10.1016/j.yapd.2021.05.011
0065-3101/21/

Table 1
Classic pediatric toxidromes

Agent category	Symptoms and signs
Alcohols	Stupor, ataxia, slurred speech, drowsiness, flushing, mydriasis, emesis, convulsion, hypoventilation, hypothermia, hypotension, coma
Anticholinergics	Delirium, agitation, mydriasis, nystagmus, dryness, flushing, urinary retention, tachycardia, hypertension, dysrhythmia
Cholinergics	Miosis, diarrhea, bronchospasm, urination, emesis, lacrimation, salivation, muscle twitching, bradycardia or tachycardia, hypotension or hypertension
Opioids	Somnolence, hypoventilation, miosis, seizure, hypotension, bradycardia
Sedative-hypnotics	Altered mental status, stupor, hypoventilation, hypotension, hypothermia
Sympathomimetics	Agitation, mydriasis, tachycardia, hypertension, diaphoresis, hyperthermia
Tricyclic antidepressants	Decreased responsiveness, seizure, dysrhythmia, hypotension, coma

Data from Calello D, Henretig F. Pediatric toxicology: specialized approach to the poisoned child. Emerg Med Clin N Am. 2014; 32(1):29-52.

adult drug prescriptions has been strongly associated with rising unintentional poisonings [3]. Nationally, the prevalence of illicit drug use (including marijuana) among adolescents age 12 years or older is 50% [4]. Polysubstance use is common, reported in up to 39% of adolescents in secondary school [5]. A potent, dose–response relationship between adverse childhood experience and the initiation of alcohol, nicotine, marijuana, and prescription opioid use in adolescence has been consistently demonstrated in large-scale studies [6–11]. Further, substance use initiation in adolescence serves as a strong predictor of persistent use and substance use disorder [12–14].

In 2018, the American Association of Poison Control Centers serving all 50 US states reported more than 2 million human exposure cases, the majority (44%) of which were in children ages 5 years or younger, although this group comprised only approximately 1% of exposure-related fatalities [15]. Among patients ages 13 to 19 years of age, fatality was primarily owing to intentional ingestion, with analgesics by far being the most common cause (41%), and "street drugs" second (18%) [13]. The American Association of Poison Control Centers report, however, does not detail the implications of common emerging recreational drugs used among pediatric and adolescent populations, which will be examined in this article. These include (Table 2):

- Nicotine-containing electronic cigarettes (vaping),
- Marijuana and "edibles,"
- Synthetic cannabinoids (SCs),

Table 2
Current and emerging pediatric toxidromes

Agent category	Symptoms and signs
Nicotine-containing electronic cigarettes	EVALI: subjective fever, fatigue, headache, myalgias, seizure, gastrointestinal (nausea, emesis, anorexia, abdominal pain), respiratory (cough, chest pain, dyspnea, respiratory failure)
Marijuana and edibles	Afebrile young child with acute onset altered mental status; older child with anxiety, dysphoria, tachycardia, psychosis, conjunctival injection; cannabis hyperemesis syndrome: recurrent bouts of intractable nausea, vomiting, and abdominal pain, improved with hot showers or baths
SCs	Inattention, altered spatial orientation, impaired memory, nausea, neuropsychiatric (acute psychosis, agitation, CNS depression, seizure), hyperthermia, tachycardia, bradycardia, hypertension, hypotension, respiratory depression; Young children: decreased muscle coordination, lethargy, seizure, obtundation
Opioids	Somnolence, hypoventilation, miosis, seizure, hypotension, bradycardia
Prescription drug misuse	Variable presentation; may have symptomatic components of acute opioid, stimulant, and/or sedative–hypnotic ingestion
Psychedelics	Nausea, vomiting, headache, seizure, hallucinations (auditory, visual, or tactile), dysphoria, aggression, hyperthermia, tachycardia, diaphoresis, mydriasis, nystagmus, hyperreflexia
Inhalants	Dizziness, cough, poor coordination, slurred speech, euphoria, slowed thinking and movement, muscle weakness, tremor, blurred vision, seizure, lethargy, stupor/coma, hypoxia
DM	Restlessness, uncontrolled laughter, mydriasis, nystagmus, disorientation, hallucinations, impaired coordination, ataxia, disassociation with agitation or somnolence

- Opioids,
- Prescription drug misuse,
- Microdose psychedelics,
- Inhalants, and
- Dextromethorphan (DM).

CLINICAL APPROACH

General history

Gathering a concise and accurate history is often a challenge in the scenario of an acutely intoxicated pediatric patient for whom the caregiver or other historian may not be present at bedside. Critical information to obtain includes identifying the specific exposure substance or class of substance, when the exposure occurred, and other potential medications and/or poisons to which the patient may have had access. The exact amount of a substance ingested may also be difficult to ascertain. When possible, the history should also include prior substance use or misuse, the setting and context of the exposure (ie, experimentation or suicide attempt; alone at home, at school, or among peers at a party), recent decline in school performance, psychiatric history, and any collateral information that is able to be obtained from present family or friends. Calling or texting peer friends and siblings can sometimes provide valuable information.

Workup

In acute exposures, there may be a wide array of possible clinical presentations depending on the specific substance, dose, concentration or potency, timing of exposure, coexposure, and/or host factors such as first-time versus chronic user. On a focused examination, critical information can be derived from the patient's vital signs, neurologic status (alertness, pupils, motor response), cardiovascular status (perfusion), respiratory examination (work of breathing, auscultated lung findings), and skin examination (moist or dry, flushing). The immediate workup may include a point-of-care blood glucose, blood gas, electrocardiogram, serum electrolytes, toxicology screen, urine pregnancy test, complete blood count, and/or chest radiograph. In the acutely agitated patient, urinalysis and creatinine kinase levels are useful to evaluate for possible rhabdomyolysis.

Treatment

Supportive care is frequently the core of acute clinical management and depends on vigilant monitoring of clinical status and vital signs, maintaining a patent and protected airway, the use of supplemental oxygen as needed, the administration of intravenous fluids, maintaining euthermia through cooling or warming techniques, benzodiazepines for agitation and/or seizure, and naloxone administration if opioids are suspected. Consultation with a toxicologist or poison control center may help to guide acute any therapeutic intervention and clinical disposition (ie, observation in the emergency department for a specified amount of time or admission with a recommended level of care).

CURRENT TOXIDROMES

Nicotine-containing electronic cigarettes

Background and epidemiology

Nicotine-containing e-cigarette use, commonly known as vaping, was introduced in 2007 as a smoking cessation tool that rapidly gained popularity among adolescents in the following decade, surpassing combustible tobacco cigarette use in this age group by 2014 [16,17]. E-cigarette use became so widespread that 35% of twelfth-grade students reported vaping in the past 12 months in 2019 [17,18]. Multiple studies have demonstrated a correlation between adolescent vaping and cigarette smoking initiation, with higher nicotine concentrated e-cigarettes linked to increased frequency and intensity of smoking [17,19–22]. The majority of middle and high school students favor pod-based, flavored e-cigarettes; however, products have a wide range of nicotine concentrations, formulations, and delivery, devices, voltages, and tank sizes [16,17].

Emergency presentation and management

Young children who ingest liquid nicotine meant for use in vaping devices may present with nausea, vomiting, abdominal pain, salivation, tachycardia, hypertension, bronchorrhea, wheezing, tremor, and fasciculations. More severe presentations include muscle paralysis, apnea, shock, seizures, coma, and death [23]. The median lethal dose for children is approximately 10 mg, which may be contained in 1 mL of liquid nicotine or less.

Patients with e-cigarette or vaping product associated lung injury (EVALI) may present initially with a myriad of symptoms, including subjective fever, fatigue, myalgias, gastrointestinal symptoms (nausea, emesis, anorexia, abdominal pain), respiratory symptoms (cough, chest pain, dyspnea), headache, and seizure [24–26]. Examination findings commonly demonstrate fever, tachycardia, tachypnea, hypoxemia, and/or bibasilar crackles [24,25]. It is important to note that, although respiratory symptoms and signs may not be predominant at the time of presentation, patients with EVALI frequently progress to respiratory failure [24,25].

A laboratory workup may show leukocytosis and elevated inflammatory markers (C-reactive protein), complicating differentiation from bacterial pneumonia [25,27]. A chest radiograph may show diffuse or bibasilar interstitial pulmonary infiltrates; however, the absence of these findings on a chest radiograph is not sufficiently sensitive to make an EVALI diagnosis early in the clinical course [24,26]. A computed tomography scan of the chest characteristically demonstrates bilateral ground-glass opacities, as well as consolidation and interlobular septal thickening [26].

EVALI therapy is largely supportive, using successively higher modalities of supplemental oxygen administration and ventilatory support as needed, with approximately one-fourth of patients requiring mechanical ventilation [24,28]. Although antibiotics targeting community-acquired pneumonia are routinely initiated early, the use of systemic glucocorticoids is typically reserved for those with severe lung disease [24,29].

Sequelae and complications

When inhaled, nicotine causes bronchoconstriction and increased airway resistance through parasympathetic stimulation that, over time, contributes to elastin degeneration and alveolar volume expansion similar to chronic obstructive pulmonary disease [17,23,30]. Among patients with EVALI, impaired diffusing capacity of the lungs on pulmonary function testing is typically noted after hospital discharge; however, long-term outcomes are not known owing to insufficient longitudinal population-based studies [31,32]. One prospective study among adult users suggested a modest risk of developing chronic respiratory disease [33].

Marijuana: Weed, wax, and edibles

Background and epidemiology

Marijuana, derived from the *Cannabis sativa* plant, is one of the most commonly abused substances among adolescents age 12 years and older, with a lifetime use of 45.20% [4]. The 2 main cannabinoids in marijuana are tetrahydrocannabinol (THC) and cannabidiol. The rapid movement toward the legalization and decriminalization of cannabis has resulted in a significant increase in pediatric exposures, both intentional and accidental [34]. Eleven states have legalized recreational cannabis use, and 4 more voted to do so in the November 2020 election. Many more states have decriminalized its use, and at least some form of medicinal use is approved in all but 2 states [35]. Legalization has resulted in increased use in young adults, including parents of young children, and contributed to a perception of marijuana and cannabis products as having minimal risk [36,37]. Studies have shown increases in emergency department visits and accidental exposures in young children related to cannabis over the last decade [34].

Common routes of exposure include inhalation, with vaping of cannabinoids increasingly common, as well as ingestion of marijuana "edibles." Inhaled cannabis exerts a peak effect in 15 to 30 minutes with duration of effect up to 4 hours, whereas edibles take 1 to 2 hours (on rare occasions up to 8 hours) to reach peak effect [34]. Sometimes novice users are impatient and consume multiple additional doses because they "do not feel anything." Edibles are usually packaged to look like candy, cookies, and other treats attractive to young children. Cannabis in dried resin extract form (hashish) may resemble a chocolate bar. The standard adult dose of 10 mg is often found in a portion size much less than a child would be expected to eat in 1 sitting (eg, a single gummy bear), and some products may contain 400 mg of THC or more [34]. The extraction of the primary psychoactive cannabinoid THC into a "wax" that can then be smoked (also known as dab, budder, shatter, and butane hash oil) results in a highly concentrated product, raising the risks for toxicity and sequelae. Additionally, the chemical extraction process creates a risk of flammability [36].

Emergency presentation and management

Although recreational cannabis users expect a pleasant relaxed effect, symptoms such as dysphoria, dizziness, anxiety, psychosis, ataxia, tremor, nystagmus, and tachycardia may occur [34]. Other common symptoms include conjunctival injection, increased appetite, dry mouth, and impaired short-term memory, concentration, reaction time, and motor coordination. Young children may present after the ingestion of edibles or cannabis products with lethargy, hypotonia, and altered mental status to the point of coma [38]. A careful history taking for possible exposure in the afebrile young child presenting with acute onset lethargy or coma may help to avoid an extensive unneeded workup, such as a lumbar puncture and brain imaging. Urine THC screen, typically part of standard urine toxicology screens, confirms the diagnosis in unintentional ingestions by naive users, but a positive screen in a chronic user may represent use as much as 1 month prior [34].

Treatment is supportive. Patients who are agitated can be kept in a low stimulus (low light and noise) room, and given benzodiazepines as needed. Very rarely do young children have significant neurologic symptoms or hypoventilation necessitating intubation. Most patients' acute symptoms will resolve over 8 to 12 hours [34].

Cannabis hyperemesis syndrome, first described in 2004, is now seen more often in emergency departments. Patients who are chronic marijuana users present with intermittent episodes of intractable vomiting and abdominal pain that is relieved by hot showers or baths [39]. A systematic review of cannabis hyperemesis patients found the median age of onset of regular cannabis use to be 16 years, with the median age of symptom onset 24 years. However, 25% of patients had been users for 1 year or less. Although 71% used cannabis on a daily basis, 19% used it only weekly [40]. Acute treatment usually involves intravenous fluid rehydration and antiemetics such as ondansetron (although nausea and vomiting are often resistant to standard antiemetics). Benzodiazepines, haloperidol, and topical capsaicin for abdominal pain have been reported to be effective [39]. The only definitive treatment, however, is stopping cannabis use completely.

Sequelae and complications

Neurodevelopmental studies of adolescents using cannabis have shown increased impulsivity and hyperactivity issues, mental health concerns such as depression and psychosis, structural brain changes, and cognitive deficits that did not recover with stopping cannabis use [36,41]. Brain development continues through the early 20s, increasing the risk of long-term neurologic impact of adolescent marijuana use [41]. Also, much of the research on neurodevelopmental effects was done before the widespread use of higher potency forms such as wax and the increased availability of high-dose edibles [38]. Higher potency forms and onset of use in adolescence increase the risk of addiction from the baseline of 9% to 17% or higher [37,41]. EVALI has been particularly associated with vaping THC products, possibly owing to the inclusion of vitamin E acetate in the cartridges [42]. Impaired coordination and judgment may result in increased injuries, especially if users drive under the influence of marijuana [41].

Synthetic cannabinoids

Background and epidemiology

SCs are potent heterogeneous chemicals intended to mimic the primary psychoactive component of cannabis (THC) with affinity for cannabinoid receptors up to 200-fold stronger than marijuana [43,44]. Commonly known as "spice" or "K2," SCs are often smoked, with a quicker time to peak onset (within minutes) and shorter duration of action compared with marijuana [45–47]. SCs can be easily accessed in convenience stores, smoke shops, or bought online [48]. Over the last decade, their use increased across all of adolescence, especially in twelfth graders, surging in 2015 before a slight decrease in subsequent years [49]. Compared with marijuana users, adolescents using SCs demonstrate riskier health behaviors related to violence, injury, mental health, sexual health, and polydrug use, including opioids and cocaine [50,51].

Emergency presentation and management

Common symptoms of SC intoxication are similar to those of marijuana, including inattention, altered spatial orientation, impaired memory, and nausea. However, patients also present with unique sympathomimetic toxicity and neuropsychiatric symptoms such as acute psychosis, agitation, central nervous system (CNS) depression and/or seizure [43,44,46,52,53]. The physical examination does not reliably demonstrate a recognizable toxidrome and may also be influenced by polydrug exposure. Hyperthermia, tachycardia or bradycardia, hypertension or hypotension, respiratory depression, and altered mental status–from impaired orientation to obtundation–have all been reported [43,44,46,54]. Young children who ingest SCs more typically present with decreased muscle coordination, lethargy, seizure, and obtundation [52].

SC intoxication requires aggressive treatment and endotracheal intubation in the case of severe altered mental status, as well as the management of agitation with benzodiazepines or antipsychotic agents, of seizures with benzodiazepines, and of dehydration with intravenous fluid resuscitation [44,52]. An electrocardiogram and troponin level should be obtained on all patients, because dysrhythmia and/or myocardial ischemia are associated complications of SC exposure [52,55]. Rhabdomyolysis and renal injury are common, and hemodialysis may be needed in severe cases [52]. Standard hospital urine drug screening has limited utility in detecting SCs owing to their wide range of chemical structures [52]. Admission is indicated in the case of CNS depression, altered mental status, seizure, rhabdomyolysis, or persistently abnormal vital signs [52].

Sequelae and complications

Life-threatening conditions induced by SCs include status epilepticus, respiratory depression, myocardial infarction, cerebral ischemic events, intracranial hemorrhage, diffuse alveolar hemorrhage, rhabdomyolysis, and acute tubular necrosis [44–46,49]. Patients may also develop transient cerebral edema with a clinical presentation mimicking anoxic brain injury [45]. Evidence shows that cannabinoid use in adolescence affects neural circuits in the prefrontal cortex and hippocampus, leading to impaired neurocognitive functioning [46,56]. Depression, marijuana use, and alcohol use have all been shown to be predictive of persistent SC use [48].

Opioids

Background and epidemiology

Opioids have become by far the most commonly abused prescription drugs among adolescents and young adults [57–59]. Pediatric opioid-related emergency department visits have increased by 101% from 2001 to 2008, accompanied by an 86% increase in admission rates [60]. Intentional exposures are a common reason for hospital admission, and oxycodone and methadone have been associated with the most pediatric deaths [57]. The overall pediatric mortality rate from opioids increased by 268% from 1999 to 2016, with the vast majority among 15- to 19-year-old males [59]. During this same period, mortality rates increased for all pediatric age groups, including infants and toddlers, in which nearly one-fourth of cases were attributed to homicide [59]. Those who abuse opioids incur high health care costs and resource use, and there is substantial evidence that this pattern is initiated in adolescence [57,61]. Additionally, parental use of opioids in the home setting impacts all stages of childhood, because it is closely associated with neglect, domestic violence, and the placement of children in the foster care system [62–64].

Prescribers themselves may also fuel persistent pediatric opioid use owing to highly variable postoperative prescribing practices, overprescribing, and use of excessive dosages, most commonly with hydrocodone and particularly among female adolescent patients, those with chronic pain, and/or previous substance use disorder [65–69]. After common pediatric surgeries, patients receiving postoperative opioid prescriptions have a more than 3-fold risk of a subsequent emergency department visit compared with those who do not [67]. Inconsistent, unregulated prescription practices also risk accidental exposure in young children; nearly one-third of children under the age of 12 years with opioid poisoning were found to have taken a household member's medication [70].

Emergency presentation and management

Opioid poisonings typically present in a bimodal fashion, with unintentional exposures accounting for the majority in younger age groups (0–5 years) and intentional in older age groups (15–19 years) [57,71]. The clinical presentation commonly consists of a combination of CNS and respiratory depression along with miosis, with possible bradycardia and hypotension. Emergency management is based on maintaining a patent airway and maximizing oxygenation and ventilation, largely by reversal of central and respiratory depression with use of naloxone. The recommended dose of naloxone is 0.1 mg/kg for children 5 years or less or up to 20 kg in weight and 2 mg for those over 20 kg, preferably intravenously although intramuscular, subcutaneous, intranasal, endotracheal, and intraosseous routes are all possible [72]. Onset is within 1 to 2 minutes with a 30- to 60-minute duration of action, and dosing may be repeated every 3 to 5 minutes as needed to maintain opioid reversal and adequate respiratory status [73]. Patients with suspected chronic opioid use may be given a smaller 0.4 mg dose to avoid opioid withdrawal, repeated as described and as needed [73]. Continuous naloxone infusions can be safely used by administering two-thirds of the dose required to reverse respiratory depression (loading dose) as an hourly infusion, mixed in a solution of 5% dextrose or normal saline [74]. Additionally, one-half of the loading dose should be given 15 minutes after initiating an infusion to avoid a transient decrease in naloxone levels [74]. Subsequently, the infusion is titrated to maintain respiratory function and can be decreased by one-half every hour over the following 6 to 12 hours until the effect of the opioid has worn off [74].

Unintentional buprenorphine exposure has also increased markedly among young children owing to its candy-like appearance. Toxicity is significant after even a single lick, and similar to methadone may have delayed or prolonged effects for up to 24 hours, often requiring hospital admission [71,75,76]. In general, emergency providers must also consider polysubstance overdose which, owing to multiple, counteracting, or synergistic effects, may be challenging to both recognize and treat [77].

Sequelae and complications

The opioid epidemic has accelerated over the last 2 decades, becoming a potent destabilizing force in childhood with significant impact on pediatric development, mental health, mortality, and substance abuse [62,78]. During this time there has been a 5-fold increase in the number of neonates born with neonatal abstinence syndrome, which has been linked to poor neurodevelopmental outcome, placing an unprecedented burden on the health care system [79,80].

Prescription drug misuse

Background and epidemiology

In recent years, adolescent prescription drug misuse has markedly increased along with medical provider prescribing practices, with more than 16.7 million US individuals ages 12 years and older reported to abuse prescription drugs in 2012, superseding alcohol and tobacco use, and now second only to marijuana [2,81–83]. Up to 10% of youth ages 14 to 20 years presenting to the emergency department report prescription drug misuse, whereas less than 15% of this group has an appropriate prescription for use [84]. The most commonly ever abused drugs among twelfth-grade students are opioids (13%), stimulants (9.5%), and sedative–hypnotics (7.5%); up to 23% of college students report ever abusing [58,81,85,86].

Nonmedical misuse describes drug use without a prescription, whereas medical misuse refers to use of a drug in a manner not intended by the prescriber [85]. Prescription drug misuse rates are higher among adolescents not in school or with poor school adjustment, and those with other substance use disorders or psychiatric illnesses [58,81,85,87]. Although adolescents may misuse prescription drugs for their intended effect (eg, to aid in sleep or treat pain), common motives include intentionally seeking to get high, decrease anxiety, or increase concentration [88]. Notably, in a national survey approximately 41% of adolescents assumed prescription medication to be safer than illicit drugs [89]. Prescription drugs are readily and often legally available to adolescents via prescription from a doctor, diversion from friends or relatives, purchase from illicit online pharmacies without a prescription, or socially in "pharm" parties, in which a mixture of pills are ingested at once [77,81,89–92]. However, the majority of known intentional prescription drug misuse exposures are within the adolescent's own home [57].

Emergency presentation and management

Although the clinical presentation depends on the medication or combination of medications taken, management is largely supportive. CNS and cardiorespiratory depression may be expected with opioids and sedative abuse, and a trial of naloxone is indicated in low dose to reverse opioid-induced depression while avoiding possible opioid withdrawal [92]. In the case of stimulants, patients may present with agitation, mydriasis, tachycardia, hypertension, diaphoresis, and/or hyperthermia and may benefit from cooling measures, intravenous rehydration, and benzodiazepines. Nearly one-half of medical providers do not ask about prescription drug abuse; however, certain key predictors may raise suspicion, particularly poor school attendance or performance, substance use disorder, mood disorder, high risk-taking levels, and/or chronic pain [93,94]. Preventing prescription drug misuse requires wide-scale collaborative action between medical providers, schools, parents, communities, and policymakers in a multifaceted approach to education and screening while decreasing the availability of prescription drugs for diversion [95].

Sequelae and complications

About 38% of all intentional adolescent prescription drug exposures are classified as suspected suicide attempts, with oxycodone and methadone accounting for the most deaths [57]. The most commonly abused prescription drugs–opioids, stimulants, and sedative-hypnotics–each have unique neuropsychiatric effects and potential for severe addiction, making adolescence a sensitive developmental risk period in drug exposure [96]. Adolescent prescription drug misuse is closely associated with future development of substance abuse, exposure to violence, delinquency, and psychiatric disorders [81,97].

Microdose psychedelics

Background and epidemiology

Although microdosing classically refers to the subpharmacologic administration of an investigational drug, in recent years it has become a trend among recreational drug users seeking perceived beneficial properties of an ingested psychedelic drug–usually lysergic acid diethylamide-25 (LSD), ketamine, or psilocybin–without an undesirable intoxication or impaired functioning [98–100]. Individuals may microdose psychedelics (between 5% and 10% of a standard dose) for various reasons in the personal, social, school, or workplace setting, including to enhance mood, cognition, creativity, and/or connection to others and environment [99–102]. In the last decade there has been a renewed interest in the clinical application of psychedelics in the treatment of anxiety, depression, and substance use disorders; however, the concurrent recreational use of hallucinogens among adolescents has also become increasingly common, with 15% of adolescents 12 years or older having experimented [4,98,102–104].

Emergency presentation and management

Although there is lack of literature on expected microdosing effects, individuals experimenting are at risk of adverse effects of psychedelic intoxication, either alone or in combination with other drugs, as well as associated risky behavior when cognition is impaired, such as physical trauma, multiple drug use, and legal offenses [99,103,105]. Symptoms may include nausea, vomiting, headache, distressing hallucinations (auditory, visual, or tactile), anxiety, panic attacks, flashbacks, insomnia, paranoia, and aggression [106]. Rare but serious effects include seizure, coma, renal injury from rhabdomyolysis, and cardiac arrest [103]. Possible examination findings are hyperthermia, tachycardia, diaphoresis, mydriasis, nystagmus, confusion, perceptual abnormality, dysphoria, or hyperreflexia [103]. Blood work may show coagulopathy, elevated creatinine kinase, elevated serum blood urea nitrogen/creatinine, and/or electrolyte abnormalities [103]. Supportive emergency care is the mainstay of treatment [103]. The majority of patients are discharged from the emergency department with a symptom duration of typically less than 24 hours, although those with end-organ damage require intensive care [103,107].

Sequelae and complications

Critical illness and mortality are most often the result of acute polydrug abuse and/or accidental physical trauma while intoxicated [108]. Long-term studies on the safety of microdosing psychedelics have not been performed, although LSD has been shown to cause aggression and hyper-reactivity in mouse models months after discontinuation [100]. Psychological dependence and tolerance may occur with habitual use when endogenous dopamine is exhausted [109,110].

Inhalants

Background and epidemiology

Inhalants are a widely available, heterogeneous collection of volatile substances that are misused to quickly achieve intoxication with rapid dissipation [111]. The most commonly used substances include gasoline, lighter fluid, glue, paints, aerosol propellants, shoe polish, and more recently, computer and electronic duster spray [112–115]. Inhalants are easily concealed in common household product containers or soaked rags and are inhaled through the nose (sniffing, snorting) and/or mouth (huffing, bagging) then rapidly absorbed through the lungs [111]. Owing to ease of access, rapid onset, and a lack of legal ramifications, inhalants are commonly the first substance used by young adolescents typically among peers, although more than one-third of adolescent users report using alone [113,116,117]. The prevalence of inhalant use by adolescents age 12 years and older has slightly increased over the last decade with a rate up to 20% [4,118,119]. Inhalant initiation has been found to peak at age 13 to 14 years and is associated with impaired family functioning, parental drug use, delinquent behavior, and multiple drug abuse [112,120]. Inhalant dependence has been linked to initiation at young age and use of multiple inhalant types, which also increases the risk for subsequent and earlier drug use [112,121].

Emergency presentation and management

Depending on the substance inhaled, symptoms of acute intoxication may consist of cough, dizziness, poor coordination, slurred speech, euphoria, slowed thinking and movement, muscle weakness, tremor, blurred vision, seizure, lethargy, stupor, coma, and skin injury ranging from swollen lips to mucocutaneous burns [115,116,122,123]. The clinical presentation can mimic ethanol intoxication, demonstrating altered mental status, hypoxia, and possible evidence of use, such as perioral or skin irritation, injected sclera, chemical breath odor, and/or staining on fingers or clothes [119]. Diagnosis relies almost entirely on history because no laboratory test detects substance inhalation, although in severe or chronic presentations, abnormalities in chest radiographs, liver enzymes, and/or serum blood urea nitrogen/creatinine may indicate end-organ damage [119]. Emergency management is supportive, with the administration of supplemental oxygen as needed and education on the dangers of continued inhalant use [119].

Sequelae and complications

Inhalant abuse may lead to death by suffocation, aspiration, anaphylaxis, suicide attempt, or accidental traumatic injury while impaired, especially given that comorbid psychiatric or behavioral disorders are commonly associated with inhalation abuse [111,117]. A phenomenon called sudden sniffing death may occur immediately or hours after inhalant use, caused by a fatal cardiac arrhythmia from superphysiologic effect of epinephrine on a sensitized myocardium [111]. Chronic use can lead to direct lung injury, renal–hepatic failure, and neurotoxic effects on white matter leading to impairments in mood, short-term memory, attention, coordination, hearing, and judgment [115,117,122,124,125].

Dextromethorphan

Background and epidemiology

Intentional abuse of DM by adolescents began in the 1980s and became rapidly popular by 2000, with an estimated prevalence of 5% among twelfth-grade students, leading to enactment of age restriction laws in multiple states by 2015 [126–129]. An active antitussive ingredient in more than 125 over-the-counter cough and cold preparations, DM may be ingested in either syrup or gelcap form, and among adolescents is used experimentally in social circles or while alone (common slang includes dexing, robo-tripping, red hots, and skittles) [127,129,130]. DM is a semisynthetic codeine analogue derivative without mu-receptor activity or analgesic properties, although its metabolites act as *N*-methyl-D-aspartate receptor antagonists [127,129,131].

Emergency presentation and management

DM is often abused by individuals seeking its euphoric and/or dissociative effects in supratherapeutic doses [127,129,132]. Clinical presentation varies depending on the ingested dose, which may mimic stimulants at a dose between 100 and 200 mg, whereas doses of 600 to 1500 mg can induce dissociative sedation similar to ketamine [127,133,134]. In minimally intoxicated patients, examination findings may include tachycardia, restlessness, uncontrolled laughter, mydriasis, and nystagmus, whereas those moderately intoxicated can exhibit disorientation, auditory or visual (closed-eye) hallucinations, impaired coordination, distortion of motion, and a so-called zombie-like plodding ataxic gait [129,133–135]. Disassociation with agitation or somnolence are the predominant findings in severe intoxication [134].

In the agitated patient, laboratory tests may demonstrate metabolic acidosis, acute kidney injury, electrolyte abnormality, and/or rhabdomyolysis, whereas the sedated patient may show respiratory acidosis. Evaluation of co-ingestants is important, especially because over-the-counter cough and cold preparations often contain acetaminophen, decongestants, and/or antihistamines, and when combined with a selective serotonin reuptake inhibitor, serotonin syndrome may ensue [133,134,136].

Emergency management is supportive, using intravenous fluids for those with dehydration and/or rhabdomyolysis and benzodiazepines for agitation, hyperthermia, hypertension, and/or tachycardia [134]. In rare circumstances, endotracheal intubation may be required for the severely altered or agitated patient, whereas naloxone has variable response for somnolence [134,135].

Sequelae and complications

Although DM is not an addictive drug, psychological dependency is common among regular users and an abstinence syndrome may include dysphoria, flashbacks, hallucinations, and intense cravings within 3 days of stopping DM [133,137]. Chronic users may exhibit cognitive deterioration and psychosis [134].

SUMMARY

An epidemic of recreational use of new drugs has accelerated and evolved over the last 2 decades, with a thorough scientific understanding and regulation both lacking. Older adolescents are particularly susceptible to drug initiation and abuse. The clinical presentation after drug exposure varies widely owing in part to the range of substances being used or combined, their concentration and specific route, and factors owing to the host (new or chronic user), as well as the relative new emergence of specific substances without substantial medical precedent. Drug exposures may range from relatively benign presentations requiring only emergency department observation to multisystemic, life-threatening complications. Targeted supportive measures are critical in the acute clinical picture, and apart from naloxone for opioid reversal, specific antidotes do not exist for the majority of these recreational drug exposures. Children are susceptible to the long-term impacts on neurocognitive and social development, in addition to future polysubstance use and persistent drug use.

CLINICS CARE POINTS

- Teens with EVALI may present with predominant gastrointestinal symptoms initially.
- Many currently available cannabis products are highly concentrated, and young children may present with altered mental status to the point of coma.

- Chronic cannabis use in older teens is also causing a cannabis hyperemesis syndrome, which entails intermittent episodes of intractable vomiting and/or abdominal pain.
- SC use may cause seizures, rhabdomyolysis, or may mimic psychiatric disorders.
- The opioid crisis has had a profound effect on children and adolescents as well as adults.
- Parents should be counseled on appropriate storage and disposal of prescription drugs to avoid misuse.
- Microdosed psychedelics, household inhalants, and over-the-counter DM products are used by teens who believe they are obtaining a safer high.

References

[1] Centers for Disease Control and Prevention, National Center for Injury Prevention and Control. Vital signs: unintentional injury deaths among persons aged 0–19 years—United States, 2000–2009. MMWR Morb Mortal Wkly Rep 2012;61:270–6.

[2] Valdez A, Mars T. Rx for injury: adolescent prescription drug misuse. J Emerg Nurs 2014;40:497–9.

[3] Burghardt L, Ayers J, Brownstein J, et al. Adult prescription drug use and pediatric medication exposures and poisonings. J Pediatr 2013;132(1):18–27.

[4] National Survey of Drug Use and Health. National Institute on Drug Abuse. 2013. Available at: https://www.drugabuse.gov/drug-topics/trends-statistics/national-drug-early-warning-system-ndews/national-survey-drug-use-health. Accessed August 5, 2020.

[5] Weinberg N, Lopez M, Compton W. Epidemiology of drug abuse: building blocks for etiologic research. In: Madras B, Kuhar M, editors. The effects of drug abuse on the human nervous system. Oxford (United Kingdom): Elsevier; 2014. p. 51–76.

[6] Dube S, Felitti V, Dong M, et al. Childhood abuse, neglect, and household dysfunction and the risk of illicit drug use: the Adverse Childhood Experiences Study. J Pediatr 2003;111(3):564–72.

[7] Stein M, Conti M, Kenney S, et al. Adverse childhood experience effects on opioid use initiation, injection drug use, and overdose among persons with opioid use disorder. Drug Alcohol Depend 2017;179(1):325–9.

[8] Allem J, Soto D, Baezconde-Garbanati L, et al. Adverse childhood experiences and substance use among Hispanic emerging adults in Southern California. Addict Behav 2015;50:199–204.

[9] Dube S, Miller J, Brown D, et al. Adverse childhood experiences and the association with ever using alcohol and initiating alcohol use during adolescence. J Adolesc Health 2006;38(4):1–10.

[10] Anda R, Croft J, Felitti V, et al. Adverse childhood experiences and smoking during adolescence and adulthood. JAMA 1999;282(17):1652–8.

[11] LeTendre M, Reed M. The effect of adverse childhood experience on clinical diagnosis of a substance use disorder: results of a nationally representative study. Subst Use Misuse 2017;52(6):689–97.

[12] McGue M, Iacono W. The adolescent origins of substance use disorders. Int J Methods Psychiatr Res 2008;17(1):30–8.

[13] Timberlake D, Haberstick B, Hopfer C, et al. Progression from marijuana use to daily smoking and nicotine dependence in a national sample of U.S. adolescents. Drug Alcohol Depend 2007;88:272–81.

[14] Palmer R, Young S, Hopfer C, et al. Developmental epidemiology of drug use and abuse in adolescence and young adulthood: evidence of generalized risk. Drug Alcohol Depend 2009;102(1):78–87.
[15] Gummin D, Mowry J, Spyker D, et al. 2018 annual report of the American Association of Poison Control Centers' National Poison Data System (NPDS): 36th annual report. Clin Toxicol (Phila) 2019;57(12):1220-1413.
[16] Cullen K, Gentzke A, Sawdey M, et al. e-Cigarette use among youth in the United States, 2019. JAMA 2019;322:2095–103.
[17] Hamberger E, Halpern-Felsher B. Vaping in adolescents: epidemiology and respiratory harm. Curr Opin Pediatr 2020;32(3):378–83.
[18] Miech R, Johnston L, O'Malley PM, et al. Trends in adolescent vaping, 2017-2019. N Engl J Med 2019;381:1490–1.
[19] Spindle T, Hiler M, Cooke M, et al. Electronic cigarette use and uptake of cigarette smoking: a longitudinal examination of U.S. College Students. Addict Behav 2017;67:66–72.
[20] Wills T, Knight R, Sargent J, et al. Longitudinal study of e-cigarette use and onset of cigarette smoking among high school students in Hawaii. Tob Control 2017;26:34–9.
[21] Miech R, Patrick M, O'Malley P, et al. E-cigarette use as a predictor of cigarette smoking: results from a 1-year follow-up of a national sample of 12th grade students. Tob Control 2017;26:106–11.
[22] Goldenson N, Leventhal A, Stone M, et al. Associations of electronic cigarette nicotine concentration with subsequent cigarette smoking and vaping levels in adolescents. JAMA Pediatr 2017;171(12):1192–9.
[23] Mishra A, Chaturvedi P, Datta S, et al. Harmful effects of nicotine. Indian J Med Paediatr Oncol 2015;36:24–31.
[24] Layden J, Ghinai I, Pray I, et al. Pulmonary illness related to E-Cigarette use in Illinois and Wisconsin - Final report. N Engl J Med 2020;382(10):903–16.
[25] Messina M, Levin T, Conrad L, et al. Vaping associated lung injury: a potentially life-threatening epidemic in US youth. Pediatr Pulmonol 2020;55:1705–11.
[26] Wang K, Jadhav S, Smitha Yenduri N, et al. E-cigarette or vaping product use-associated lung injury in the pediatric population: imaging features at presentation and short-term follow-up. Pediatr Radiol 2020;50:1231–9.
[27] Khanijo S, Lou B, Makaryus M, et al. Coagulopathy and inflammatory dysregulation with E-Cigarette use. Am J Med 2020;133(5):530–1.
[28] Maddock S, Cirulis M, Callahan S, et al. Pulmonary lipid-laden macrophages and vaping. N Engl J Med 2019;381(15):1488–9.
[29] Triantafyllou G, Tiberio P, Zou R, et al. Vaping-associated acute lung injury: a case series. Am J Respir Crit Care Med 2019;200(11):1430–1.
[30] Beck E, Taylor R, Lee L, et al. Bronchoconstriction and apnea induced by cigarette smoke: nicotine dose dependence. Lung 1986;164:293–301.
[31] Corcoran A, Carl J, Rezaee F. The importance of anti-vaping vigilance-EVALI in seven adolescent pediatric patients in Northeast Ohio. Pediatr Pulmonol 2020;55(7):1719–24.
[32] Carroll B, Kim M, Hemyari A, et al. Impaired lung function following e-cigarette or vaping product use associated lung injury in the first cohort of hospitalized adolescents. Pediatr Pulmonol 2020;55(7):1712–8.
[33] Bhatta D, Glantz S. Association of E-cigarette use with respiratory disease among adults: a longitudinal analysis. Am J Prev Med 2019;58:182–90.
[34] Wong K, Baum C. Acute Cannabis Toxicity. Pediatr Emerg Care 2019;35(11):799–804.
[35] "Legality of Cannabis by U.S. Jurisdiction." Wikipedia, Wikimedia Foundation. 2020. Available at: https://en.wikipedia.org/wiki/Legality_of_cannabis_by_U.S._jurisdiction. Accessed November 18, 2020.
[36] Blohm E, Sell P, Neavyn M. Cannabinoid toxicity in pediatrics. Curr Opin Pediatr 2019;31(2):256–61.

[37] Dirisu O, Shickle D, Elsey H. Influence of legal status on the uptake of cannabis in young people. Curr Opin Psychiatry 2016;29(4):231–5.
[38] Richards J, Smith N, Moulin A. Unintentional Cannabis ingestion in children: a systematic review. J Pediatr 2017;190:142–52.
[39] Richards J, Gordon B, Danielson A, et al. Pharmacologic treatment of Cannabinoid hyperemesis syndrome: a systematic review. Pharmacotherapy 2017;37(6):725–34.
[40] Sorensen C, DeSanto K, Borgelt L, et al. Cannabinoid hyperemesis syndrome: diagnosis, pathophysiology, and treatment-a systematic review. J Med Toxicol 2017;13(1):71–87.
[41] Ryan S, Ammerman S, Committee on Substance Use and Prevention. Counseling parents and teens about Marijuana use in the era of legalization of Marijuana. J Pediatr 2017;139(3):e20164069.
[42] Aldy K, Cao D, Weaver M, et al. E-cigarette or vaping product use-associated lung injury (EVALI) features and recognition in the emergency department. J Am Coll Emerg Physicians Open 2020;1:1090–6.
[43] Gilley M, Brent J, Calello D, et al, Toxicology Investigators Consortium. Synthetic cannabinoid exposure in adolescents presenting for emergency care. Pediatr Emerg Care 2021;37(1):13–6.
[44] Katz K, Leonetti A, Bailey B, et al. Case series of synthetic cannabinoid intoxication from one toxicology center. West J Emerg Med 2016;17(3):290–4.
[45] Kourouni I, Mourad B, Khouli H, et al. Critical illness secondary to synthetic cannabinoid ingestion. JAMA Netw Open 2020;3(7):1–11.
[46] Dharmapuri S, Miller K, Klein J. Marijuana and the pediatric population. J Pediatr 2020;146(2):279–89.
[47] Foster BC, Abramovici H, Harris CS. Cannabis and cannabinoids: kinetics and interactions. Am J Med 2019;132(11):1266–70.
[48] Ninnemann A, Choi HJ, Stuart G, et al. Longitudinal predictors of synthetic cannabinoid use in adolescents. J Pediatr 2017;139(4):1–7.
[49] Keyes K, Rutherford C, Hamilton A, et al. Age, period, and cohort effects in synthetic cannabinoid use among US adolescents, 2011-2015. Drug Alcohol Depend 2016;166:159–67.
[50] Clayton H, Lowry R, Ashley C, et al. Health risk behaviors with synthetics cannabinoids versus marijuana. J Pediatr 2017;139(4):1–10.
[51] Palamar J, Barratt M, Coney L, et al. Synthetic cannabinoid use among high school seniors. J Pediatr 2017;140(4):1–9.
[52] Kelly B, Nappe T. Cannabinoid toxicity. Treasure Island (FL): StatPearls Publishing; 2020.
[53] Anderson SA, Oprescu A, Calello D, et al. Neuropsychiatric sequelae in adolescents with acute synthetic cannabinoid toxicity. J Pediatr 2019;144(2):1–7.
[54] Cohen J, Morrison S, Greenberg J, et al. Clinical presentation of intoxication due to synthetic cannabinoids. J Pediatr 2012;129(4):1064–7.
[55] Mir A, Obafemi A, Young A, et al. Myocardial infarction associated with use of the synthetic cannabinoid K2. J Pediatr 2011;128(6):1622–7.
[56] Rubino T, Realini N, Braida D, et al. Changes in hippocampal morphology and neuroplasticity induced by adolescent THC treatment are associated with cognitive impairment in adulthood. Hippocampus 2009;19(8):763–72.
[57] Zosel A, Bartelson B, Bailey E, et al. Characterization of adolescent prescription drug abuse and misuse using the researched abuse diversion and addiction-related surveillance (RADARS) system. J Am Acad Child Adolesc Psychiatry 2013;52(2):196–204.
[58] McCabe S, West B, Teter C, et al. Medical and nonmedical use of prescription opioids among high school seniors in the United States. Arch Pediatr Adolesc Med 2012;166(9):797–802.
[59] Gaither J, Shabanova V, Leventhal J. US national trends in pediatric deaths from prescription and illicit opioids. JAMA Netw Open 2018;1(8):e186558.

[60] Gugelmann H, Nelson L. The prescription opioid epidemic: repercussions on pediatric emergency medicine. Clin Pediatr Emerg Med 2012;13(4):260–8.
[61] Strassels S. Economic burden of prescription opioid misuse and abuse. J Manag Care Spec Pharm 2009;15(7):556–62.
[62] Spehr M, Coddington J, Ahmed A, et al. Parental opioid abuse: barriers to care, policy, and implications for primary care pediatric providers. J Pediatr Health Care 2017;31(6):695–702.
[63] Smith V, Wilson C. Families affected by parental substance use. J Pediatr 2016;138(2): 1–13.
[64] Child Welfare Information Gateway. Parental substance use and the child welfare system. Washington, DC: Children's Bureau; 2014. Available at: https://www.childwelfare.gov/pubPDFs/parentalsubabuse.pdf. Accessed September 10, 2020.
[65] Mazer-Amirshahi M, Mullins P, Rasooly I, et al. Trends in prescription opioid use in pediatric emergency department patients. Pediatr Emerg Care 2014;30(4):230–5.
[66] Horton J, Munawar S, Corrigan C, et al. Inconsistent and excessive opioid prescribing after common pediatric surgical operations. J Pediatr Surg 2019;54(7):1427–31.
[67] Anderson K, Bartz-Kurycki M, Ferguson D, et al. Too much of a bad thing: discharge opioid prescriptions in pediatric appendectomy patients. J Pediatr Surg 2018;53(12):2374–7.
[68] Harbaugh C, Lee J, Hu H, et al. Persistent opioid use among pediatric patients after surgery. J Pediatr 2018;141(1):e20172439.
[69] Hill MV, Mcmahon ML, Stucke RS, et al. Wide variation and excessive dosage of opioid prescriptions for common general surgical procedures. Ann Surg 2017;265(4):709–14.
[70] Allen J, Casavant M, Spiller H, et al. Prescription opioid exposures among children and adolescents in the United States: 2000–2015. J Pediatr 2017;139(4):e20163382.
[71] Tadros A, Layman S, Davis S, et al. Emergency department visits by pediatric patients for poisoning by prescription opioids. Am J Drug Alcohol Abuse 2016;42(5):550–5.
[72] Committee on Drugs. Naloxone dosage and route of administration for infants and children: addendum to emergency drug doses for infants and children. J Pediatr 1990;86(3):484–5.
[73] Chamberlain J, Klein B. A comprehensive review of naloxone for the emergency physician. Am J Emerg Med 1994;12(6):650–60.
[74] Goldfrank L, Weisman R, Errick J, et al. A dosing nomogram for continuous infusion intravenous naloxone. Ann Emerg Med 1986;15(5):566–70.
[75] Lovegrove M, Hampton LM, Budnitz DS, et al. Notes from the Field: Emergency Department Visits and Hospitalizations for Buprenorphine Ingestion by Children — United States, 2010–2011. Morbidity and Mortality Weekly Report (MMWR). Available at: http://www.cdc.gov/mmwr/preview/mmwrhtml/%20mm6203a5.htm.
[76] Pedapati E, Bateman S. Toddlers requiring pediatric intensive care unit admission following at-home exposure to buprenorphine/naloxone. Pediatr Crit Care Med 2011;12(2):102–7.
[77] Solecki S, Turchi R. Pharming: pill parties can be deadly for teens. Contemp Pediatr 2014;31(11):24–7.
[78] Simmons L, Havens J, Whiting J, et al. Illicit drug use among women with children in the United States 2002-2003. Ann Epidemiol 2009;19(3):187–93.
[79] Patrick S, Schumacher R, Benneyworth B, et al. Neonatal abstinence syndrome and associated health care expenditures. JAMA 2012;307(18):1934–40.
[80] McGlone L, Mactier H. Infants of opioid-dependent mothers: neurodevelopment at six months. Early Hum Dev 2014;91(1):19–21.
[81] McHugh RK, Nielsen S, Weiss R. Prescription drug abuse: from epidemiology to public policy. J Subst Abuse Treat 2015;48(1):1–7.
[82] Howard M, Weiler R, Haddox J. Development and reliability of items measuring the nonmedical use of prescription drugs for the Youth Risk Behavior Survey: results from an initial pilot test. J Sch Health 2009;79:554–60.

[83] Warner M, Chen L, Makuc D, et al. Drug poisoning deaths in the United States, 1980–2008. NCHS data brief, No. 81. Hyattsville (MD): National Center for Health Statistics; 2011. Available at: http://www.cdc.gov/nchs/data/databriefs/db81.pdf.
[84] Whiteside L, Walton M, Bohnert A, et al. Nonmedical prescription opioid and sedative use among adolescents in the emergency department. J Pediatr 2013;132(5):825–32.
[85] Schepis T, Teter C, McCabe S. Prescription drug use, misuse and related substance use disorder symptoms vary by educational status and attainment in US adolescents and young adults. Drug Alcohol Depend 2018;189:172–7.
[86] Johnston L, O'Malley P, Bachman J, et al. Monitoring the Future national survey results on drug use, 195-2006. Volume II: college students and adults ages 19-45. NIH Publication 07-6206. Bethesda (MD): National Institute on Drug Abuse; 2007.
[87] Huang D, Dawson D, Stinson F, et al. Prevalence, correlates, and comorbidity of nonmedical prescription drug use and drug use disorders in the United States: results of the National Epidemiologic Survey on Alcohol and related conditions. J Clin Psychiatry 2006;67(7):1062–73.
[88] Boyd C, McCabe S, Cranford J, et al. Adolescents' motivations to abuse prescription medications. J Pediatr 2006;118(6):2472–80.
[89] Taylor O. The cultural influence of adolescent prescription drug abuse. Hum Behav Macro Social Environ 2015;25(4):304–11.
[90] Joffe A. Your role in curbing prescription and OTC drug abuse by adolescents. Contemp Pediatr 2006;23:97–101.
[91] Katsuki T, Mackey T, Cuomo R. Establishing a link between prescription drug abuse and illicit online pharmacies: analysis of Twitter data. J Med Internet Res 2015;17(12):e280.
[92] Levine D. 'Pharming': the abuse of prescription and over-the-counter drugs in teens. Curr Opin Pediatr 2007;19:270–4.
[93] Elliott E, Souder C, Privette T, et al. The scope of adolescent prescription drug abuse. Emerg Med 2009;41(1):16–22.
[94] Schepis T, Krishnan-Sarin S. Characterizing adolescent prescription misusers: a population-based study. J Am Acad Child Adolesc Psychiatry 2008;47(7):745–54.
[95] Jones B, Fullwood H, Hawthorn M. Preventing prescription drug abuse in adolescence: a collaborative approach. Prev Res 2012;19(1):13–6.
[96] Caplan J, Epstein L, Quinn D, et al. Neuropsychiatric effects of prescription drug abuse. Neuropsychol Rev 2007;17:363–80.
[97] Drazdowski T, Jaggi L, Borre A, et al. Use of prescription drugs and future delinquency among adolescent offenders. J Subst Abuse Treat 2015;48(1):28–36.
[98] Bornemann J. The viability of microdosing psychedelics as a strategy to enhance cognition and well-being - an early review. J Psychoactive Drugs 2020;52(4):300–8.
[99] Johnstad P. Powerful substances in tiny amounts: an interview study of psychedelic microdosing. Nordisk Alkohol Nark 2018;35(1):39–51.
[100] Kuypers K, Ng L, Erritzoe D, et al. Microdosing psychedelics: more questions than answers? An overview and suggestions for future research. J Psychopharmacol 2019;33:1039–57.
[101] Lea T, Amada N, Jungaberle H, et al. Microdosing psychedelics: motivations, subjective effects and harm reduction. Int J Drug Policy 2020;75:102600.
[102] Fadiman J, Korb S. Might microdosing psychedelics be safe and beneficial? An initial exploration. J Psychoactive Drugs 2019;51(2):118–22.
[103] Leonard J, Anderson B, Klein-Schwartz W. Does getting high hurt? Characterization of cases of LSD and psilocybin-containing mushroom exposures to national poison centers between 2000 and 2016. J Pschopharmacol 2018;32(12):1286–94.
[104] Ni A, Cantrell L, Clark R. Ketamine exposure demographics and outcome over 16 years as reported to US poison centers. Am J Emerg Med 2018;36:1459–62.
[105] Degenhardt L, Copeland J, Dillon P. Recent trends in the use of "club drugs": an Australian review. Subst Use Misuse 2005;40:1241–56.

[106] Schwartz R. LSD: its rise, fall, and renewed popularity among high school students. Pediatr Clin North Am 1995;42(2):403–12.
[107] Weiner A, Vieira L, McKay C, et al. Ketamine abusers presenting to the emergency department: a case series. J Emerg Med 2000;18(4):447–51.
[108] Bearn J, O'Brien M. "Addicted to Euphoria": the history, clinical presentation, and management of party drug misuse. Int Rev Neurobiol 2015;120:205–33.
[109] Copeland J, Dillon P. The health and psycho-social consequences of ketamine use. Int J Drug Policy 2005;16(2):122–31.
[110] Kalsi S, Wood D, Dargan P. The epidemiology and patterns of acute and chronic toxicity associated with recreational ketamine use. Emerg Health Threats J 2011;4:7107–16.
[111] Williams J, Storck M, Committee on Substance Abuse and Committee on Native American Child Health. Inhalant abuse. J Pediatr 2007;119(5):1009–17.
[112] Wu L, Pilowsky D, Schlenger W, et al. Inhalant abuse and dependence among adolescents in the United States. J Am Acad Child Adolesc Psychiatry 2004;43(10):1206–14.
[113] McGarvey E, Clavet G, Mason W, et al. Adolescent inhalant abuse: environments of use. Am J Drug Alcohol Abuse 1999;25(4):731–41.
[114] Kurtzman R, Otsuka K, Wahl R. Inhalant abuse by adolescents. J Adolesc Health 2001;28(3):170–80.
[115] Forrester M. Computer and electronic duster spray inhalation (huffing) injuries managed at emergency departments. Am J Drug Alcohol Abuse 2020;46(2):180–3.
[116] Cazzell M. Linking theory, evidence, and practice in assessment of adolescent inhalant use. J Addict Nurs 2008;19(1):17–25.
[117] Nguyen J, O'Brien C, Schapp S, et al. Adolescent inhalant use prevention, assessment, and treatment: a literature synthesis. Int J Drug Policy 2016;31:15–24.
[118] Johnston L, O'Malley P, Bachman J, et al. Monitoring the future national survey results on drug use, 1975–2008. Volume I: secondary school students (NIH Publication No. 09–7402). Bethesda (MD): National Institute on Drug Abuse; 2009.
[119] Anderson C, Loomis G. Recognition and prevention of inhalant abuse. Am Fam Physician 2003;68(5):869–74.
[120] Nonnemaker J, Crankshaw E, Shive D, et al. Inhalant use initiation among US adolescents: evidence from the National Survey of Parents and Youth using discrete-time survival analysis. Addict Behav 2011;36:878–81.
[121] Crossin R, Cairney S, Lawrence A, et al. Adolescent inhalation abuse leads to other drug use and impaired growth; implications for diagnosis. Aust N Z J Public Health 2017;41(1):99–104.
[122] Howard M, Bowen S, Garland E, et al. Inhalant use and inhalant use disorders in the United States. Addict Sci Clin Pract 2011;6(1):18–31.
[123] Plumb J, Thomas R. Sudden severe perioral swelling in an adolescent boy. Clin Toxicol 2013;51:379–80.
[124] Mermiri D, Papdopoulou A, Xristianakis E, et al. Severe lung injury due to chronic volatile hydrocarbon (VHC) inhalation in an adolescent. Eur Respir J 2016;48(suppl 60):PA3914.
[125] Baird C, Furek M. Adolescents and inhalant abuse: how huffing affects the myelin sheath. J Addict Nurs 2012;23(2):129–31.
[126] Wilson M, Ferguson R, Mazer M, et al. Monitoring trends in dextromethorphan abuse using the National Poison Data System: 2000–2010. Clin Toxicol 2011;49:409–15.
[127] Karami S, Major J, Calderon S, et al. Trends in dextromethorphan cough and cold products: 2000-2015 National Poison Data System intentional abuse exposure calls. Clin Toxicol 2018;56(7):656–63.
[128] Consumer Healthcare Products Association. Dextromethorphan: preventing teen cough medicine abuse. Washington, DC: Consumer Healthcare Products Association; 2017. Available at: http://www.chpa.org/Dex.aspx. Accessed 10 November 2020.
[129] Falck R, Li L, Carlson R, et al. The prevalence of dextromethorphan abuse among high school students. J Pediatr 2006;118(5):2267–9.

[130] Akerman S, Hammel J, Brunette M. Dextromethorphan abuse and dependence in adolescents. J Dual Diagn 2010;6:266–78.
[131] Silvasti M, Karttunen P, Tukiainen H, et al. Pharmacokinetics of dextromethorphan and dextrorphan: a single dose comparison of three preparations in human volunteers. Int J Clin Pharmacol Ther Toxicol 1987;25(9):493–7.
[132] Romanelli F, Smith K. Dextromethorphan abuse: clinical effects and management. J Am Pharm Assoc 2009;49:20–7.
[133] Antoniou T, Juurlink D. Dextromethorphan abuse. CMAJ 2014;186(16):E631.
[134] Boyer E. Dextromethorphan abuse. Pediatr Emerg Care 2004;20(12):858–63.
[135] Schwartz R. Adolescent abuse of dextromethorphan. Clin Pediatr 2005;44(7):565–8.
[136] Helfer J, Kim O. Psychoactive abuse potential of Robitussin-DM. Am J Psychiatry 1990;147(5):672–3.
[137] Ziaee V, Hamed E, Hoshmand A, et al. Side effects of dextromethorphan abuse, a case series. Addict Behav 2005;30(8):1607–13.

FSC
www.fsc.org
MIX
Papier | Fördert
gute Waldnutzung
FSC® C083411

Kolibri 360 GmbH
Ferdinand-Jühlke-Straße 7
99095 Erfurt, Deutschland
produktsicherheit@kolibri360.de